Neurologic Emergencies

Editors

JONATHAN A. EDLOW
MICHAEL K. ABRAHAM

EMERGENCY MEDICINE CLINICS OF NORTH AMERICA

www.emed.theclinics.com

Consulting Editor
AMAL MATTU

November 2016 • Volume 34 • Number 4

ELSEVIER

1600 John F. Kennedy Boulevard • Suite 1800 • Philadelphia, Pennsylvania, 19103-2899

http://www.theclinics.com

EMERGENCY MEDICINE CLINICS OF NORTH AMERICA Volume 34, Number 4
November 2016 ISSN 0733-8627, ISBN-13: 978-0-323-47681-2

Editor: Patrick Manley
Developmental Editor: Casey Jackson

Emergency Medicine Clinics of North America (ISSN 0733-8627) is published quarterly by Elsevier Inc., 360 Park Avenue South, New York, NY, 10010-1710. Months of issue are February, May, August, and November. Business and Editorial Offices: 1600 John F. Kennedy Boulevard, Suite 1800, Philadelphia, PA 19103-2899. Customer Service Office: 6277 Sea Harbor Drive, Orlando, FL 32887-4800. Periodicals postage paid at New York, NY, and additional mailing offices. Subscription prices are $100.00 per year (US students), $320.00 per year (US individuals), $579.00 per year (US institutions), $220.00 per year (international students), $450.00 per year (international individuals), $711.00 per year (international institutions), $220.00 per year (Canadian students), $385.00 per year (Canadian individuals), and $711.00 per year (Canadian institutions). International air speed delivery is included in all *Clinics'* subscription prices. All prices are subject to change without notice. **POSTMASTER:** Send address changes to *Emergency Medicine Clinics of North America*, Elsevier Periodicals Customer Service, 11830 Westline Industrial Drive, St. Louis, MO 63146. Customer Service (orders, claims, online, change of address): Elsevier Periodicals **Customer Service, 11830 Westline Industrial Drive, St. Louis, MO 63146. Tel: 1-800-654-2452 (U.S. and Canada); 314-453-7041 (outside U.S. and Canada). Fax: 314-453-5170. E-mail: journalscustomerservice-usa@elsevier.com (for print support); journalsonlinesupport-usa@elsevier.com (for online support).**

Reprints. For copies of 100 or more of articles in this publication, please contact the Commercial Reprints Department, Elsevier Inc., 360 Park Avenue South, New York, NY 10010-1710. Tel.: 212-633-3874; Fax: 212-633-3820; E-mail: reprints@elsevier.com.

Emergency Medicine Clinics of North America is covered in *MEDLINE/PubMed (Index Medicus), Current Contents/Clinical Medicine, EMBASE/Excerpta Medica, BIOSIS, SciSearch, CINAHL, ISI/BIOMED*, and *Research Alert*.

Contributors

CONSULTING EDITOR

AMAL MATTU, MD, FAAEM, FACEP
Professor and Vice Chair, Department of Emergency Medicine, University of Maryland School of Medicine, Baltimore, Maryland

EDITORS

JONATHAN A. EDLOW, MD
Vice Chair, Department of Emergency Medicine, Beth Israel Deaconess Medical Center, Professor of Medicine and Emergency Medicine, Harvard Medical School, Boston, Massachusetts

MICHAEL K. ABRAHAM, MD, MS
Clinical Assistant Professor, Department of Emergency Medicine, University of Maryland School of Medicine, Baltimore, Maryland

AUTHORS

MICHAEL K. ABRAHAM, MD, MS
Clinical Assistant Professor, Department of Emergency Medicine, University of Maryland School of Medicine, Baltimore, Maryland

EVERETT W. AUSTIN, MD
Emergency Medicine Resident, Department of Emergency Medicine, University of Virginia, Charlottesville, Virginia

WAN-TSU WENDY CHANG, MD
Assistant Professor, Department of Emergency Medicine, University of Maryland School of Medicine, Baltimore, Maryland

MAIA DORSETT, MD, PhD
Division of Emergency Medicine, Washington University School of Medicine, St Louis, Missouri

ANDREA DUCA, MD
Department of Emergency Medicine, Università Vita-Salute San Raffaele, Milan, Italy

ANDREA G. EDLOW, MD, MSc
Division of Maternal-Fetal Medicine, Department of Obstetrics and Gynecology, Tufts Medical Center; Assistant Professor, Tufts University School of Medicine, Boston, Massachusetts

BRIAN L. EDLOW, MD
Division of Neurocritical Care and Emergency Neurology, Department of Neurology, Massachusetts General Hospital; Instructor of Neurology, Harvard Medical School, Boston, Massachusetts

JONATHAN A. EDLOW, MD
Vice Chair, Department of Emergency Medicine, Beth Israel Deaconess Medical Center, Professor of Medicine and Emergency Medicine, Harvard Medical School, Boston, Massachusetts

LATHA GANTI, MD, MS, MBA, FACEP
Professor of Emergency Medicine & Neurology, University of Central Florida College of Medicine, Orlando, Florida

JOSHUA N. GOLDSTEIN, MD, PhD
J. P. Kistler Stroke Research Center; Department of Emergency Medicine, Massachusetts General Hospital, Harvard Medical School, Boston, Massachusetts

J. STEPHEN HUFF, MD
Professor of Emergency Medicine and Neurology, Department of Emergency Medicine, University of Virginia, Charlottesville, Virginia

ANDY JAGODA, MD, FACEP
Professor and Chair, Department of Emergency Medicine, Icahn School of Medicine at Mount Sinai, New York, New York

DANYA KHOUJAH, MBBS
Assistant Professor, Department of Emergency Medicine, University of Maryland School of Medicine, Baltimore, Maryland

STEPHEN Y. LIANG, MD, MPHS
Division of Emergency Medicine; Division of Infectious Diseases, Washington University School of Medicine, St Louis, Missouri

ANDREA MOROTTI, MD
J. P. Kistler Stroke Research Center, Massachusetts General Hospital, Harvard Medical School, Boston, Massachusetts

LAUREN M. NENTWICH, MD, FACEP
Assistant Professor of Emergency Medicine, Boston University School of Medicine; Attending, Department of Emergency Medicine, Boston Medical Center, Boston, Massachusetts

VAIBHAV RASTOGI, MD
Department of Internal Medicine, North Florida Regional Medical Center, Gainesville, Florida

MATTHEW S. SIKET, MD, MS, FACEP
Co-Director, Rhode Island Hospital, The Miriam Hospital Stroke Centers; Assistant Professor of Emergency Medicine, The Warren Alpert Medical School of Brown University, Providence, Rhode Island

JENNIFER SINGLETON, MD
Instructor, Department of Emergency Medicine, Beth Israel Deaconess Medical Center, Harvard Medical School, Boston, Massachusetts

STUART P. SWADRON, MD, FRCPC, FACEP, FAAEM
Professor of Clinical Emergency Medicine and Medical Education; LAC+USC Emergency Medicine Residency, LAC+USC Medical Center, Keck School of Medicine of USC, Los Angeles, California

RAMIN R. TABATABAI, MD, FACEP
Assistant Professor of Clinical Emergency Medicine; Assistant Program Director, LAC+USC Emergency Medicine Residency, LAC+USC Medical Center, Keck School of Medicine of USC, Los Angeles, California

STEPHEN J. TRAUB, MD
Associate Professor of Emergency Medicine, Mayo Clinic Arizona, Phoenix, Arizona

EELCO F. WIJDICKS, MD
Professor of Neurology, Mayo Clinic, Rochester, Minnesota

Contents

There are a number of dangerous secondary causes of headaches that are
life, limb, brain, or vision threatening that emergency physicians must
consider in patients presenting with acute headache. Careful history and
physical examination targeted at these important secondary causes of headache will help to avoid misdiagnosis in these patients. Patients with acute
thunderclap headache have a differential diagnosis beyond subarachnoid
hemorrhage. Considering the "context" of headache "PLUS" some other
symptom or sign is one strategy to help focus the differential diagnosis.

Dizziness is a common chief complaint in emergency medicine. The differential diagnosis is broad and includes serious conditions, such as stroke,
cardiac arrhythmia, hypovolemic states, and acute toxic and metabolic disturbances. Emergency physicians must distinguish the majority of patients
who suffer from benign self-limiting conditions from those with serious illnesses that require acute treatment. Misdiagnoses are frequent and diagnostic test costs high. The traditional approach does not distinguish benign
from dangerous causes and is not consistent with best current evidence.
This article presents a new approach to the diagnosis of acutely dizzy patients that highly leverages the history and the physical examination.

Acute back pain is a common presenting complaint in the emergency
department that leads to a great deal of resource utilization. The differential diagnosis is long and most cases are caused by benign pathology that
will resolve on its own. Imaging is over-used and rarely helps. This article
presents an algorithmic approach using red flags in the history and physical examination that will help physicians better identify the small of patients with serious conditions that, if untreated, will result in significant
neurological damage.

The emergent evaluation and treatment of generalized convulsive status epilepticus presents challenges for emergency physicians. This disease is one of the few in which minutes can mean the difference between life and significant morbidity and mortality. It is imperative to use parallel processing and have multiple treatment options planned in advance, in case the current treatment is not successful. There is also benefit to exploring, or initiating, treatment algorithms to standardize the care for these critically ill patients.

Coma represents a true medical emergency. Drug intoxications are a leading cause of coma; however, other metabolic disturbances and traumatic brain injury are also common causes. The general emergency department approach begins with stabilization of airway, breathing, and circulation, followed by a thorough physical examination to generate a limited differential diagnosis that is then refined by focused testing. Definitive treatment is ultimately disease-specific. This article presents an overview of the pathophysiology, causes, examination, and treatment of coma.

Weakness is a common complaint in the emergency department, and a most challenging one, because before the emergency physician can proceed with an evaluation, the complaint of weakness must be fully clarified to determine about what the patient is actually complaining. This article will focus on causes of acute generalized nontraumatic bilateral weakness. Evaluation begins with the history and physical examination, followed by diagnostic testing in some cases.

The definition of a transient ischemic attack (TIA) has evolved over the past decade from a clinical diagnosis to a tissue-based definition based on neuroimaging results. TIA shares the same pathophysiology as stroke, which occurs in up to 5% of patients within 48 hours of the TIA and 10% within 90 days. This rate is decreasing, likely due to improved diagnostic and management strategies. Decision support scores have been developed to risk stratify patients, which include clinical and radiological elements. Antiplatelet and anticoagulant therapy, as well as carotid endarterectomy/stenting have been shown to reduce the stroke occurrence after TIA.

Acute ischemic stroke is a challenging and time-sensitive diagnosis. Diagnosis begins with rapid detection of acute stroke symptoms by the patient, their family or caregivers, or bystanders. If acute stroke is suspected, EMS providers should be called for rapid assessment. EMS providers will utilize prehospital stroke tools to diagnose and determine potential stroke severity. Once at the hospital, the stroke team works rapidly to solidify the patient history, perform a focused neurologic examination and obtain necessary laboratory tests and brain imaging to accurately diagnose acute ischemic stroke and properly treat the patient.

Matthew S. Siket

Although stroke declined from the third to fifth most common cause of death in the United States, the annual incidence and overall prevalence continue to increase. Since the available US Food and Drug Administration–approved treatment options are time dependent, improving early stroke care may have more of a public health impact than any other phase of care. Timely and efficient stroke treatment should be a priority for emergency department and prehospital providers. This article discusses currently available and emerging treatment options in acute ischemic stroke focusing on the preservation of salvageable brain tissue, minimizing complications, and secondary prevention.

Andrea Morotti and Joshua N. Goldstein

Intracerebral hemorrhage (ICH) is the deadliest type of stroke and up to half of patients die in hospital. Blood pressure management, coagulopathy reversal, and intracranial pressure control are the mainstays of acute ICH treatment. Prevention of hematoma expansion and minimally invasive hematoma evacuation are promising therapeutic strategies under investigation. This article provides an updated review on ICH diagnosis and management in the emergency department.

Michael K. Abraham and Wan-Tsu Wendy Chang

Aneurysmal subarachnoid hemorrhage (SAH) is a neurological emergency with high risk of neurological decline and death. Although the presentation of a thunderclap headache or the worst headache of a patient's life easily triggers the evaluation for SAH, subtle presentations are still missed. The gold standard for diagnostic evaluation of SAH remains noncontrast head computed tomography (CT) followed by lumbar puncture if the CT is negative for SAH. Management of patients with SAH follows standard resuscitation of critically ill patients with the emphasis on reducing risks of rebleeding and avoiding secondary brain injuries.

Maia Dorsett and Stephen Y. Liang

Central nervous system (CNS) infections, including meningitis, encephalitis, and brain abscess, are rare but time-sensitive emergency department (ED) diagnoses. Patients with CNS infection can present to the ED with nonspecific signs and symptoms, including headache, fever, altered mental status, and behavioral changes. Neuroimaging and CSF fluid analysis can appear benign early in the course of disease. Delaying therapy negatively impacts outcomes, particularly with bacterial meningitis and herpes simplex virus encephalitis. Therefore, diagnosis of CNS infection requires vigilance and a high index of suspicion based on the history and physical examination, which must be confirmed with appropriate imaging and laboratory evaluation.

Andrea G. Edlow, Brian L. Edlow, and Jonathan A. Edlow

Acute neurologic symptoms in pregnant and postpartum women may be caused by exacerbation of a preexisting neurologic condition, the initial presentation of a non–pregnancy-related problem, or a new neurologic problem. Pregnant and postpartum patients with headache and neurologic symptoms are often diagnosed with preeclampsia or eclampsia; however, other etiologies must also be considered. A team approach with close communication between emergency physicians, neurologists, maternal–fetal medicine specialists, and radiologists is the key to obtaining best outcomes. This article reviews the clinical features and differential diagnosis of acute serious neurologic conditions in pregnancy and the puerperium, focusing on diagnosis.

J. Stephen Huff and Everett W. Austin

Understanding the anatomy and physiology of the eye, the orbit, and the central connections is key to understanding neuro-ophthalmologic emergencies. Anisocoria is an important sign that requires a systematic approach to avoid misdiagnosis of serious conditions, including carotid dissection (miosis) and aneurysmal third nerve palsy (mydriasis). Ptosis may be a sign of either Horner syndrome or third nerve palsy. An explanation should be pursued for diplopia since the differential diagnosis ranges from the trivial to life-threatening causes.

EMERGENCY MEDICINE
CLINICS OF NORTH AMERICA

THE CLINICS ARE NOW AVAILABLE ONLINE!
Access your subscription at:
www.theclinics.com

PROGRAM OBJECTIVE
The goal of *Emergency Medicine Clinics of North America* is to keep practicing emergency medicine physicians and emergency medicine residents up to date with current clinical practice in emergency medicine by providing timely articles reviewing the state of the art in patient care.

LEARNING OBJECTIVES
Upon completion of this activity, participants will be able to:
1. Review the evaluation of headache and dizziness in the emergency department.
2. Recognize emerging strategies in the diagnosis and treatment of both acute ischemic and hemorrhagic strokes.
3. Discuss the initial diagnosis and management of neurological emergencies such as coma and epilepsy, among others.

ACCREDITATION
The Elsevier Office of Continuing Medical Education (EOCME) is accredited by the Accreditation Council for Continuing Medical Education (ACCME) to provide continuing medical education for physicians.

The EOCME designates this enduring material for a maximum of 15 *AMA PRA Category 1 Credit*(s)™. Physicians should claim only the credit commensurate with the extent of their participation in the activity.

All other health care professionals requesting continuing education credit for this enduring material will be issued a certificate of participation.

DISCLOSURE OF CONFLICTS OF INTEREST
The EOCME assesses conflict of interest with its instructors, faculty, planners, and other individuals who are in a position to control the content of CME activities. All relevant conflicts of interest that are identified are thoroughly vetted by EOCME for fair balance, scientific objectivity, and patient care recommendations. EOCME is committed to providing its learners with CME activities that promote improvements or quality in healthcare and not a specific proprietary business or a commercial interest.

The planning committee, staff, authors and editors listed below have identified no financial relationships or relationships to products or devices they or their spouse/life partner have with commercial interest related to the content of this CME activity:
Michael K. Abraham, MD, MS; Everett W. Austin, MD; Wan-Tsu Wendy Chang, MD; Maia Dorsett, MD, PhD; Andrea Duca, MD; Jonathan A. Edlow, MD; Andrea G. Edlow, MD, MSc; Brian L. Edlow, MD; Anjali Fortna; Latha Ganti, MD, MS, MBA, FACEP; J. Stephen Huff, MD; Danya Khoujah, MBBS; Indu Kumari; Stephen Y. Liang, MD, MPHS; Amal Mattu, MD, FAAEM, FACEP; Andrea Morotti, MD; Lauren M. Nentwich, MD, FACEP; Katie Pfaff; Vaibhav Rastogi, MD; Erin Scheckenbach; Matthew S. Siket, MD, MS; Jennifer Singleton, MD; Stuart P. Swadron, MD, FRCPC, FACEP, FAAEM; Ramin R. Tabatabai, MD, FACEP; Stephen J. Traub, MD; Eelco F. Wijdicks, MD.

The planning committee, staff, authors and editors listed below have identified financial relationships or relationships to products or devices they or their spouse/life partner have with commercial interest related to the content of this CME activity:
Joshua N. Goldstein, MD, PhD is a consultant/advisor for CSL Behring and Bristol-Myers Squibb Company, and has research support from Portola Pharmaceuticals, Inc.
Andy Jagoda, MD, FACEP is a consultant/advisor for Banyan Biomarkers, Inc.; Pfizer Inc.; AstraZeneca; Daiichi Sankyo Company, Limited; Teva Pharmaceutical Industries Ltd; and Emergency Medicine Practice.

UNAPPROVED/OFF-LABEL USE DISCLOSURE
The EOCME requires CME faculty to disclose to the participants:
1. When products or procedures being discussed are off-label, unlabelled, experimental, and/or investigational (not US Food and Drug Administration [FDA] approved); and
2. Any limitations on the information presented, such as data that are preliminary or that represent ongoing research, interim analyses, and/or unsupported opinions. Faculty may discuss information about pharmaceutical agents that is outside of FDA-approved labelling. This information is intended solely for CME and is not intended to promote off-label use of these medications. If you have any questions, contact the medical affairs department of the manufacturer for the most recent prescribing information.

TO ENROLL

To enroll in the *Emergency Medicine Clinics* Continuing Medical Education program, call customer service at 1-800-654-2452 or sign up online at http://www.theclinics.com/home/cme. The CME program is available to subscribers for an additional annual fee of $235 USD.

METHOD OF PARTICIPATION

In order to claim credit, participants must complete the following:

1. Complete enrolment as indicated above.
2. Read the activity.
3. Complete the CME Test and Evaluation. Participants must achieve a score of 70% on the test. All CME Tests and Evaluations must be completed online.

CME INQUIRIES/SPECIAL NEEDS

For all CME inquiries or special needs, please contact elsevierCME@elsevier.com.

Foreword

Neurologic Emergencies

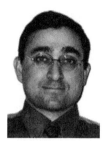

Amal Mattu, MD, FAAEM, FACEP
Consulting Editor

If you were to ask emergency physicians which organ system they feel least comfortable managing in times of emergency, the majority are likely to mention the neurologic system. This system, and in particular the brain, has been considered the "black box" of the human body for generations. I believe that the reasons for this difficulty is fairly simple: basic science training of the neurologic system in medical school is often considered complicated, and clinical training in most medical schools in neurology is very brief compared with other areas in medicine. In addition, the neurologic system cannot be seen, felt, or auscultated. Yet, neurologic complaints and emergencies are common, and their complications are devastating. Physician discomfort and worry regarding the proper management of many neurologic conditions lead to an excess in radiologic testing and even a false sense of security when the imaging is normal.

Almost every continuing medical education conference focused on emergency medicine or risk management includes teaching sessions on neurologic emergencies. Despite this, litigation for misdiagnosed neurologic conditions such as stroke, spinal cord disorders, and intracranial hemorrhage continues to be common. We as educators clearly are not doing enough to spread the knowledge of proper diagnosis and treatment of such conditions.

I was, therefore, thrilled to welcome Drs Jonathan Edlow and Michael Abraham to serve as Guest Editors of this issue of *Emergency Medicine Clinics of North America*. Both of these educators have dedicated their careers to educating emergency physicians in the improved care of patients with neurologic emergencies. In this issue, they have assembled an outstanding team to discuss a wide range of conditions, from the common to the catastrophic. Common neurologic presentations are addressed, including headache, dizziness, weakness, back pain, and coma. Authors discuss how to identify red flags in the history and physical exam that can help identify the needle in the haystack of these patients. Other authors discuss cerebrovascular conditions, including transient ischemic attack and stroke, both ischemic and hemorrhagic. Status epilepticus is addressed and includes a discussion of some

Emerg Med Clin N Am 34 (2016) xv–xvi
http://dx.doi.org/10.1016/j.emc.2016.09.003
0733-8627/16/© 2016 Published by Elsevier Inc.

emed.theclinics.com

newer therapies. Final articles address neurologic conditions in the pregnant patient, and there is a special article on neuro-ophthalmology in emergency medicine.

The Guest Editors and authors are to be commended for their hard work. This issue of *Emergency Medicine Clinics of North America* represents an invaluable addition to the emergency neurology literature and should be considered required reading in the curriculum for all emergency care providers and trainees. In this issue, I'm happy to say that the Guest Editors and authors have certainly shed some light on the "black box" of the neurologic system.

Amal Mattu, MD, FAAEM, FACEP
Department of Emergency Medicine
University of Maryland School of Medicine
Baltimore, MD 21201, USA

E-mail address:
amalmattu@comcast.net

Preface

Neurologic Emergencies— Making the Diagnosis and Treating the Life Threats

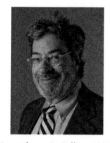 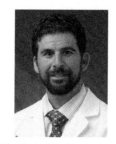

Jonathan A. Edlow, MD   Michael K. Abraham, MD, MS
Editors

When Dr Amal Mattu asked us to consider organizing and editing this issue of *Emergency Medicine Clinics of North America*, we both had to say yes. This is, in part, due to our respect for him, but also to our interest in and commitment to improving the care of our patients who present to the emergency department with acute neurologic problems. This group of patients is not an insignificant number, and most estimates suggest that between 5% and 8% of all patients seen in an emergency department have neurologic issues. If you need confirmation, simply think about your last shift and consider how many patients had back pain or headache or dizziness or altered mentation. Most of these patients have fairly trivial and often self-limited problems. However, as with emergency medicine in general, there are the needles in the haystack.

Several decades ago, when one of us started practicing emergency medicine, the range of diagnostic imaging was quite limited and the menu of various therapeutic options for patients with neurologic problems even more so. Computed Tomography (CT) scan was available, but often only during daytime hours. MRI was still on the drawing board. TPA was a couple of decades away. The notion that treating patients with transient ischemic attack (TIA) within the first couple of days could reduce the outcome of stroke did not exist. Phenobarbital was a common treatment for patients with status epilepticus, and the probability of getting an EEG in the emergency department was essentially zero. My younger counterpart wasn't so lucky.

For quite some time, a spirit of therapeutic nihilism existed for patients with neurologic emergencies. Neurologic emergencies incite fear into emergency physicians as they can be more complicated than many of the other critical issues that confront emergency physicians every day. But the range of diagnostic modalities and the various treatments that are now available for these patients have markedly expanded

Emerg Med Clin N Am 34 (2016) xvii–xviii
http://dx.doi.org/10.1016/j.emc.2016.09.002
0733-8627/16/© 2016 Published by Elsevier Inc.   emed.theclinics.com

in the last two decades and therapeutic nihilism is no longer an option. Not surprisingly, this group of patients is an important source of medicolegal liability for the clinician.

We have therefore organized this issue to cover the common neurologic symptoms that emergency physicians encounter regularly (back pain, visual symptoms, headache, weakness, and altered mental status) as well as the important areas of central nervous system infections, and the recognition and treatment of patients with acute cerebrovascular emergencies (ischemic and hemorrhagic stroke, TIA, and subarachnoid hemorrhage). We've also included an article about neurologic conditions affecting pregnant and postpartum women because of its special high-risk nature. We believe that we have recruited an all-star list of authors for this issue. We believe that the result is a truly cutting-edge issue that will help emergency clinicians better diagnose and treat their patients with these neurologic conditions. We hope that the content of this issue helps to improve patient safety and patient outcomes.

When possible, we have tried to include illustrations, tables, and algorithms to help clarify the clinical approach to these patients.

We would both like to thank our families for their understanding, our colleagues for their support, and most of all, our patients for their inspiration. We would also like to thank the editorial staff at Elsevier for their important contributions to this issue. All of these individuals have helped to make this issue of *Emergency Medicine Clinics of North America* the success that we believe it is.

Jonathan A. Edlow, MD
Department of Emergency Medicine
Beth Israel Deaconess Medical Center
Harvard Medical School
Boston, MA 02215, USA

Michael K. Abraham, MD, MS
Department of Emergency Medicine
University of Maryland School of Medicine
110 South Paca Street, 6th Floor
Suite 200
Baltimore, MD 21201, USA

E-mail addresses:
jedlow@bidmc.harvard.edu (J.A. Edlow)
mabraham@umem.org (M.K. Abraham)

Headache in the Emergency Department
Avoiding Misdiagnosis of Dangerous Secondary Causes

Ramin R. Tabatabai, MD*, Stuart P. Swadron, MD, FRCPC

KEYWORDS

- Primary headache • Secondary headache • Thunderclap headache
- Headache misdiagnosis

KEY POINTS

- There are a number of dangerous secondary causes of headaches that are life, limb, brain, or vision threatening that emergency physicians must consider in patients presenting with acute headache.
- Careful history and physical examination targeted at these important secondary causes of headache will help to avoid misdiagnosis in these patients.
- Patients with acute thunderclap headache have a differential diagnosis beyond subarachnoid hemorrhage.
- Considering the "context" of headache "PLUS" some other symptom or sign is one strategy to help focus the differential diagnosis.

NATURE OF THE PROBLEM/DEFINITION

Headache is the fourth most common chief complaint in the emergency department (ED), comprising approximately 3% of all ED visits in the United States.[1,2] Depending on its underlying cause, headache can be broadly categorized as either primary or secondary. The International Classification of Headache Disorders identifies primary headaches as migraine, tension-type, cluster, or one of the other trigeminal autonomic cephalgias.[3] These comprise the vast majority of headaches.[4] Secondary headaches are defined as those due to a distinctive underlying disorder, such as trauma, infection, or malignancy.[3] Evaluation of the patient with headache in the ED is focused on the alleviation of pain and the consideration of dangerous secondary causes.

Disclosures: None.
LAC+USC Emergency Medicine Residency, LAC+USC Medical Center, Keck School of Medicine of USC, 1200 North State Street, Room 1060E, Los Angeles, CA 90033, USA
* Corresponding author.
E-mail address: tabatabai.usc@gmail.com

Emerg Med Clin N Am 34 (2016) 695–716
http://dx.doi.org/10.1016/j.emc.2016.06.003
0733-8627/16/© 2016 Elsevier Inc. All rights reserved.
emed.theclinics.com

A sophisticated clinical approach must be used to determine which patients require expedited neuroimaging or further diagnostic evaluation for potential secondary headache. An in-depth understanding of several specific pathologic entities, many of them rare, is necessary to identify serious disease without the overuse of diagnostic resources in patients with primary and benign presentations. Moreover, in some cases, misdiagnosis of a particular type of secondary headache may lead to treatment that is deleterious to the patient.

GENERAL APPROACH TO THE PATIENT WITH HEADACHE

The first goal of the emergency physician (EP), if the patient is stable, will be targeted at relieving the patient's pain and discomfort. It is important to note that primary and secondary headaches cannot reliably be differentiated based on response to analgesic therapy. A multitude of life-threatening causes of secondary headache, including subarachnoid hemorrhage (SAH) and cervical artery dissection (CeAD), have been reported to respond to simple analgesic and antimigraine medications.[5–12] As the patient's pain is being addressed, the EP considers secondary causes that warrant further workup and intervention. **Table 1** illustrates the most critical secondary diagnoses to consider in the patient with undifferentiated headache, along with key clinical features, and diagnostic and treatment considerations.

The 2009 American College of Emergency Physician (ACEP) clinical policy on acute headache evaluation describes 4 specific groups that deserve special attention and may warrant neuroimaging in the ED setting (**Table 2**).[13] Although we advocate adherence to these guidelines, we aim to highlight additional high-risk presentations and diagnoses. In this article, we identify 10 important clinical scenarios. Not all scenarios necessarily mandate neuroimaging or other testing; each case should be evaluated within its own unique clinical context. Following the discussion of high-risk scenarios, the specific diagnoses of greatest importance to the practicing EP are examined further.

HIGH-RISK CLINICAL SCENARIOS
Scenario 1: Headache + Sudden/Severe Onset

The quintessential dangerous headache presentation is that of the patient with severe, sudden onset of symptoms. Although cases of "thunderclap headache" may ultimately be attributed to primary or benign causes, emergent causes must be considered. A patient presenting with the new onset of a severe and sudden headache will require neuroimaging in the ED to detect hemorrhagic stroke, including SAH.[13–16] Best practices for ruling out SAH in this clinical setting continue to evolve as new data emerge. Cranial computed tomography (CT) without intravenous (IV) contrast does not demonstrate bleeding in all cases and a complete workup currently includes a lumbar puncture (LP) to detect the presence of xanthochromia or red blood cells.[17–19]

Although SAH is a critical to identify, a broader differential of life-threatening diagnoses exists in these patients.[16,20,21] In addition to hemorrhagic stroke, any vascular origin of headache in the arterial or venous system can cause a sudden onset of symptoms. For example, other potential underlying pathologies, such as CeAD and cerebral venous thrombosis (CVT), may present with a thunderclap, and may be clinically indistinguishable from SAH. Severe unilateral symptoms in the head and neck, particularly when accompanied by neurologic deficits, raise concern for CeAD.[22–25] Although CVT more often presents as a gradual-onset headache with other associated visual or neurologic symptoms, a significant proportion (2%–13%) also can present with a thunderclap.[26,27]

The patient with severe-onset headache, ocular pain, and visual complaints should alert the physician to the possibility of acute angle closure glaucoma (AACG), prompting a more thorough ophthalmologic examination that includes visual acuity and intraocular pressure measurement. Careful inspection of the patient's eyes may reveal a mid-fixed dilated pupil along with conjunctival injection. An intraocular pressure measurement greater than 21 mm Hg is considered abnormal and any pressure greater than 30 mm Hg is highly concerning for AACG. Other important diagnoses in this category include pituitary apoplexy, spontaneous intracranial hypotension, reversible cerebral vasoconstriction syndrome (RCVS), and hypertensive encephalopathy.[28–31] Although it is important to maintain high vigilance for SAH in the patient with headache of sudden onset, simple awareness and consideration of these other secondary causes can help avoid misdiagnoses.

Scenario 2: Headache + Focal Neurologic Deficits and Altered Mental Status

There should be no hesitation to obtain neuroimaging in patients with headache and new neurologic deficits, including any alteration in mental status. The presence of focal neurologic findings has the single highest predictive value for intracranial pathology.[32]

Neurologic findings can result from a variety of dangerous secondary causes, including malignancies, trauma, infection, and any disease state resulting in increased intracranial pressure (ICP). Vascular causes should also be considered, such as CeAD and CVT. Toxic/metabolic causes, notably carbon monoxide (CO) poisoning, may also manifest with neurologic deficits. All such clinical presentations require further diagnostic evaluation.

Headache is a primary feature of acute cerebrovascular disease, most commonly in patients with hemorrhagic stroke or SAH. However, patients with ischemic stroke also may present with headache at time of onset. The frequency of headache in ischemic stroke is higher in women, younger patients, and those with posterior circulation ischemia and infarction.[33] It is important, therefore, to avoid making a diagnosis of hemiplegic migraine in young patients without a complete and thorough evaluation.

Anterior circulation stroke symptoms in the setting of unilateral headache, facial pain, or neck pain should prompt consideration of carotid artery dissection, particularly if seen in the setting of sudden onset retinal ischemic symptoms or Horner syndrome. Posterior circulation stroke symptoms with unilateral head, face, or neck pain should similarly prompt suspicion for vertebral artery dissection.[22] It should be emphasized that in both carotid and vertebral dissection, there may be a significant time interval between the onset of headache and any focal neurologic findings, often several days. Although the diagnosis may be a difficult one at this stage, this presents an important opportunity to prevent potentially devastating complications that may ensue.

Finally, specific cranial nerve deficits in the setting of headache should trigger alarm. A cranial nerve II (optic nerve) palsy may indicate cerebral ischemia, temporal arteritis, or primary ocular pathology. A cranial nerve III (oculomotor nerve) palsy in the setting of headache has several potential dangerous and benign causes, but is most concerning for a posterior communicating aneurysm in the subarachnoid space. More than 90% of patients with SAH with a posterior communicating aneurysm will present with a cranial nerve III palsy.[34] In the setting of severe head trauma, a cranial nerve

Table 1
Dangerous causes of secondary headache

Diagnosis	Clinical Features	Diagnostic Testing	Interventions	Additional Comments
Subarachnoid hemorrhage (SAH)	Severe, sudden onset headache Different from other headaches	CT head Lumbar puncture	Neurosurgical consultation Blood pressure control Nimodipine Ventriculostomy	CT has extremely high sensitivity in first 6 h, then decreases after that Important to consider other causes of thunderclap headache
Cervical artery dissection (CeAD) Internal carotid artery dissection (ICAD) OR Vertebral artery dissection (VAD)	New-onset head, neck, or facial pain ICAD: Anterior circulation ischemia, Horner syndrome, cranial nerve abnormalities, or monocular vision loss VAD: Posterior circulation ischemia	CT head/neck angiography	Anticoagulation vs antiplatelet Consider thrombolytics in early ischemic stroke and extracranial dissection	Neurologic symptoms can be delayed after headache onset Rule out concomitant SAH before initiating anticoagulation Traumatic mechanism in 40%
Giant cell arteritis (GCA)	Headache in age >50 Polymyalgia rheumatica association Temporal artery abnormalities on examination Jaw claudication Visual loss (mainly monocular) Fevers	ESR (cannot rule out if normal) Temporal artery biopsy	Systemic glucocorticoid therapy	When suspicion high, start steroid therapy while awaiting ESR/biopsy results Consider GCA and perform thorough scalp and ophthalmologic examination in elderly patients with fever of unknown source
Cerebral venous thrombosis (CVT)	Headache + signs of increased ICP or focal neurologic deficits	CT or MR venogram	Anticoagulation Endovascular thrombectomy if progressive symptoms despite anticoagulation	Highest risk if history of oral contraceptive, pregnancy/post-partum, thrombophilia

Condition	Clinical features	Diagnostics	Treatment	Comments
Idiopathic intracranial hypertension (IIH)	Most common in young, obese women in 3rd or 4th decade of life. Headache, vision loss, papilledema, transient visual obscurations (TVO), pulsatile tinnitus	Neuroimaging to rule out other space-occupying lesions. Lumbar puncture with opening pressure >20 mm Hg	Weight loss. Acetazolamide or furosemide. Optic nerve fenestration or CNS shunt if progressive vision loss	Cranial VI (abducens) palsy in at-risk patient population is suggestive. Treat to prevent visual loss in 25% of patients
Acute angle closure glaucoma (AACG)	Acute-onset monocular pain, headache, redness, decreased vision ± nausea vomiting. Mid-fixed dilated pupil, "steamy cornea"	Ocular pressure >21 mm Hg (most often >30 mm Hg)	Ophthalmologic consultation. Pressure-lowering eye drops. Systemic osmotic therapy	Perform an eye examination on alert patients with dilated pupil and sudden-onset severe headache (can mimic SAH with PCOM aneurysm)
Bacterial meningitis	Fever, headache, altered mental status, nuchal rigidity	Lumbar puncture (+/− CT head) see 2008 ACEP Clinical Policy on Acute Headache)	IV antibiotics. Consider IV dexamethasone	Jolt accentuation, Brudzinki sign, Kernig sign, nuchal rigidity all are poorly sensitive physical examination findings
Preeclampsia	Headache in pregnancy >20 ± visual symptoms, abdominal pain, chest pain, shortness of breath, vomiting	SBP >140 mm Hg or DBP >110 on 2 occasions + any of the following: proteinuria, thrombocytopenia, renal insufficiency, impaired liver function, pulmonary edema, cerebral or visual disturbances	Obstetric consultation. Urgent delivery if severe symptoms. Blood pressure management. IV magnesium	Must consider diagnosis up to 6 wk postpartum, highest risk in 1st week postdelivery

(continued on next page)

Table 1
(continued)

Diagnosis	Clinical Features	Diagnostic Testing	Interventions	Additional Comments
Pituitary apoplexy	Severe headache Visual complaints, vomiting +/– hypopituitarism	CT head noncontrast for hemorrhage MRI for pituitary mass	Neurosurgical consultation Systemic glucocorticoids for any adrenal insufficiency	Ocular paresis can occur, affecting CN III, IV, or VI (most commonly CN III)
Carbon monoxide poisoning	Flulike illness; worse each morning Mild: headache, nausea, myalgia, dizzy Severe: confusion, syncope, neurologic deficits, death	Arterial blood gas co-oximetry	Non-rebreather oxygen +/– Hyperbaric oxygen chamber therapy	Consider when multiple patients from same household have similar symptoms Hyperbaric oxygen therapy is indicated for neurologic or cardiovascular signs and above certain cutoffs
Space-occupying lesions	Progressively worsening headache History of malignancy Worse in morning or in head-down position	CT Head MRI	Neurosurgical consultation ICP-lowering therapies Lesion-specific therapies	Emergent ICP-lowering therapies may include elevating head of bed, diuretics, and hyperventilation Lesion-specific therapies may include operative intervention, corticosteroids, and antimicrobial agents
Occult trauma	Signs of abuse or neglect Anticoagulation or coagulopathy	CT head	Neurosurgical consultation	Patients in at-risk populations (eg, abuse) may not volunteer a history of trauma
Reversal cerebral vasoconstriction syndrome (RCVS)	Thunderclap headaches resolving within minutes or hours Multiple recurrent sudden, severe exacerbations are highly suggestive	CT or MR angiography	Supportive care, monitoring in neurosurgical ICU	Ischemic or hemorrhagic strokes can occur in 20% of patients Postpartum period is a risk factor (occurs in other patient populations as well)
Cerebellar infarction	Headache with dizziness Cerebellar signs Cranial nerve abnormalities	CT head MRI	Neurologic/neurosurgical consultation	Although CT head is insensitive for infarction, it is helpful initially to rule out hemorrhage and identify life-threatening edema and mass effect

Abbreviations: ACEP, American College of Emergency Physicians; CN, cranial nerve; CNS, central nervous system; CT, computed tomography; DBP, diastolic blood pressure; ESR, erythrocyte sedimentation rate; ICP, intracranial pressure; ICU, intensive care unit; IV, intravenous; SBP, systolic blood pressure.

Table 2
2008 American College of Emergency Physicians Clinical Policy: Which patients with headache require neuroimaging in the ED?

Patient Presentation	Recommendation Level
Headache + new abnormal findings in a neurologic examination (eg, focal deficit, altered mental status, altered cognitive function)	Level B Recommendation (emergent noncontrast head CT)[a]
New sudden-onset severe headache	Level B Recommendation (emergent noncontrast head CT)[a]
HIV-positive patients with a new type of headache	Level B Recommendation (emergent noncontrast head CT)[a]
Age >50 with new headache but with normal neurologic examination	Level C Recommendation (urgent noncontrast head CT)[b]

Abbreviations: CT, computed tomography; ED, emergency department; HIV, human immunodeficiency virus.

Routine studies are indicated when the study is not considered necessary to make a disposition in the ED.

[a] *Emergent studies* are those essential for a timely decision regarding potentially life-threatening or severely disabling entities.

[b] *Urgent studies* are those that are arranged before discharge from the ED (scan appointment is included in the disposition).

Data from Edlow JA, Panagos PD, Godwin SA, et al; American College of Emergency Physicians. Clinical policy: critical issues in the evaluation and management of adult patients presenting to the emergency department with acute headache. Ann Emerg Med 2008;52(4):407–36.

III palsy also can indicate uncal (transtentorial) herniation. Cranial nerve VI (abducens nerve) has a long intracranial course before exiting the skull and is sensitive to any pathology that causes an increase or decrease in ICP. Moreover, any involvement of a combination of cranial nerves III, IV, and VI can indicate serious pathology of the cavernous sinus. Finally, the involvement of multiple cranial nerves may also indicate the presence of brainstem disease. Thus, the presence of new neurologic deficits in the setting of headache is a true "red flag" for serious pathology and neuroimaging should be pursued without delay.

Scenario 3: Headache + Human Immunodeficiency Virus or Other Immunocompromised State

Patients with a history of immunosuppression and headache should immediately raise suspicion for intracranial pathology. Patients with human immunodeficiency virus (HIV) and headaches have substantially higher rates of intracranial disease when compared with the general population, 24% to 36% in 2 separate studies.[35,36] Key considerations of headache in patients with HIV include infectious causes, such as cryptococcal meningitis and toxoplasmosis, and noninfectious causes, most notably lymphomas.

Similarly, patients on immunosuppressive therapy, such as those on posttransplantation medications, have a broad range of potential complications. Bacterial, fungal, viral, and parasitic infections of the brain or meninges account for 4% to 29% of central nervous system (CNS) lesions in organ transplant recipients and are associated with high mortality. After transplantation, patients can similarly develop several other noninfectious neurotoxic complications, including de novo CNS malignancies and posterior reversible encephalopathy (PRES).[37,38] The increased prevalence of both infectious and noninfectious neurologic complications in immunosuppressed patients underscores the importance of a more comprehensive workup in this patient subgroup.

Scenario 4: Headache + Advanced Age

The ACEP specifically advocates for advanced imaging in patients older than 50 years with a new-type headache (Level C Recommendation, see **Table 2**). Elderly patients are at higher risk for several concerning secondary causes of headache, such as intracranial hemorrhage, occult trauma, giant cell arteritis, and malignancy.[32,39–41] One review of patients with headache revealed a 15% incidence of dangerous secondary headaches in patients older than 65 years.[42] Another large study examining all available risk factors for headache found that patients older than 50 years demonstrated 4 times the rate of pathology compared with younger patients.[43] Given the increased likelihood of secondary headache in this age population, further diagnostic testing should be strongly considered in the elderly patient with new headache. In patients older than 60 years with a new headache, especially if accompanied by polymyalgia rheumatic (PMR) or symptoms such as scalp tenderness, jaw claudication, or visual symptoms, consider giant cell arteritis (see later in this article).

Scenario 5: Headache + Pregnancy

The most likely etiologies of headache in patients who are pregnant or postpartum are similar to the general population with primary headaches, such as tension-type and migraines, being most common.[44,45]

However, patients are at increased risk for secondary headaches during pregnancy, warranting a meticulous evaluation for etiologies such as preeclampsia, cerebral venous thrombosis, and pituitary apoplexy. A particularly high index of suspicion should be maintained for the diagnoses of preeclampsia and eclampsia.[46] These etiologies must be considered in pregnant women at greater than 20 weeks' gestation up through 6 weeks postpartum, with the highest risk in the first week postdelivery.[47] Patients with eclampsia are often found to have had headaches preceding their seizures by more than a day, thus a low threshold for initiating diagnostic workup is necessary even in the absence of symptoms beyond headache.[48]

The prothrombotic state associated with pregnancy also increases the risk for stroke and CVT, particularly in the third trimester and postpartum period.[49] From an endocrine perspective, pregnancy may cause a 139% size increase of the pituitary gland, increasing the risk for pituitary apoplexy.[50,51]

Postpuncture dural headaches and RCVS should also be considered in the postpartum patient. Postpuncture dural headaches can occur in patients receiving epidural injections. Postpartum RCVS is a rare but potentially serious cause of headache that occurs in the early postpartum period and is characterized by acute-onset, severe headaches due to prolonged vasoconstriction of medium and large cerebral arteries. Recurrent episodes of a thunderclap headache are highly suggestive of RCVS.[52] The symptoms of RCVS are often recurrent and can lead to life-threatening emergencies, such as intracranial hemorrhage, cerebral infarction, and vasogenic brain edema.[53]

Other causes of secondary headache in pregnancy occur with approximately similar prevalence as the general population and workup should be guided by the patient's clinical presentation.[46,54]

Scenario 6: Headache + Coagulopathy

Any patient with hematologic disturbances due to hypercoagulability or an anticoagulated state has an increased likelihood of serious pathology associated with his or her headache. Prothrombotic disorders can be inherited or acquired and account for approximately 34% of patients diagnosed with CVT.[55] Patients with antithrombin deficiency, protein C/S deficiency, factor V Leiden mutations, use of oral contraceptives, and hyperhomocysteinemia all have increased risk for CVT.[56]

On the other hand, in patients with bleeding disorders, several risk factors can lead to an increased probability of spontaneous intracranial hemorrhage. Patients with both acquired and congenital disorders, such as hemophilia A/B and von Willebrand disease, are at higher risk for intracranial hemorrhage, particularly after trauma.[57–59] Patients on anticoagulant medications are of particular concern, as they account for 12% to 20% of patients with intracranial hemorrhage.[60] Hematoma expansion also can occur more aggressively in these patients with rapid neurologic deterioration, further emphasizing the importance of expedited diagnosis, workup, and intervention.[61]

Scenario 7: Headache + Malignancy

Headache in the patient with history of malignancy can occur from a variety of causes, including the mass effect of the tumor itself or as a result of the therapy.[62] Although traditional teaching holds that a morning or nocturnal headache can be suggestive of intracranial malignancy, this pattern is actually uncommon in adult patients, with nausea, vomiting, and neurologic abnormalities being far more common.[62,63] Both primary and metastatic tumors are equally likely to cause headache at a rate of approximately 60%.[64] The most common primary sites for metastases to the brain are as follows: lung (19.9%), melanoma (6.9%), renal (6.5%), breast (5.1%), and colorectal (1.8%).[65] It is important to note that brain cancer rarely presents with headache as its sole presenting feature, occurring in only 2% to 8% of patients.[66] Most patients with primary or metastatic disease will demonstrate concomitant neurologic deficits, neuropsychiatric disorders, or seizures.

In addition to pain caused by the tumor itself, patients with intracranial malignancy are at risk for intracranial hemorrhage. Approximately 1% to 11% of intracranial hemorrhage cases are secondary to malignancy, most commonly from metastatic solid tumors. Therefore, new headaches in patients with identified tumors should be further investigated.[67] Finally, patients receiving chemotherapeutic agents or radiation therapy and those who have received a craniotomy can all present with the onset of a new type of headache. In such patients, the clinician should first evaluate the possibility of other more serious causes before attributing the symptoms to therapeutic interventions.

Scenario 8: Headache + Fever

Fever in the setting of headache can occur secondary to a CNS infection as well as systemic disease. In the toxic patient with fever and altered mental status, it can be particularly difficult to differentiate CNS infection from other systemic causes, such as septicemia, serotonin syndrome, or other potential pathologies. If other systemic etiologies are not readily apparent, the diagnostic study of choice to evaluate for meningitis or meningoencephalitis is an LP; however, certain patient subsets are at increased risk for elevated ICP, and these patients should likely undergo neuroimaging before LP (ACEP Level C Recommendation, see **Table 2**). Specifically, cranial CT prior to LP should be considered in any patient with any of the following features: 60 years or older, immune-compromised, history of CNS disease, recent seizures, altered mental status, focal neurologic deficit, or papilledema, as these patients may have a higher potential risk of brain herniation with LP.[68,69]

Brain abscess is another uncommon but important primary CNS infection to be considered. It is very rarely associated with meningitis. Potential mechanisms for development of brain abscess include contiguous spread from surrounding structures, hematogenous spread, and after neurosurgical manipulation. The most common is via direct spread from surrounding sinusitis, otitis media, or dental infections.[70] Alternatively, hematogenous seeding from sources such as lung abscess or infective endocarditis can also lead to brain abscess. Approximately 70% of patients with brain abscess will report headache, but only 50% are febrile.[70,71] In fact, the triad of headache, fever, and focal neurologic deficits occurs in only 20% of patients; the only clue may be a new headache in an at-risk patient (eg, recent neurosurgical instrumentation). Lastly, brain abscess should be a special consideration in patients who are immunosuppressed from acquired immune deficiency syndrome (AIDS) or posttransplantation.

Other important noninfectious causes of headache that may present with fever include SAH, pituitary apoplexy, and giant cell arteritis (GCA). Fever in the setting of SAH tends to occur in the days following the event and is associated with increased mortality and functional disability.[72] Fever in SAH can be attributed to both a systemic inflammatory reaction and a loss of central thermoregulatory control.[73] Pituitary apoplexy also can pose a diagnostic challenge with a meningitis/encephalitis-type clinical presentation. Of 12 patients examined in a case series of pituitary apoplexy, 33% presented with fever and 83% had signs of meningeal irritation.[74] Further complicating matters, cerebrospinal fluid (CSF) samples can show inflammatory changes resembling meningitis.[75] Finally, vasculitic diseases, such as GCA, may lead to various systemic manifestations, including febrile illness, and should remain in the provider's differential diagnosis.

The spectrum of severity in patients with headache and fever can range from benign to high risk with increased mortality. A patient with fever and headache will therefore require a careful and thorough evaluation for systemic pathology as well as consideration of primary CNS infectious and noninfectious causes.

Scenario 9: Headache + Visual Deficits

Patients with a clinical presentation of headache and visual complaints warrant further consideration for the possibility of secondary etiologies. Clarifying the nature of the patient's visual symptoms is paramount in determining the likelihood of serious disease. For example, a migraine headache commonly presents with a visual aura that is clinically distinct from visual symptoms due to dangerous causes such as vascular disease. Patients with migraine classically describe visual complaints involving colors, scintillations, and scotomata. The aura in migraine will usually develop gradually over 5 to 20 minutes and resolve within 60 minutes, often preceding the onset of headache.[76] Distinguishing these more benign features in the setting of the patient's typical headaches from concerning new visual features such as sudden-onset monocular visual loss or visual field defects can prevent misidentification of more concerning pathology.

Patients presenting with headache and transient monocular vision loss should undergo evaluation for underlying secondary headache. Carotid artery dissection can result in retinal ischemia but this presentation occurs in only 2% of patients.[77] Other causes of monocular vision loss include optic neuritis, GCA, and AACG. Rarely, "retinal migraines" have been described with transient monocular vision loss, although this diagnosis should be considered only in consultation and only after all other dangerous causes have been ruled out.[78] In the case of headache and binocular visual loss, idiopathic intracranial hypertension and intracranial masses should be strongly considered.

A visual field examination should be conducted on all patients with headache and visual complaints. The presence of headache with visual field disturbance, such as homonymous hemianopsia, is highly concerning for a dangerous underlying cause. Most cases of hemianopsia in adults are secondary to vascular pathology, including cerebral infarction and intracranial hemorrhage, followed by trauma and brain tumor.[79] A fundoscopic examination is another key component of evaluation. The presence of papilledema suggests increased ICP from any cause, including idiopathic intracranial hypertension, cerebral venous thrombosis, malignancy, or infection.[80] Patients with headache and papilledema require expedited workup to prevent ischemia and subsequent permanent optic nerve damage.

Scenario 10: Headache + Loss of Consciousness

A headache associated with loss of consciousness is worrisome. In some cases, it can be difficult to discern whether the patient experienced a syncopal episode or a seizure. Both scenarios, however, justify further investigation. In the case of loss of consciousness with headache, vascular etiologies should be considered primarily and ruled out. Subarachnoid hemorrhage can present with syncope in 5% of cases and should be a leading consideration.[81] Another consideration of note for patients presenting with headache and syncope is an intracranial mass obstructing the third ventricle, such as a colloid cyst.[82] A presentation of headache and seizure may indicate dangerous disease including eclampsia, CNS infection, intracranial hemorrhage, CNS malignancy, and increased ICP. In subarachnoid hemorrhage, the presence of seizures alone predicts worsening clinical disability.[83] Regardless of the underlying cause for unconsciousness, patients with a headache in this setting merit a thorough diagnostic evaluation.

DANGEROUS CAUSES OF SECONDARY HEADACHE
Subarachnoid Hemorrhage

SAH is among the most important considerations in patients presenting with headache. Onset can occur during physical exertion, such as exercise or during coitus, but such a trigger is noted in only approximately 20% of cases.[84] The classic clinical picture is one of sudden and severe headache that is maximal at onset.[85] Other important clinical features include vomiting, neck stiffness, seizure, neurologic deficits, and alteration in mental status or coma.

Currently, the gold standard in the diagnosis of SAH is by CSF analysis. Recently, some investigators have concluded that it may be reasonable to rule out SAH without LP if a third-generation CT scan is performed within 6 hours of symptom onset and interpreted by a radiologist experienced with cranial CT.[86–88] This 6-hour approach has been challenged by others and would apply only to patients with normal levels of consciousness and no focal neurologic deficits.[89] It should be noted that the 2012 American Heart Association/American Stroke Association (AHA/ASA) guidelines on the management of aneurysmal SAH continue to recommend LP if a noncontrast CT of the head is nondiagnostic.[90] CT angiography also has been proposed as an alternative diagnostic approach, potentially identifying more than 99% of aneurysmal SAH; however, this approach has the unintended consequence of identifying asymptomatic aneurysms that do not require neurosurgical intervention.[91–93] "Nonculprit" aneurysms (eg, those that have not bled) do not carry the same risk of bleeding as those that have resulted in SAH. The authors recommend that if the LP is omitted for any reason, that a shared decision-making model informing the patient of potential risk of missed SAH be used.

Carotid/Vertebral Artery Dissection

CeAD is an important but difficult cause of headache to diagnose in the ED. Cervical artery dissection includes both internal carotid artery dissection (ICAD) and vertebral artery dissection (VAD). ICAD is estimated as the underlying cause of 2% of all cases of stroke and up to 24% of strokes in children and young adults.[94–96] Both subtypes of CeAD are linked to preceding cervical trauma, such as vigorous physical activity, coughing, sneezing, or chiropractic manipulation in approximately 40% of cases.[97] Headache in CeAD is a prominent symptom in approximately 70% of cases, but patients also may present with isolated neck or facial pain.[98,99] Perhaps the biggest obstacle to prompt and precise diagnosis of CeAD is the delayed onset of neurologic symptoms, with median times ranging from 4 days in patients with ICAD and 14.5 hours in patients with VAD.[99]

In the large, observational Cervical Artery Dissection and Ischemic Stroke Patients (CADISP) study, patients with ICAD presented with cerebral ischemic symptoms 73% of the time and patients with VAD presented with cerebral ischemic symptoms in 90% of cases.[98] Patients with ICAD typically present with anterior circulation ischemic symptoms, whereas VAD classically presents with posterior circulation ischemic deficits. Additional clinical findings in ICAD may include a complete or partial Horner syndrome, cranial nerve palsies, pulsatile tinnitus, and permanent or transient monocular vision loss secondary to ischemia.[100] Cranial nerve palsies are less common, but also may occur in ICAD with the hypoglossal (XII) nerve most frequently affected in isolation or in combination with other lower cranial nerves IX to XI.[101] CeAD that presents with headache, or facial or neck pain alone is especially challenging. In these cases, the only clinical clues may lie in a concerning mechanism and a typical pattern of pain. Diagnosis is confirmed via MRI/magnetic resonance angiography (MRA) or CT angiography (CTA).[102] The sensitivity for ultrasound in the diagnosis of CeAD ranges from 70% to 86% and therefore the provider should pursue more advanced CTA or MRA studies if clinical suspicion exists.[103] Ideally, if the diagnosis can be made before the development of neurologic deficits, a window of opportunity exists to prevent a poor clinical outcome.

Giant Cell Arteritis

GCA, or temporal arteritis, is a vasculitis of medium and large vessels and is the most common cause of systemic vasculitis in patients older than 50 in North America and Europe.[104] The most important risk factor in GCA is age, as disease almost never develops in patients younger than 50, with most patients developing GCA after 70 years of age.[105,106]

Headache is the most critical clinical feature, occurring in 83% of patients with GCA. Other important features include the presence of Polymyalgia rheumatica (PMR), temporal artery abnormalities (tender, nodular, swollen, thickened arteries, and/or decreased pulse), jaw claudication, fevers, and visual loss.[107] PMR is characterized by aching morning stiffness in the shoulder, hip girdle, and neck muscles and is associated with approximately half of all cases of GCA.[108] The presence of unexplained anemia or constitutional symptoms of fever, weight loss, or malaise also may provide additional clues. In a review of elderly patients with fever of unknown origin, GCA was the most frequent specific ultimate diagnosis, accounting for 17% of cases.[109] Transient monocular visual impairment or diplopia can be an early manifestation of GCA, although in 10% of patients, binocular visual changes are present.[110]

The feared complication of permanent visual loss in GCA most commonly results from optic or retinal ischemia, occurring in 15% of patients.[110,111] If GCA is strongly suspected, empiric treatment with corticosteroids should be started and temporal artery biopsy should be considered. Elevated erythrocyte sedimentation rate (ESR) levels may suggest the presence of GCA but 5% of patients with biopsy-confirmed GCA can have normal ESR levels and a negative ESR cannot reliably rule out the disease.[106,112]

Initiation of steroid therapy should not be delayed in awaiting temporal biopsy if suspicion for GCA is high, as biopsy results will not be affected for at least 1 week.[113]

Cerebral Vein and Sinus Thrombosis

Cerebral vein and sinus thrombosis (CVT) is a rare form of stroke that can occur at any age with a mean age of 39 years.[55] Oral contraceptive use and thrombophilia are the most common risk factors for development of CVT. Several additional risk factors have been identified, including pregnancy and postpartum states, as well as infections, particularly those involving the ears, sinus, mouth, face, and neck.[55]

Headache is the most common presenting complaint in cases of CVT, occurring in more than 90% of cases. It is the sole symptom, however, in only 25% of cases.[55,114] The headache is most typically slow and progressive in onset but may have a thunderclap presentation in a minority of patients.[26,27] The average time delay from presentation to diagnosis is 7 days and a careful evaluation for signs of increased ICP or focal brain injury is needed to identify patients with CVT.[55] Signs of increased ICP, such as papilledema or a cranial nerve VI (abducens) palsy, may suggest superior sagittal sinus thrombosis, the most commonly affected location in CVT.[56] A wide range of additional focal neurologic deficits can develop depending on the location of infarction or secondary hemorrhage, including aphasia, unilateral or bilateral weakness, and altered mental status. Rapid neurologic deterioration with stupor and coma has been noted in 14% of cases, whereas seizures are found in approximately 40% of patients.[55] Finally, one-third of patients with CVT develop intracerebral hemorrhage, placing them at risk for worse outcomes.[115]

Initial neuroimaging will often include CT or MRI of the brain. Unfortunately, neither CT nor MRI effectively rules out CVT and further workup with CT or MR venography is recommended when clinical suspicion is high.

Idiopathic Intracranial Hypertension

Idiopathic intracranial hypertension (IIH) is characterized by an elevation of ICP (ICP >20 cm H_2O), with normal ventricles and CSF analysis and in the absence of space-occupying lesions.[116] It is most common in young, obese women in the third or fourth decade of life.[117]

Headaches in IIH can be severe and disabling, and there is a risk of permanent visual loss in the absence of therapeutic intervention.[118] Headaches occur in most patients with IIH with variable, nonspecific headache features. Associated symptoms include transient visual obscurations, pulsatile tinnitus, photopsia, and occasional radicular shoulder and arm pains.[117] Transient visual obscurations are described as brief episodes of monocular or binocular visual loss followed by full recovery.[119] Pulsatile tinnitus is seen in approximately one-half of patients and is likely due to turbulent blood flow through a stenotic venous sinus.[117] Physical examination should involve a search for papilledema, peripheral visual field defects, and unilateral or bilateral cranial nerve VI (abducens) palsy. Any other physical findings suggest another diagnosis. The key to diagnosis in IIH is an elevated opening pressure by LP in the absence of space-occupying lesions on neuroimaging. There is a link between IIH and CVT; a negative CT or MRI in combination with elevated opening pressures may warrant further workup with venography to evaluate for potential CVT.

Acute Angle Closure Glaucoma

AACG develops when the anterior chamber angle is narrowed, obstructing the flow of aqueous humor and leading to increased intraocular pressure (IOP). Patients older than 50 years are at risk for AACG, and its peak incidence occurs in patients older than 70.[120] Pupillary dilation resulting from any cause (eg, a dimly lit room) can precipitate an attack.

Clinically, patients present with abrupt-onset eye pain, blurry vision, and headache. They may additionally complain of nausea and vomiting. The typical physical examination reveals a mid-fixed dilated pupil with decreased visual acuity, injected conjunctiva, and a steamy (ie, edematous) cornea.[121] Ocular pressures greater than 21 mm Hg are necessary to make the diagnosis and IOP is typically 30 mm Hg or higher. Once identified, medical and surgical therapy should be targeted at reducing the IOP to prevent permanent visual loss.[122]

Bacterial Meningitis

Meningitis can result from a bacterial, viral, fungal, parasitic, or noninfectious cause. Of these, bacterial meningitis is of particular concern and is associated with a high mortality (approximately 15%).[123]

The classic triad of headache, fever, and neck stiffness is present in only 44% of cases.[124] However, 99% of patients with bacterial meningitis will have at least 1 of these 3 classic symptoms and 95% present with 2 of the following: headache, fever, neck stiffness, altered mental status.[124] Many patients with bacterial meningitis have preceding ear, sinus, or lung infections.[125]

Physical examination findings for bacterial meningitis have included the Kernig sign, Brudzinski sign, nuchal rigidity, and jolt accentuation.[126] A prospective analysis of these tests for meningitis found that jolt accentuation has a sensitivity of 21% with a specificity of 82%. Nuchal rigidity was found to have a sensitivity of 13% with a specificity of 80%. Kernig and Brudzinski signs both were found to have very low sensitivities of 2% with specificities of 97% and 98%, respectively.[127] Although these findings may help suggest the diagnosis of bacterial meningitis, the absence of these findings cannot rule out the disease, and CSF analysis is necessary for appropriate evaluation. Treatment with antimicrobials should not be delayed for LP or CSF results.[128]

Preeclampsia

Preeclampsia is considered in the newly hypertensive patient after 20 weeks' gestation up to 6 weeks postpartum and affects approximately 5% of all pregnancies.[129] A systolic blood pressure greater than 140 mm Hg or diastolic blood pressure greater than 90 mm Hg on 2 occasions in combination with either proteinuria or end-organ damage is diagnostic.[130] The American College of Obstetricians and Gynecologists (ACOG) updated their criteria in 2013, and proteinuria is no longer an essential component for diagnosis if new onset of any of the following findings are present: thrombocytopenia, renal insufficiency, impaired liver function, pulmonary edema, or cerebral or visual disturbance.[130] Therefore, any patient at greater than 20 weeks' gestation meeting the ACOG criteria with new-onset headache should be identified as having preeclampsia, and urgent consultation and treatment should be considered.

Pituitary Apoplexy

Pituitary apoplexy is an acute ischemic or hemorrhagic infarction of the pituitary gland, occurring in patients with pituitary adenomas.[131] Underlying risk factors for apoplexy are identified in only 25% to 40% of patients, and they include pregnancy, head trauma, pituitary radiation, major surgery, and treatment with dopamine agonists.[131–133]

The clinical presentation of pituitary apoplexy is widely variable, from benign to catastrophic. The typical patient complains of severe headache, vomiting, and visual complaints. The headache can often present as sudden and severe in its onset, mimicking SAH.[28] Patients also may present with infectious-type symptoms of fever, meningeal irritation, and alteration in mental status. The visual symptoms can manifest as decreased visual acuity or visual field defects in 75% of patients, with ocular paresis occurring in approximately 70%.[133] Ocular paresis can develop as a result of compression of the cavernous sinus and associated cranial nerves III, IV, and VI. Of these, cranial nerve III (oculomotor) is most susceptible to compression.[134] Finally, at time of presentation, patients may demonstrate evidence of hypopituitarism and any evidence of glucocorticoid deficiency in the form of hypoglycemia, hypotension, or hyponatremia will require replacement with IV hydrocortisone.[133] The initial diagnostic test for evaluation of pituitary apoplexy will often be a noncontrast CT of the head to rule out SAH. Although noncontrast CT is sensitive for acute hemorrhage, MRI should be pursued if CT is negative to detect infarction.[135,136]

Carbon Monoxide Poisoning

CO poisonings account for approximately 50,000 ED visits per year in the United States.[137] CO poisoning is a dangerous underlying cause of headache; most cases are related to smoke inhalation, but faulty furnaces, inadequate ventilation of heating sources, and exposure to engine exhaust are also important causes.[138] Mild exposures may cause headaches, myalgias, dizziness, and neuropsychological impairment.[139,140] More severe exposures can result in alteration of mental status, focal neurologic deficits, loss of consciousness, or death.[138] Delayed neurologic sequelae and neuropsychiatric effects also may result.[141,142]

In the ED, the patient with headache and recent potential exposure must be evaluated for CO poisoning, particularly when multiple household members or pets also are ill. Pulse oximetry (SpO2) is unable to distinguish between oxyhemoglobin and carboxyhemoglobin and thus cannot reliably screen for CO exposure.[143] Therefore, co-oximetry via serum blood gas analysis is needed to measure elevated carboxyhemoglobin levels. Once identified, oxygen by non-rebreather mask should be initiated and consideration given to hyperbaric oxygen treatment.[144]

REFERENCES

1. Pitts SR, Niska RW, Xu J, et al. National Hospital Ambulatory Medical Care Survey: 2006 emergency department summary. Natl Health Stat Rep 2008;(7):1–38.
2. Available at: http://www.cdc.gov/nchs/data/ahcd/nhamcs_emergency/2011_ed_web_tables.pdf. Accessed November 27, 2015.
3. Headache Classification Committee of the International Headache Society (IHS). The International Classification of Headache Disorders, 3rd edition (beta version). Cephalalgia 2013;33(9):629–808.
4. Morgenstern LB, Huber JC, Luna-Gonzales H, et al. Headache in the emergency department. Headache 2001;41(6):537–41.
5. Pope JV, Edlow JA. Favorable response to analgesics does not predict a benign etiology of headache. Headache 2008;48:944.
6. Pfadenhauer K, Schonsteiner T, Keller H. The risks of sumatriptan administration in patients with unrecognized subarachnoid haemorrhage (SAH). Cephalalgia 2006;26:320.
7. Lipton RB, Mazer C, Newman LC, et al. Sumatriptan relieves migraine-like headaches associated with carbon monoxide exposure. Headache 1997;37:392.
8. Abisaab J, Nevadunsky N, Flomenbaum N. Emergency department presentation of bilateral carotid artery dissections in a postpartum patient. Ann Emerg Med 2004;44:484.

9. Leira EC, Cruz-Flores S, Leacock RO, et al. Sumatriptan can alleviate headaches due to carotid artery dissection. Headache 2001;41:590.

10. Prokhorov S, Khanna S, Alapati D, et al. Subcutaneous sumatriptan relieved migraine-like headache in two adolescents with aseptic meningitis. Headache 2008;48:1235.

11. Rosenberg JH, Silberstein SD. The headache of SAH responds to sumatriptan. Headache 2005;45:597.

12. Barclay CL, Shuaib A, Montoya D, et al. Response of non-migrainous headaches to chlorpromazine. Headache 1990;30:85.

13. Edlow JA, Panagos PD, Godwin SA, et al, American College of Emergency Physicians. Clinical policy: critical issues in the evaluation and management of adult patients presenting to the emergency department with acute headache. Ann Emerg Med 2008;52(4):407–36.

14. Suarez JI, Tarr RW, Selman WR. Aneurysmal subarachnoid hemorrhage. N Engl J Med 2006;354(4):387–96.

15. Edlow JA, Caplan LR. Avoiding pitfalls in the diagnosis of subarachnoid hemorrhage. N Engl J Med 2000;342(1):29–36.

16. Harling DW, Peatfield RC, Van Hille PT, et al. Thunderclap headache: is it migraine? Cephalalgia 1989;9(2):87–90.

17. Lledo A, Calandre L, Martinez-Menendez B, et al. Acute headache of recent onset and subarachnoid hemorrhage: a prospective study. Headache 1994; 34(3):172–4.

18. Sidman R, Connolly E, Lemke T. Subarachnoid hemorrhage diagnosis: lumbar puncture is still needed when the computed tomography scan is normal. Acad Emerg Med 1996;3(9):827–31.

19. Perry JJ, Spacek A, Forbes M, et al. Is the combination of negative computed tomography result and negative lumbar puncture result sufficient to rule out subarachnoid hemorrhage? Ann Emerg Med 2008;51(6):707–13.

20. Landtblom AM, Fridriksson S, Boivie J, et al. Sudden onset headache: a prospective study of features, incidence and causes. Cephalalgia 2002;22(5): 354–60.

21. Linn FH, Wijdicks EF, van der Graaf Y, et al. Prospective study of sentinel headache in aneurysmal subarachnoid haemorrhage. Lancet 1994;344(8922):590–3.

22. Debette S, Leys D. Cervical-artery dissections: predisposing factors, diagnosis, and outcome. Lancet Neurol 2009;8(7):668–78.

23. Arnold M, Cumurciuc R, Stapf C, et al. Pain as the only symptom of cervical artery dissection. J Neurol Neurosurg Psychiatry 2006;77(9):1021–4.

24. Maruyama H, Nagoya H, Kato Y, et al. Spontaneous cervicocephalic arterial dissection with headache and neck pain as the only symptom. J Headache Pain 2012;13(3):247–53.

25. Mitsias P, Ramadan NM. Headache in ischemic cerebrovascular disease. Part I: clinical features. Cephalalgia 1992;12(5):269–74.

26. Cumurciuc R, Crassard I, Sarov M, et al. Headache as the only neurological sign of cerebral venous thrombosis: a series of 17 cases. J Neurol Neurosurg Psychiatry 2005;76(8):1084–7.

27. de Bruijn SF, Stam J, Kappelle LJ. Thunderclap headache as first symptom of cerebral venous sinus thrombosis. CVST Study Group. Lancet 1996;348(9042): 1623–5.

28. Dodick DW, Wijdicks EF. Pituitary apoplexy presenting as a thunderclap headache. Neurology 1998;50(5):1510–1.

29. Embil JM, Kramer M, Kinnear S, et al. A blinding headache. Lancet 1997; 350(9072):182.
30. Garza I, Kirsch J. Pituitary apoplexy and thunderclap headache. Headache 2007;47(3):431–2.
31. Dodick DW. Thunderclap headache. Headache 2002;42(4):309–15.
32. Locker TE, Thompson C, Rylance J, et al. The utility of clinical features in patients presenting with nontraumatic headache: an investigation of adult patients attending an emergency department. Headache 2006;46(6):954–61.
33. Tentschert S, Wimmer R, Greisenegger S, et al. Headache at stroke onset in 2196 patients with ischemic stroke or transient ischemic attack. Stroke 2005; 36(2):e1–3.
34. Prasad S, Volpe NJ. Paralytic strabismus: third, fourth, and sixth nerve palsy. Neurol Clin 2010;28(3):803–33.
35. Lipton RB, Feraru ER, Weiss G, et al. Headache in HIV-1 related disorders. Headache 1991;31:518–22.
36. Rothman RE, Keyl PM, McAruthur JC, et al. A decision guideline for emergency department utilization of noncontrast head computed tomography in HIV-infected patients. Acad Emerg Med 1999;6:1010–9.
37. Pruitt AA, Graus F, Rosenfeld MR. Neurologic complications of solid organ transplantation. Neurohospitalist 2013;3(3):152.
38. Pustavoitau A, Bhardwaj A, Stevens R. Neurological complications of transplantation. J Intensive Care Med 2011;26(4):209–22.
39. Ramirez-Lassepas M, Espinosa CE, Cicero JJ, et al. Predictors of intracranial pathologic findings in patients who seek emergency care because of headache. Arch Neurol 1997;54:1506–9.
40. Kahn CE, Sanders GD, Lyons EA, et al. Computed tomography for nontraumatic headache: current utilization and cost-effectiveness. Can Assoc Radiol J 1993; 44:189–93.
41. Duarte J, Sempere AP, Delgado JA, et al. Headache of recent onset in adults: a prospective population-based study. Acta Neurol Scand 1996;94:67–70.
42. Pascual J, Berciano J. Experience in the diagnosis of headaches that start in elderly people. J Neurol Neurosurg Psychiatry 1994;57(10):1255–7.
43. Goldstein JN, Camargo CA Jr, Pelletier AJ, et al. Headache in United States emergency departments: demographics, work-up and frequency of pathological diagnoses. Cephalalgia 2006;26:684–90.
44. Dixit A, Bhardwaj M, Sharma B. Headache in pregnancy: a nuisance or a new sense? Obstet Gynecol Int 2012;2012:697697.
45. MacGregor EA. Headache in pregnancy. Neurol Clin 2012;30(3):835–66.
46. Schoen JC, Campbell RL, Sadosty AT. Headache in pregnancy: an approach to emergency department evaluation and management. West J Emerg Med 2015; 16(2):291–301.
47. Al-Safi Z, Imudia AN, Filetti LC, et al. Delayed postpartum preeclampsia and eclampsia: demographics, clinical course, and complications. Obstet Gynecol 2011;118(5):1102–7.
48. Shah AK, Rajamani K, Whitty JE. Eclampsia: a neurological perspective. J Neurol Sci 2008;271:158.
49. Bousser MG, Crassard I. Cerebral venous thrombosis, pregnancy and oral contraceptives. Thromb Res 2012;130(Suppl 1):S19–22.
50. Karaca Z, Tanriverdi F, Unluhizarci K, et al. Pregnancy and pituitary disorders. Eur J Endocrinol 2010;162(3):453–75.

51. Piantanida E, Gallo D, Lombardi V, et al. Pituitary apoplexy during pregnancy: a rare, but dangerous headache. J Endocrinol Invest 2014;37(9):789–97.

52. Edlow JA, Caplan LR, O'Brien K, et al. Diagnosis of acute neurological emergencies in pregnant and post-partum women. Lancet Neurol 2013;12(2): 175–85.

53. Skeik N, Porten BR, Kadkhodayan Y, et al. Postpartum reversible cerebral vasoconstriction syndrome: review and analysis of the current data. Vasc Med 2015; 20(3):256–65.

54. Huna-Baron R, Kupersmith MJ. Idiopathic intracranial hypertension in pregnancy. J Neurol 2002;249(8):1078–81.

55. Ferro JM, Canhão P, Stam J, et al, ISCVT Investigators. Prognosis of cerebral vein and dural sinus thrombosis: results of the International Study on Cerebral Vein and Dural Sinus Thrombosis (ISCVT). Stroke 2004;35(3):664–70.

56. Saposnik G, Barinagarrementeria F, Brown RD Jr, et al, American Heart Association Stroke Council and the Council on Epidemiology and Prevention. Diagnosis and management of cerebral venous thrombosis: a statement for healthcare professionals from the American Heart Association/American Stroke Association. Stroke 2011;42(4):1158–92.

57. Witmer CM, Raffini LJ, Manno CS. Utility of computed tomography of the head following head trauma in boys with haemophilia. Haemophilia 2007;13(5):560–6.

58. Fang MC, Go AS, Chang Y, et al. Death and disability from warfarin-associated intracranial and extracranial hemorrhages. Am J Med 2007;120(8):700–5.

59. Fogelholm R, Eskola K, Kiminkinen T, et al. Anticoagulant treatment as a risk factor for primary intracerebral haemorrhage. J Neurol Neurosurg Psychiatry 1992; 55:1121–4.

60. Hemphill JC 3rd, Greenberg SM, Anderson CS, et al, American Heart Association Stroke Council, Council on Cardiovascular and Stroke Nursing, Council on Clinical Cardiology. Guidelines for the management of spontaneous intracerebral hemorrhage: a guideline for healthcare professionals from the American Heart Association/American Stroke Association. Stroke 2015;46(7):2032–6.

61. Cucchiara B, Messe S, Sansing L, et al, CHANT Investigators. Hematoma growth in oral anticoagulant related intracerebral hemorrhage. Stroke 2008; 39(11):2993–6.

62. Kirby S, Purdy RA. Headache and brain tumors. Curr Neurol Neurosci Rep 2007;7(2):110–6.

63. Forsyth PA, Posner JB. Headaches in patients with brain tumors: a study of 111 patients. Neurology 1993;43(9):1678–83.

64. Schankin CJ, Ferrari U, Reinisch VM, et al. Characteristics of brain tumour-associated headache. Cephalalgia 2007;27(8):904–11.

65. Barnholtz-Sloan JS, Sloan AE, Davis FG, et al. Incidence proportions of brain metastases in patients diagnosed (1973 to 2001) in the Metropolitan Detroit Cancer Surveillance System. J Clin Oncol 2004;22(14):2865–72.

66. Kirby S, Purdy RA. Headaches and brain tumors. Neurol Clin 2014;32(2): 423–32.

67. Navi BB, Reichman JS, Berlin D, et al. Intracerebral and subarachnoid hemorrhage in patients with cancer. Neurology 2010;74(6):494–501.

68. Gopal AK, Whitehouse JD, Simel DL, et al. Cranial computed tomography before lumbar puncture: a prospective clinical evaluation. Arch Intern Med 1999;159(22):2681–5 [Erratum appears in Arch Intern Med 2000;160(21):3223].

69. Hasbun R, Abrahams J, Jekel J, et al. Computed tomography of the head before lumbar puncture in adults with suspected meningitis. N Engl J Med 2001; 345(24):1727-33.
70. Brouwer MC, Coutinho JM, van de Beek D. Clinical characteristics and outcome of brain abscess: systematic review and meta-analysis. Neurology 2014;82(9): 806-13.
71. Muzumdar D, Jhawar S, Goel A. Brain abscess: an overview. Int J Surg 2011; 9(2):136-44.
72. Fernandez A, Schmidt JM, Claassen J, et al. Fever after subarachnoid hemorrhage: risk factors and impact on outcome. Neurology 2007;68:1013-9.
73. Dorhout Mees SM, Luitse MJ, van den Bergh WM, et al. Fever after aneurysmal subarachnoid hemorrhage: relation with extent of hydrocephalus and amount of extravasated blood. Stroke 2008;39(7):2141-3.
74. Vidal E, Cevallos R, Vidal J, et al. Twelve cases of pituitary apoplexy. Arch Intern Med 1992;152(9):1893-9.
75. Winer JB, Plant G. Stuttering pituitary apoplexy resembling meningitis. J Neurol Neurosurg Psychiatr 1990;53:440.
76. Foroozan R. Visual dysfunction in migraine. Int Ophthalmol Clin 2009;49(3): 133-46.
77. Arnold M, Kappeler L, Georgiadis D, et al. Gender differences in spontaneous cervical artery dissection. Neurology 2006;67(6):1050-2.
78. Hill DL, Daroff RB, Ducros A, et al. Most cases labeled as "retinal migraine" are not migraine. J Neuroophthalmol 2007;27(1):3-8.
79. Zhang X, Kedar S, Lynn MJ, et al. Homonymous hemianopias: clinical-anatomic correlations in 904 cases. Neurology 2006;66(6):906-10.
80. Lee AG, Wall M. Papilledema: are we any nearer to a consensus on pathogenesis and treatment? Curr Neurol Neurosci Rep 2012;12(3):334-9.
81. Perry JJ, Stiell IG, Sivilotti ML, et al. Clinical decision rules to rule out subarachnoid hemorrhage for acute headache. JAMA 2013;310(12):1248-55.
82. Goldberg EM, Schwartz ES, Younkin D, et al. Atypical syncope in a child due to a colloid cyst of the third ventricle. Pediatr Neurol 2011;45(5):331-4.
83. Butzkueven H, Evans AH, Pitman A, et al. Onset seizures independently predict poor outcome after subarachnoid hemorrhage. Neurology 2000;55(9):1315-20.
84. Anderson C, Ni Mhurchu C, Scott D, et al, Australasian Cooperative Research on Subarachnoid Hemorrhage Study Group. Triggers of subarachnoid hemorrhage: role of physical exertion, smoking, and alcohol in the Australasian Cooperative Research on Subarachnoid Hemorrhage Study (ACROSS). Stroke 2003; 34(7):1771-6.
85. van Gijn J, Kerr RS, Rinkel GJ. Subarachnoid haemorrhage. Lancet 2007; 369(9558):306-18.
86. Dubosh NM, Bellolio MF, Rabinstein AA, et al. Sensitivity of early brain computed tomography to exclude aneurysmal subarachnoid hemorrhage: a systematic review and meta-analysis. Stroke 2016;47(3):750-5.
87. Perry JJ, Stiell IG, Sivilotti ML, et al. Sensitivity of computed tomography performed within six hours of onset of headache for diagnosis of subarachnoid haemorrhage: prospective cohort study. BMJ 2011;343:d4277.
88. Blok KM, Rinkel GJ, Majoie CB, et al. CT within 6 hours of headache onset to rule out subarachnoid hemorrhage in nonacademic hospitals. Neurology 2015;84(19):1927-32.
89. Mark DG, Hung YY, Offerman SR, et al, Kaiser Permanente CREST Network Investigators. Nontraumatic subarachnoid hemorrhage in the setting of negative

cranial computed tomography results: external validation of a clinical and imaging prediction rule. Ann Emerg Med 2013;62(1):1–10.e1.

90. Connolly ES Jr, Rabinstein AA, Carhuapoma JR, et al, American Heart Association Stroke Council, Council on Cardiovascular Radiology and Intervention, Council on Cardiovascular Nursing, Council on Cardiovascular Surgery and Anesthesia, Council on Clinical Cardiology. Guidelines for the management of aneurysmal subarachnoid hemorrhage: a guideline for healthcare professionals from the American Heart Association/American Stroke Association. Stroke 2012; 43(6):1711–37.

91. McCormack RF, Hutson A. Can computed tomography angiography of the brain replace lumbar puncture in the evaluation of acute-onset headache after a negative noncontrast cranial computed tomography scan? Acad Emerg Med 2010;17(4):444–51.

92. Carstairs SD, Tanen DA, Duncan TD, et al. Computed tomographic angiography for the evaluation of aneurysmal subarachnoid hemorrhage. Acad Emerg Med 2006;13(5):486–92.

93. Edlow JA. What are the unintended consequences of changing the diagnostic paradigm for subarachnoid hemorrhage after brain computed tomography to computed tomographic angiography in place of lumbar puncture? Acad Emerg Med 2010;17(9):991–5 [discussion: 996–7].

94. Nedeltchev K, der Maur TA, Georgiadis D, et al. Ischaemic stroke in young adults: predictors of outcome and recurrence. J Neurol Neurosurg Psychiatry 2005;76(2):191–5.

95. Putaala J, Metso AJ, Metso TM, et al. Analysis of 1008 consecutive patients aged 15 to 49 with first-ever ischemic stroke: the Helsinki young stroke registry. Stroke 2009;40(4):1195–203.

96. Schievink WI. Spontaneous dissection of the carotid and vertebral arteries. N Engl J Med 2001;344(12):898–906.

97. Engelter ST, Grond-Ginsbach C, Metso TM, et al, Cervical Artery Dissection and Ischemic Stroke Patients Study Group. Cervical artery dissection: trauma and other potential mechanical trigger events. Neurology 2013;80(21):1950–7.

98. Debette S, Grond-Ginsbach C, Bodenant M, et al, Cervical Artery Dissection Ischemic Stroke Patients (CADISP) Group. Differential features of carotid and vertebral artery dissections: the CADISP study. Neurology 2011;77(12): 1174–81.

99. Silbert PL, Mokri B, Schievink WI. Headache and neck pain in spontaneous internal carotid and vertebral artery dissections. Neurology 1995;45(8):1517–22.

100. Biousse V, Touboul PJ, D'Anglejan-Chatillon J, et al. Ophthalmologic manifestations of internal carotid artery dissection. Am J Ophthalmol 1998;126(4):565–77.

101. Sturzenegger M, Huber P. Cranial nerve palsies in spontaneous carotid artery dissection. J Neurol Neurosurg Psychiatry 1993;56(11):1191–9.

102. Provenzale JM, Sarikaya B. Comparison of test performance characteristics of MRI, MR angiography, and CT angiography in the diagnosis of carotid and vertebral artery dissection: a review of the medical literature. AJR Am J Roentgenol 2009;193(4):1167–74.

103. Benninger DH, Baumgartner RW. Ultrasound diagnosis of cervical artery dissection. Front Neurol Neurosci 2006;21:70–84.

104. González-Gay MA, García-Porrúa C. Epidemiology of the vasculitides. Rheum Dis Clin North Am 2001;27(4):729–49.

105. Gonzalez-Gay MA, Miranda-Filloy JA, Lopez-Diaz MJ, et al. Giant cell arteritis in northwestern Spain: a 25-year epidemiologic study. Medicine (Baltimore) 2007; 86(2):61-8.

106. Salvarani C, Crowson CS, O'Fallon WM, et al. Reappraisal of the epidemiology of giant cell arteritis in Olmsted County, Minnesota, over a fifty-year period. Arthritis Rheum 2004;51(2):264-8.

107. Gonzalez-Gay MA, Vazquez-Rodriguez TR, Lopez-Diaz MJ, et al. Epidemiology of giant cell arteritis and polymyalgia rheumatica. Arthritis Rheum 2009;61(10): 1454-61.

108. Gonzalez-Gay MA, Barros S, Lopez-Diaz MJ, et al. Giant cell arteritis: disease patterns of clinical presentation in a series of 240 patients. Medicine(Baltimore) 2005;84(5):269-76.

109. Tal S, Guller V, Gurevich A, et al. Fever of unknown origin in the elderly. J Intern Med 2002;252(4):295-304.

110. Hayreh SS, Podhajsky PA, Zimmerman B. Occult giant cell arteritis: ocular manifestations. Am J Ophthalmol 1998;125(4):521-6 [Erratum appears in Am J Ophthalmol 1998;125(6):893].

111. González-Gay MA, García-Porrúa C, Llorca J, et al. Visual manifestations of giant cell arteritis. Trends and clinical spectrum in 161 patients. Medicine (Baltimore) 2000;79(5):283-92.

112. Smetana GW, Shmerling RH. Does this patient have temporal arteritis? JAMA 2002;287(1):92-101.

113. Achkar AA, Lie JT, Hunder GG, et al. How does previous corticosteroid treatment affect the biopsy findings in giant cell (temporal) arteritis? Ann Intern Med 1994;120(12):987-92.

114. Crassard I, Bousser MG. Headache in patients with cerebral venous thrombosis. Rev Neurol (Paris) 2005;161(6-7):706-8.

115. Girot M, Ferro JM, Canhão P, et al, ISCVT Investigators. Predictors of outcome in patients with cerebral venous thrombosis and intracerebral hemorrhage. Stroke 2007;38(2):337-42.

116. Friedman DI, Jacobson DM. Diagnostic criteria for idiopathic intracranial hypertension. Neurology 2002;59(10):1492-5.

117. Wall M, Kupersmith MJ, Kieburtz KD, et al, NORDIC Idiopathic Intracranial Hypertension Study Group. The idiopathic intracranial hypertension treatment trial: clinical profile at baseline. JAMA Neurol 2014;71(6):693-701.

118. Corbett JJ, Savino PJ, Thompson HS, et al. Visual loss in pseudotumor cerebri. Follow-up of 57 patients from five to 41 years and a profile of 14 patients with permanent severe visual loss. Arch Neurol 1982;39(8):461-74.

119. Giuseffi V, Wall M, Siegel PZ, et al. Symptoms and disease associations in idiopathic intracranial hypertension (pseudotumor cerebri): a case-control study. Neurology 1991;41(2 Pt 1):239-44.

120. Bonomi L, Marchini G, Marraffa M, et al. Epidemiology of angle-closure glaucoma: prevalence, clinical types, and association with peripheral anterior chamber depth in the Egna-Neumarket Glaucoma Study. Ophthalmology 2000; 107(5):998-1003.

121. Saw SM, Gazzard G, Friedman DS. Interventions for angle-closure glaucoma: an evidence-based update. Ophthalmology 2003;110(10):1869-78 [quiz: 1878-9], 1930.

122. Choong YF, Irfan S, Menage MJ. Acute angle closure glaucoma: an evaluation of a protocol for acute treatment. Eye (Lond) 1999;13(Pt 5):613-6.

123. Thigpen MC, Whitney CG, Messonnier NE, et al, Emerging Infections Programs Network. Bacterial meningitis in the United States, 1998-2007. N Engl J Med 2011;364(21):2016–25.
124. Van de Beek D, de Gans J, Spanjaard L, et al. Clinical features and prognostic factors in adults with bacterial meningitis. N Engl J Med 2004;351(18):1849–59.
125. Brouwer MC, Thwaites GE, Tunkel AR, et al. Dilemmas in the diagnosis of acute community-acquired bacterial meningitis. Lancet 2012;380(9854):1684–92.
126. Attia J, Hatala R, Cook DJ, et al. The rational clinical examination. Does this adult patient have acute meningitis? JAMA 1999;282(2):175–81.
127. Nakao JH, Jafri FN, Shah K, et al. Jolt accentuation of headache and other clinical signs: poor predictors of meningitis in adults. Am J Emerg Med 2014;32(1):24–8.
128. Tunkel AR, Hartman BJ, Kaplan SL, et al. Practice guidelines for the management of bacterial meningitis. Clin Infect Dis 2004;39(9):1267–84.
129. Abalos E, Cuesta C, Grosso AL, et al. Global and regional estimates of pre-eclampsia and eclampsia: a systematic review. Eur J Obstet Gynecol Reprod Biol 2013;170(1):1–7.
130. American College of Obstetricians and Gynecologists, Task Force on Hypertension in Pregnancy. Hypertension in pregnancy. Report of the American College of Obstetricians and Gynecologists' task force on hypertension in pregnancy. Obstet Gynecol 2013;122(5):1122–31.
131. Lubina A, Olchovsky D, Berezin M, et al. Management of pituitary apoplexy: clinical experience with 40 patients. Acta Neurochir (Wien) 2005;147(2):151–7 [discussion: 157].
132. Sibal L, Ball SG, Connolly V, et al. Pituitary apoplexy: a review of clinical presentation, management and outcome in 45 cases. Pituitary 2004;7(3):157–63.
133. Nawar RN, AbdelMannan D, Selman WR, et al. Pituitary tumor apoplexy: a review. J Intensive Care Med 2008;23(2):75–90.
134. Bahmani Kashkouli M, Khalatbari MR, Yahyavi ST, et al. Pituitary apoplexy presenting as acute painful isolated unilateral third cranial nerve palsy. Arch Iran Med 2008;11(4):466–8.
135. L'Huillier F, Combes C, Martin N, et al. MRI in the diagnosis of so-called pituitary apoplexy: seven cases. J Neuroradiol 1989;16(3):221–37.
136. Piotin M, Tampieri D, Rüfenacht DA, et al. The various MRI patterns of pituitary apoplexy. Eur Radiol 1999;9(5):918–23.
137. Hampson NB, Weaver LK. Carbon monoxide poisoning: a new incidence for an old disease. Undersea Hyperb Med 2007;34(3):163–8.
138. Weaver LK. Clinical practice. Carbon monoxide poisoning. N Engl J Med 2009; 360(12):1217–25.
139. Amitai Y, Zlotogorski Z, Golan-Katzav V, et al. Neuropsychological impairment from acute low-level exposure to carbon monoxide. Arch Neurol 1998;55(6):845–8.
140. Heckerling PS, Leikin JB, Terzian CG, et al. Occult carbon monoxide poisoning in patients with neurologic illness. J Toxicol Clin Toxicol 1990;28(1):29–44.
141. Jasper BW, Hopkins RO, Duker HV, et al. Affective outcome following carbon monoxide poisoning: a prospective longitudinal study. Cogn Behav Neurol 2005;18(2):127–34.
142. Choi IS. Delayed neurologic sequelae in carbon monoxide intoxication. Arch Neurol 1983;40(7):433–5.
143. Bozeman WP, Myers RA, Barish RA. Confirmation of the pulse oximetry gap in carbon monoxide poisoning. Ann Emerg Med 1997;30(5):608–11.
144. Buckley NA, Juurlink DN, Isbister G, et al. Hyperbaric oxygen for carbon monoxide poisoning. Cochrane Database Syst Rev 2011;(4):CD002041.

A New Approach to the Diagnosis of Acute Dizziness in Adult Patients

Jonathan A. Edlow, MD

KEYWORDS

- Dizziness • Vertigo • BPPV • Vestibular neuritis • Nystagmus
- Posterior circulation stroke

KEY POINTS

- Use timing and triggers to identify which vestibular syndrome a patient has.
- Use the physical examination to differentiate vestibular neuritis from posterior circulation stroke in patients with the acute vestibular syndrome (AVS).
- Diagnose and treat benign paroxysmal positional vertigo (BPPV) at the bedside.

INTRODUCTION

Approximately 3.5% of emergency department (ED) visits are for dizziness.[1,2] Numerous conditions, some benign and self-limiting and others extremely serious, can present with dizziness. This is classic emergency medicine — sorting out the large majority of patients with a given chief complaint who have a self-limiting or easily treatable condition from the smaller number who have life-threatening, limb-threatening, or brain-threatening problems. Increasingly, physicians are charged with performing this diagnostic process using fewer resources. As of 2013, the direct ED-related costs of care for patients with dizziness in the United States was estimated to approach $4 billion.[3] In addition to economic cost, there is additional cost in terms of patient-experienced anxiety and falls, attributed to dizziness, with their resultant morbidity.

Compared with patients without dizziness, in the ED, dizzy patients undergo more testing and more imaging, have longer ED lengths of stay, and are more likely to be admitted. The large majority of brain imaging is CT, which has little diagnostic value in patients with dizziness. In 2011, approximately 12% of the estimated $4 billion is related to brain imaging, three-quarters of which was due to CT.[3]

The existing paradigm for diagnosing dizziness is based on symptom quality (ie, asking the question, "What do you mean 'dizzy'?"). This approach is taught in nearly

Department of Emergency Medicine, Beth Israel Deaconess Medical Center, Harvard Medical School, 1 Deaconess Place, Boston, MA 02215, USA
E-mail address: jedlow@bidmc.harvard.edu

Emerg Med Clin N Am 34 (2016) 717–742
http://dx.doi.org/10.1016/j.emc.2016.06.004
0733-8627/16/© 2016 Elsevier Inc. All rights reserved.
emed.theclinics.com

all review articles and textbooks across specialties; however, newer research has shown that its scientific basis and its internal logic lack foundation.

Currently, misdiagnosis in patients with dizziness is a problem in an environment that is paying increasing attention to diagnostic errors.[4] Misdiagnosis of patients with cerebellar stroke can have disastrous consequences.[5] This article reviews the differential diagnosis of acute dizziness in adult patients, analyzes the origin of the traditional symptom quality approach to dizziness, reviews newer data on an approach to diagnosis of dizziness, and suggests a new approach.

The new approach places a heavy emphasis on history and physical examination. Using these techniques, emergency physicians can improve the care of patients with dizziness by more frequently and confidently making a specific diagnosis. When a confident diagnosis is made of a peripheral problem, time-consuming consultation, expensive imaging, and hospitalization become unnecessary. When the evaluation suggests a central problem, especially stroke, steps can be taken to diagnose and treat the offending vascular lesion and institute secondary prevention measures.

This new approach to the ED patients with dizziness should improve diagnostic accuracy, reduce length of stay and resource utilization, and likely improve overall patient outcomes.

DIFFERENTIAL DIAGNOSIS OF ACUTE DIZZINESS

Part of the problem is that numerous disorders and conditions that span multiple organ systems can present with acute dizziness. Many of these diagnoses are benign whereas others are life threatening. A study from the National Hospital Ambulatory Medical Care Survey (NHAMCS) database of patients seen in all varieties of hospitals over a 13-year period identified 9472 patients with dizziness.[2] These data suggest that most patients have general medical (including cardiovascular) diagnoses (approximately 50%), otovestibular diagnoses (approximately 33%), and neurologic (including stroke) diagnoses (approximately 11%).[2,6] This breakdown has some face validity to practicing emergency physicians, for whom general medical conditions outnumber vestibular and neurologic diagnoses in real-life practice.

Studies done on large administrative databases have the limitation that the accuracy of the charted diagnosis is unknown. In the NHAMCS study, 22% of patients received a symptom-only diagnosis (eg, dizziness, not otherwise specified). Although assigning a diagnosis of the presenting symptom is not uncommon in emergency medicine practice, a symptom-only diagnosis was almost 2 times more common in dizzy patients than in all other patients (22.1% vs 8.4%, odds ratio [OR] = 3.1, $P<.001$). In addition, even if a specific vestibular diagnosis is made, such as BPPV or an acute peripheral vestibulopathy, use of imaging and treatment with medications is not in accordance with best evidence.[7]

In the NHAMCS study, prospectively defined "dangerous" diagnoses (various cardiovascular, cerebrovascular, toxic, metabolic and infectious conditions in which the possibility of a poor outcome without treatment was likely) were found in 15% of patients and the proportion increased with age (21% dangerous diagnoses in patients >50 years vs 9.35 in patients ≤50, $P<.001$).[2] Among 15 dangerous causes analyzed, the most commonly recorded were fluid and electrolyte disturbances (5.6%), cerebrovascular diseases (4.0%), cardiac arrhythmias (3.2%), acute coronary syndromes (1.7%), anemia (1.6%), and hypoglycemia (1.4%).[2] Some dangerous causes of dizziness, such as adrenal insufficiency,[8] aortic dissection,[9] carbon monoxide intoxication,[10] pulmonary embolus,[11] and thiamine deficiency,[12] are treatable causes that are important but rare.[2]

How does this study compare to others? One older single-institution study analyzed 125 patients prospectively identified over a 16-month period[13]; 43% had a diagnosis of a peripheral vestibular problem and 30% had a "serious" diagnosis. Another much larger prospective single-institution Chinese study of adult ED patients with dizziness reported results of 413 patients recruited over just 1 month.[1] A central nervous system (CNS) cause was found in 23 patients (6%).

Two retrospective studies also provide relevant data. One study was done in a German ED of 475 consecutive dizzy patients who were seen by a neurologist during the index ED visit.[14] The initial diagnoses assigned by the neurologists were benign in 73% of cases and serious (mostly cerebrovascular and inflammatory CNS disease) in 27% of cases. Overall, the 2 most common diagnoses were BPPV (22%) and stroke (20%). In follow-up by a neurologist blinded to the ED diagnosis, 44% of diagnoses (previously made by a neurologist in the ED) were changed. More than half of these diagnostic changes were from a serious to a benign diagnosis, which errs toward patient safety but is more resource intensive than necessary. In approximately 1 patient in 7, the error was from benign to serious (5 patients diagnosed with vestibular neuritis and 1 with vestibular migraine, all reassigned to stroke), a dangerous misdiagnosis.

The other study analyzed patients who had an ED triage diagnosis of dizziness, vertigo, or imbalance as a primary symptom, collected over a 3-year period, and identified 907 patients (only 0.8% of all ED patients over that period of time), suggesting a very targeted selection compared with other large studies.[15] Of the 907 patients, 1 in 5 was admitted (68% to an ICU). The most common admitting services were medicine (41% of admissions), cardiology (32%), and neurology (24%). Of the 907 patients, most had either benign conditions, such as peripheral vestibular problems (32%), orthostatic hypotension (13%), and migraine (4%) and in a full 22% could not be specifically diagnosed. Serious neurologic disease was found in 49 patients (5%), of which 37 were cerebrovascular. Finally, only 2 patients with serious neurologic disease presented with isolated dizziness.

Many of these studies were based on the emergency physician diagnosis. In a Swiss study of 951 patients referred (not all from an ED) to a multidisciplinary dizziness clinic, there was a significant change in the final diagnoses of dizzy patients.[16] The final diagnosis of "undetermined" fell by 60% and BPPV, multisensory dizziness, and vestibular migraine were all significantly underdiagnosed by the referring doctors. This, coupled with the fact that emergency physicians often assign a symptom-only diagnosis, suggests an inherent, but unknown, incorrect diagnosis rate of dizzy patients in the ED.

The incidence of important CNS disease in adult ED patients with dizziness is approximately 5%. The high-end outlier is Royl and colleagues' study[14] that reported that 27% of patients have serious CNS causes, skewed by the fact that the study was conducted in a neurologic ED.[14] Various studies have tried to identify risk factors for ED dizzy patients with CNS causes.[1,15,17–20] One ED study of dizzy patients found that abnormal gait and subtle neurologic deficits on neurologic examination were associated with a CNS cause.[17] Overall, the risk factors include increasing age, vascular risk factors, history of previous stroke, complaint of "instability," and focal neurologic findings (**Table 1**).

Taken as a whole, these data suggest the following conclusions:

1. Most adult patients who present to the ED with acute dizziness have general medical or cardiac conditions.
2. Although benign vestibular diseases are much more common than CNS causes of dizziness, when emergency physicians make these (benign) diagnoses, their use of imaging and meclizine is not in accordance with best available evidence.

Table 1
Risk factors for a central nervous system cause in emergency department patients with dizziness

Risk Factor	Newman-Toker,[2] 2008	Cheung,[1] 2010	Navi,[15] 2012	Chase,[17] 2012	Kerber,[20] 2015
Age in years	Age >50	6.15 for age >65	5.7 for age >60	—	—
Symptom of imbalance or ataxia	—	11.39 for "ataxia"	5.9 for "imbalance"	9.3 for "gait instability"	—
Focal neurologic symptoms	—	11.78	5.9	—	—
History of previous stroke	—	3.89	—	—	—
Vascular risk factors	—	3.57 for diabetes	—	—	0.48 (CI crossed 1)
ABCD2 score	—	—	—	—	1.74 (scored as a continuous variable)
HINTS testing	—	—	—	—	2.82
Other neurologic deficits	—	—	—	8.7 for "subtle" neurologic finding	2.54

Numbers are ORs (when reported).

3. Of the CNS causes, acute cerebrovascular disease (ischemic stroke or transient ischemic attack [TIA]) is the most common cause and misdiagnosis in the ED is not uncommon in these patients.

Because some of the underlying reasons for this situation have to do with the use of the prevailing traditional symptom quality approach to dizziness, an in-depth analysis of its origin is important to this discussion.

ORIGIN OF THE SYMPTOM QUALITY APPROACH TO DIAGNOSING DIZZINESS

Prior to the publication of their article in 1972 (by a neurologist, David Drachman, and an ear, nose, and throat surgeon, Cecil Hart),[14] there was no well-accepted organized algorithmic approach to the diagnosis of an acutely dizzy patient.[21] Drachman and Hart created an outpatient dizziness clinic. Over a 2-year period, they enrolled 125 patients who had to be available to return to their clinic for 4 half days of testing. The study suffers from several shortcomings (**Box 1**).

The small number of subjects enrolled over a 2-year period suggests a highly select group of individuals. These were not representative ED patients with acute blood loss, ectopic pregnancy, sepsis, pneumonia, dehydration acute strokes, arrhythmias, and

---

Box 1
Shortcomings of the Drachman and Hart article

Methodological issues

Tautological hypothesis
   Their methods placed patients into 1 of 4 categories of dizziness by design.
   Related "appropriate" questions were only asked once the dizziness category was assigned.
   A diagnosis of a "peripheral vestibular disorder was typically applied to a patient who complained of unmistakable rotational vertigo."

Lack of independent verification and blinding
   A single individual assigned the final diagnosis; there was no independent verification of the diagnoses.
   The individual assigning the diagnoses was not blinded to the data or the categories of symptom quality.

Small number of subjects with 25% dropout rate after enrollment
   125 Total patients were enrolled (but 25.6% were excluded).
   12 (16.8%) Were excluded due to "inadequate data" obtained.
   9 (7.2%) Were excluded because of "uncertain diagnosis."
   2 (1.6%) Were excluded because they were "inappropriate referrals."

Selection bias
   Only 125 patients were enrolled over a 2-year period.
   They had to be available to return on 4 different days for testing.
   They had to be fluent in English.

Lack of long-term follow-up of patients
   There was no long-term follow-up to verify accuracy of diagnosis.

Unavoidable issues related to era in which study was performed

Lack of modern imaging
   When the study was done, neither CT nor MRI was available.

Lack of some diagnoses being established
   Vestibular migraine (a common cause of s-EVS) had not yet been described.
   Posterior circulation TIA presenting as isolated dizziness was not recognized.

other symptoms due to toxic, metabolic, or infectious conditions. One-quarter of the 125 enrolled patients were rejected for various reasons (see **Box 1**).

The patients were first asked questions to describe their "subjective experience of dizziness" to separate and classify "all complaints of dizziness into 4 types: (1) a definite rotational sensation, (2) a sensation of impending faint or loss of consciousness, (3) disequilibrium or loss of balance without head sensation and (4) ill defined 'lightheadedness' other than vertigo, syncope or disequilibrium." The methods then state, "Once the type of complaint has been sorted out, secondary inquiries were sought to identify related neurological, otological, cardiac, psychiatric, gastrointestinal, visual or other symptoms."

Patients were then asked about positional triggers and the timing of their dizziness. Finally, a comprehensive battery of physical examination testing occurred, including detailed vital sign testing; neurologic, otologic, and ophthalmologic examinations; and a variety of tests to provoke the dizziness at the clinic. Given the era, the only brain imaging that was done was plain films of the skull. At the end of the process and unblinded to the data and dizziness category, the first author made a final diagnosis.

There was no long-term follow-up or validation of the final diagnoses, which were intrinsically linked to the dizziness category that the patients were assigned at the onset. Once the type of dizziness was known, so too was its differential diagnosis. There were other issues related to diagnoses not recognized at the time the research was done (see **Box 1**). Although this was a landmark study published in a prominent journal in 1972, it has important limitations to current use in undifferentiated patients. In fairness, the investigators concluded, "this study should serve as the point of departure for further investigation." The medical world, however, largely accepted this symptom quality approach by perpetuating that the first question to be asked of the dizzy patient should be, "What do you mean, 'dizzy'?" and that the response generated a particular differential diagnosis (eg, vestibular problems if vertigo, cardiovascular disorders if lightheadedness or near-syncope, neurologic issues for disequilibrium, and largely psychiatric causes if other).

REASONS WHY THE SYMPTOM QUALITY APPROACH LACKS SCIENTIFIC VALIDITY

For the symptom quality approach to work, 2 facts must be true. First, patients should be able to reliably and consistently chose 1 (and only 1) dizziness type. Secondly, each symptom type should be tightly linked with a given differential diagnosis. Both facts are demonstrably false.[22]

Patients do not chose a single dizziness type. Sensory symptoms are difficult for many patients to describe. Patients with dizziness may use words like, "dizzy," "lightheaded," "spinning," "rocking," "vertigo," "giddy," "like I'm going to faint," "off balance," "spacey," and others to describe what they feel. For this article, I use the word *dizziness* in a general way (incorporating all of these descriptors).

In 2007, researchers published a study about how dizzy patients in an ED respond when asked a series of questions related to symptom quality.[23] Research assistants asked a series of ED patients with dizziness a battery of questions aimed at determining symptom quality and timing and triggers of the dizziness. The questions were asked and then reasked an average of 6 minutes later (the second time in a different sequence). More than 60% of the patients chose more than 1 dizziness type. In response to the same questions (the second time), more than 50% of the patients changed their primary dizziness type. The responses to timing and triggers of dizziness were more consistent and reliable between the first and second responses.

This 1 study severely undercuts the logic of a diagnostic process based on symptom quality. How should a patient be evaluated who endorses both lightheadedness and vertigo? If a patient answers "vertigo" the first time, then "disequilibrium" the second time, how should the work-up proceed?

A patient with chest pain is not evaluated differently if the pain is described as "sharp," "dull," "discomfort," or "pressure."[22] Pain described as "sharp" may be more likely to be pulmonary embolism or pleurisy and "dull" more likely an acute coronary syndrome, but the descriptor of the pain is not used in a binary way. In a patient with chest pain, it is the timing and triggers that are more important in rank-ordering a differential diagnosis.

Pain that is brought on by exercise and rapidly resolves with rest suggests angina (or aortic stenosis or right-sided heart strain due to obstruction from a pulmonary embolism). Pain that is constant for 10 hours is more likely to be a myocardial infarction (or an aortic dissection or a pulmonary infarction) rather than unstable angina. Chest pain regularly triggered by swallowing is more likely an esophageal problem than a cardiac or pulmonary one. I take histories of virtually all chief complaints using the concept of timing and triggers.

Another concept that physicians use regularly to construct a differential diagnosis is that of context. The presence of associated symptoms is also important. Patients are thought of differently with chest pain associated with (1) leg swelling and dyspnea, (2) productive cough and fever, or (3) hypotension, unilaterally diminished breath sounds, and distended neck veins. The same logic applies for patients with headache, abdominal pain, or dyspnea. It is not simply the word that the patient uses that informs a differential diagnosis but also the timing, triggers, and associated symptoms and epidemiologic context. It should be no different with dizziness.

Finally, the differential diagnosis is not tightly linked with a given use of the descriptors. The use of the word "vertigo" was not associated with a higher incidence of stroke in a large series of ED patients with dizziness.[24] Patients with a cardiovascular cause of dizziness do endorse "vertigo" in almost 40% of cases.[25] Patients with BPPV often say they feel lightheaded and not vertiginous, especially elderly patients.[26] The reality is that the differential diagnosis should NOT be based on the word but rather on the timing, triggers, associated symptoms, and epidemiologic context. Yet physicians often use a generalized approach to a patient with "vertigo" without considering the timing and triggers.[6,7]

For all these reasons, the symptom quality approach to dizziness is not based on strong science. Nevertheless, it is the predominant paradigm used across specialties. Despite this, or to some extent, because of it, significant misdiagnosis of dizzy patients exists.

MISDIAGNOSIS OF PATIENTS WITH DIZZINESS AND RESOURCE UTILIZATION

Misdiagnosis of patients with dizziness is common. In the German ED study, neurologists seeing patients made diagnostic errors in 44% of patients. The investigators of that study found 3 factors that contributed to misdiagnosis.[14] First, subsequent clinical course evolved, making the ultimate diagnosis more clear. This factor played a role in 70% of misdiagnoses. This is a regular event in emergency medicine, in which patients whose symptoms evolve in a variable way are seen. What is obvious the next day, or even a few hours later, is not always clear on initial presentation. The other 2 factors were insufficient brain imaging (mostly MRI, found to be a factor in half of cases) and failure to screen for vascular risk factors using advanced testing, such as echocardiography, long-term telemetry, or Doppler ultrasound of cervical arteries (24% of cases). There has never been a head-to-head comparison of emergency physicians versus neurologists diagnosing patients with dizziness at the same phase of care (and likely never will be), but this German study clearly shows that dizziness is complicated, even to those with specialized training and focus.

In another study of 1091 dizzy patients in US EDs, emergency physicians documented comments about nystagmus in 887 (80%), of whom nystagmus was documented to be present in 185 (21%).[27] No other information beyond presence or absence was recorded in 26% of the 185 patients and sufficient information to be diagnostically useful was only recorded in 10 patients (5.4%). Of patients given a peripheral vestibular diagnosis, the description of the nystagmus conflicted with that diagnosis. This illustrates a knowledge gap in emergency physicians' understanding of nystagmus: what to look for, how to report it, and, most importantly, how to use the findings to their advantage.

Reporting presence or absence of nystagmus in a dizzy patient is akin to reporting simple presence or absence of electrocardiographic abnormalities in a chest pain patient. The mere presence or absence of abnormalities is not the key finding. In the latter example, 3 patients with chest pain, 1 with sinus tachycardia and new right bundle branch block, another with PR segment depression with diffuse ST segment elevations, and a third with focal ST segment elevations in leads 2, 3, and aVF with reciprocal changes laterally all have very different abnormalities that have a different significance. Similarly, in a patient with an AVS (**Table 2**), the findings of direction-fixed horizontal nystagmus versus direction-fixed vertical nystagmus versus direction-changing nystagmus have different significance (discussed later). A recent review illustrates how to use the physical examination in dizzy patients.[28]

Table 2
Timing and trigger–based vestibular[a] syndromes in acute dizziness

Syndrome	Description	Common Causes
AVS	Rapid onset of acute dizziness that lasts days, often associated with nausea, vomiting and head motion intolerance	Benign: vestibular neuritis and labyrinthitis Serious: cerebellar stroke
t-EVS	Episodic dizzy episodes triggered[b] by some specific obligate event, usually head movement or standing up and usually last <1 min	Benign: BPPV Serious: serious causes of orthostatic hypotension and CPPV
s-EVS	Episodic dizzy episodes that occur spontaneously, are not triggered, and usually last minutes to hours	Benign: vestibular migraine, Meniere disease Serious: TIA
CVS	Chronic dizziness lasting weeks to months (or longer)	Benign: medication side effects, anxiety and depression Serious: posterior fossa mass

Abbreviation: CVS, chronic vestibular syndrome.
This table lists the more common causes of these presenting syndromes and is not intended to be encyclopedic.
[a] Note that the use of the word, *vestibular*, here connotes vestibular symptoms (dizziness or vertigo or imbalance or lightheadedness, etc.) rather than underlying vestibular causes (eg, BPPV and vestibular neuritis).
[b] Dizziness is triggered when it is brought on from a baseline of no symptoms, as in positional vertigo due to BPPV. This must be distinguished from dizziness that is exacerbated from a milder baseline state; such exacerbations are common in AVS, whether peripheral (neuritis) or central (stroke).

Multiple studies find that patients with an AVS that superficially appears to be a peripheral process in fact have posterior circulation strokes.[29–31] In 1 study, almost 3% of patients referred to a ear, nose, and throat clinic for vertigo had a missed cerebellar stroke.[30] There are 2 major reasons that missed stroke is an important misdiagnosis. The first is that the underlying vascular mechanism goes untreated, leaving the patient vulnerable to another stroke and the second is that some patients develop posterior fossa edema that can be fatal.[5] Although lost opportunity for thrombolysis is often suggested as a third negative consequence of missing a posterior circulation stroke, many of these patients have minor deficits and are not thrombolysis candidates. Some even have an National Institutes of Health Stroke Scale score of zero.[32]

Younger age and dissection as a cause were found risk factors for missed cerebellar stroke.[33] Posterior circulation location is a risk factor for stroke misdiagnosis in general.[34–36] To put these data into some context, only a small number (0.18%–0.63%) of patients who are seen in the ED, diagnosed with a benign or peripheral vestibular diagnosis, return to the ED within 30 days and are hospitalized with a cerebrovascular diagnosis.[37–39] On a relative basis, this is a small number. Because dizziness is so common, however, this small fraction of a large number suggests that many thousands of patients have a missed diagnosis of an acute cerebrovascular syndrome (stroke TIA) each year.

The other side of the coin is a lack of recognition of common peripheral vestibular problems, the most common of which are BPPV and vestibular neuritis (or labyrinthitis if hearing is also involved). Lack of familiarity with these diagnoses may lead to undertreatment, incorrect treatment, and resource overutilization. In addition, rarely, a patient who seems to have BPPV actually has a central mimic, called central paroxysmal positional vertigo (CPPV), discussed later.

A recent review of misdiagnosis of patients with dizziness suggested 5 common pitfalls.[40] These are over-reliance on a symptom quality approach to diagnosis, underuse of a timing and triggers approach, lack of familiarity with key physical examination findings, overweighting traditional factors such as age and vascular risk factors to screen patients, and over-reliance on CT. Although stroke is more common in older individuals, young patients do have strokes, a fact that may contribute to misdiagnosis.[5,41,42]

A NEW PARADIGM TO DIAGNOSE PATIENTS WITH ACUTE DIZZINESS ATTEST

A new diagnostic paradigm is based on the timing, triggers and context of the dizzy symptoms. It is possible that this new paradigm will reduce misdiagnosis. Although the use of this new paradigm has not been proved to reduce misdiagnosis, I have been using and teaching it for 6 years, and my experience is that it allows confidently making a specific diagnosis more frequently than the traditional paradigm (for which there are also no quality data that it helps make a specific diagnosis). Different mnemonics have been used but the basic idea is that it is the timing, triggers, evolution, and context of symptoms that should drive the work-up rather than the specific words that a patient uses to describe dizziness.[6,22] I currently favor the mnemonic, ATTEST – A (associated symptoms), TT (timing and triggers), ES (bedside examination signs), and T (additional testing as needed).

This new paradigm may seem like a radically new way of approaching a dizzy patient, but this is only because the traditional symptom quality approach is so deeply engrained in how this subject has been taught.[22] Using a timing and triggers approach is no different from taking a history in any other patient, for example, someone with chest pain. A differential diagnosis is not created based only on the descriptor of the pain (dull, sharp, pressure, or tightness) but rather on timing and triggers of the pain: "Is the pain intermittent or continuous?" "Did the pain start abruptly or gradually?" "Does the pain increase with deep breath?" and "Is it triggered by physical exertion, or by eating?" These are some of the components of the history that drives the differential diagnosis. It is no different with a dizzy patient.

Using this paradigm, there are 4 timing and triggers categories that are important for emergency physicians (see **Table 2**). In the traditional paradigm, a patient who endorsed "vertigo" would get an evaluation to try to diagnose peripheral vestibular CNS causes of dizziness. This has led to confusion, for example, using imaging for diagnosis and meclizine for treatment no matter what the diagnosis is.[7] That is, the traditional paradigm tend to treat all patients with peripheral vertigo the same whereas the 2 most common by far being BPPV and vestibular neuritis should be treated differently.[7] The following sections review the presentation, differential diagnosis, and appropriate testing to make a specific diagnosis for each of the timing and triggers categories.

ACUTE VESTIBULAR SYNDROME

Spontaneous AVS is defined as the acute onset of persistent dizziness in association with nausea or vomiting, gait instability, nystagmus, and head-motion intolerance that lasts days or weeks.[6,22,43] Patients are usually symptomatic at the time of assessment and focused physical examination is often diagnostic. The most common cause is an acute peripheral vestibulopathy known as vestibular neuritis (dizziness only) or labyrinthitis (dizziness plus hearing loss or tinnitus).[43] The most frequent dangerous cause is posterior circulation ischemic stroke, generally in the cerebellum or lateral brainstem.[43] A distant third most common cause is multiple sclerosis.[44,45] Uncommon causes of an isolated AVS include cerebellar hemorrhage and several rare, but often treatable, autoimmune, infectious, or metabolic conditions.[44,46] The spontaneous AVS is to be distinguished from a triggered AVS, which is not discussed further in this article because the cause is usually obvious, such as posttraumatic dizziness or diphenylhydantoin toxicity.

An important concept is that patients with an AVS generally experience worsening of their symptoms with head movement or during provocative testing (such as if performing a Dix-Hallpike maneuver). These exacerbating features should not be mistaken for head movement triggers that facilitate diagnosis in episodic vestibular syndrome (EVS) patients. Confusion on this point probably contributes to difficulty differentiating BPPV from vestibular neuritis.[6,7,47] Acute BPPV patients occasionally complain of more persistent symptoms that may be due to repeated triggering symptoms with small, inadvertent head movements or anticipatory anxiety about moving. This can usually be teased out by careful history taking. When such patients lack obvious features of vestibular neuritis or stroke, the Dix-Hallpike and supine roll tests should be performed to assess for an atypical, AVS-like presentation of BPPV.[48]

Vestibular neuritis is a benign, self-limited, presumed viral or postviral inflammatory condition affecting the vestibular nerve and causing spontaneous AVS. This can be thought of as similar to Bell palsy but involving the vestibular portion of the 8th nerve rather than the 7th nerve. Some cases are associated with inflammatory disorders (eg, multiple sclerosis or sarcoidosis), but most are idiopathic and possibly linked to herpes simplex infections.[49] The idiopathic form is generally monophasic, although 25% have a single, brief prodrome in the week prior to the attack, and approximately 16% recur months or years later.[50,51] High-field-strength MRI with high-dose gadolinium has demonstrated vestibular nerve enhancement in select cases,[52] but typical vestibular neuritis shows no abnormality on routine MRI with contrast.[53] The diagnosis is, therefore, clinical and requires excluding other causes. A related condition, herpes zoster oticus (Ramsay Hunt syndrome type 2), may present with AVS, usually in conjunction with hearing loss, facial palsy, and a vesicular eruption in the ear or palate.[54]

Posterior fossa strokes may present with spontaneous AVS mimicking vestibular neuritis (or labyrinthitis if auditory symptoms are present).[55] The prevalence of cerebrovascular disease in patients presenting to the ED with dizziness is 3% to 6%,[1,2,13,24] but among AVS presentations it is estimated at approximately 25%.[43] Almost all (96%) are ischemic strokes, rather than hemorrhages.[43,46] CT sensitivity for acute ischemic stroke is low (perhaps as low as 16% in the first 24 hours, possibly less in the posterior fossa).[56–58] Therefore, CT cannot rule out ischemic stroke in AVS, a fact often contributing to misdiagnosis.[5,40,47] Even MRI with diffusion-weighted imaging misses 10% to 20% of strokes in spontaneous AVS during the first 24 to 48 hours after symptom onset, and repeat delayed imaging (3–7 days post–symptom onset) may be required to confirm the presence of a new infarct.[43,59,60]

Fortunately, a physical examination can help make the distinction between vestibular neuritis and posterior circulation stroke with greater sensitivity than early MRI.[59,60] These 2 studies were done by neuro-otologists performing a targeted oculomotor examination consisting of 3 components — the head impulse test (HIT) and testing for nystagmus and skew deviation (head impulse, nystagmus, and test of skew [HINTS]). One other study showed similar accuracy when performed by stroke neurologists (not neuro-otologists).[61] Preliminary evidence suggests that components of this approach (nystagmus testing and HIT) can be successfully used by specially trained emergency physicians.[62,63] My own anecdotal experience also suggests that with some training, emergency physicians can perform and interpret this examination. Because this approach has not been fully validated when used by nonspecialists, I have added 2 additional components that should be a part of the basic evaluation of the acutely dizzy patient — the general neurologic examination and testing of gait.

I do not perform these tests in the order of the HINTS mnemonic but rather in the following order:

1. Nystagmus testing
2. Skew deviation
3. HIT
4. General neurologic examination, focusing on cranial nerves, including hearing, cerebellar testing, and long-tract signs
5. Gait testing

There are 2 reasons for my preferred sequence. First, I try to start with the least intrusive parts of the examination and, second, nystagmus testing is the component that helps the most, in part by its presence or absence and in part by its quality. Once any 1 component tests positive for a central cause, then the patient's disposition (admission for further neurologic evaluation) is clear. Although all 5 components are part of a complete examination for a patient with an AVS, worsening a patient's symptoms with further intrusive testing (eg, testing gait that provokes vomiting) does not change the disposition but causes the patient's worst symptoms.

Furthermore, nystagmus helps to anchor and inform the rest of the process. All or nearly all patients with an AVS due to a vestibular cause have nystagmus if examined within the first days, so its absence should make 1 question a peripheral or central vestibular process. To be sure that nystagmus is truly absent, it should be tested with visual fixation removed. Experts state that the absence of nystagmus in a patient examined with visual fixation removed essentially rules out a vestibular cause for the dizziness.[64] Subspecialists typically use Frenzel lenses to remove visual fixation, neither available nor common practice in emergency medicine practice. There are, however, easy bedside alternatives for emergency physicians to take away visual fixation. A newly described one uses a new less bulky set of glass lenses.[65] Another method is to use a penlight to reduce visual fixation.[66] To do this, cover 1 eye and intermittently shine a light close to and directly at the other eye, telling the patient not to look at the light, just to stare off in the distance. Observe for nystagmus appearing when the light is blocking fixation. Finally, simply take a piece of white paper and place it close to the patient's eyes (telling the patient to "look through the paper") and examine the nystagmus from the side. Note that these other steps are only needed if there is no nystagmus with the basic examination.

If nystagmus is truly absent, then this is unlikely to be a vestibular process and, therefore, HIT is probably not useful and may yield false information.

Another potential issue is that the degree (or amplitude) of nystagmus can fluctuate markedly over hours. To some extent, this may represent the natural history of the underlying pathology as the CNS accommodates to the abnormal physiology from vestibular neuritis. Medications that are often (appropriately) used in the ED, however, to reduce symptoms, such as ondansetron or a benzodiazepine, may affect the rate at which the nystagmus dampens.

With all that said, the basic clinical test for nystagmus is simple. Have the patient look straight in neutral or primary gaze and observe for eye movements. By convention, the direction of nystagmus is named by the direction of the fast component. For example, if the eyes drift leftward and snap back horizontally to the right, this is termed right-beating horizontal nystagmus. With some practice this is easy to see and describe because it is the details of the nystagmus, not simply its presence, that is most diagnostically important. After observing for nystagmus in primary gaze, test for gaze-evoked nystagmus by having the patient look to the right and then to the left, each for several seconds, and observe for the presence of nystagmus and the direction of its fast-beating component. The patient only needs to move the eyes 15° to 20° off center when testing for gaze-evoked nystagmus because many normal individuals have a few beats of horizontal nystagmus on full end gaze. This physiologic nystagmus is generally very low amplitude and extinguishes quickly. **Table 3** shows the typical findings for patients with the oculomotor examination for patients with the AVS. Direction-changing gaze-evoked nystagmus or nystagmus that is pure torsional or vertical should be considered central in origin (and in the setting of a AVS, a stroke).

Skew deviation (a vertical misalignment of the eyes due to imbalance in the gravity sensing pathways) is not sensitive (30%) but is specific (98%) for a brainstem lesion.[43] For this examination, the examiner uses the alternate cover test. With the patient looking directly at the examiner's nose, the physician alternately covers the right eye, then the left eye, and continues alternating back and forth, approximately every 2 seconds. In patients with skew deviation, each time the covered eye is uncovered, there is a slight vertical correction (1 side corrects upward and the other corrects downward). The amplitude of correction is small — 1 mm to 2 mm; therefore, it is key for the examiner to focus on 1 eye (either one), rather than following the uncovered eye. A normal response is no vertical correction, and an abnormal response should be considered a stroke in patients with an AVS.

The next component is the HIT, a test of the vestibuloocular reflex (VOR) that was only described in 1988.[67] Standing in front of the patient, the examiner holds the patient's head by each side, instructs the patient to maintain focus on the examiner's nose and to keep the head and neck loose. Then the examiner quickly turns the

Table 3 Acute vestibular syndrome oculomotor physical findings		
Oculomotor Examination Component	**Peripheral (Usually Vestibular Neuritis)**	**Central (Usually Posterior Circulation Stroke)**
Nystagmus (neutral gaze and gaze to the right and left)	Dominantly horizontal, direction-fixed, beating away from the affected side	Direction-changing horizontal or dominantly vertical and/or torsional, then central[a] (Often mimics peripheral)
Test of skew (alternate cover test)	Normal vertical eye alignment (ie, no skew deviation)	Often mimics peripheral; if skew deviation is present, then central[b]
HIT	Unilaterally abnormal toward the affected side (presence of a corrective saccade)	Usually bilaterally normal (no corrective saccade)

Note: Strokes in the AICA territory may produce a unilaterally HIT that mimics vestibular neuritis, but hearing loss is usually present as a clue. If a patient has bilaterally abnormal HIT, this is also suspicious for a central lesion if nystagmus is present (AICA stroke or Wernicke's syndrome).

[a] Inferior branch vestibular neuritis presents with down-beat–torsional nystagmus, but this is a rare disorder. From the emergency medicine perspective, vertical nystagmus in a patient with an AVS patient should be considered to be central (a stroke).

[b] Skew deviation evident by bedside alternate cover testing is rare in peripheral vestibular cases; its presence should be considered to be central (a stroke, often in the brainstem).

patient's head approximately 10° to 20°, using a lateral to center motion. The normal (individuals with normal vestibular function) response is that the patient's focus stays locked on the examiner's nose. The presence of a corrective saccade (the eyes move with the head, then snap back in a fast corrective movement to the examiner's nose) is a positive test (abnormal VOR), which generally indicates a peripheral process, usually vestibular neuritis. The absence of a corrective saccade in AVS is consistent with a stroke. It may seem counterintuitive that a normal finding predicts a dangerous disease. This is why the HIT is only useful in patients with the AVS and nystagmus. If an acutely dizzy patient with an AVS does not have nystagmus, it is unlikely to be vestibular and, therefore, the HIT (which is meant to distinguish neuritis from stroke) becomes far less useful and usually misleading. Similarly, if the HIT were done in a patient with dizziness from urosepsis or dehydration, the test is negative, that is, worrisome for a stroke.

Patients with cerebellar stroke have a negative (normal) HIT.[31,68] This is because the circuit of the VOR does not loop through the cerebellum. On the other hand, occasional patients with posterior circulation stroke have a falsely positive (abnormal) HIT, usually from a lateral brainstem infarct involving the location where the vestibular nerve enters the brainstem. These strokes are uncommon and involve the anterior inferior cerebellar artery (AICA) stroke territory or an infarction directly involving the inner ear (labyrinthine stroke) itself. In both situations, hearing is usually acutely lost. Adding a bedside test of hearing (HINTS plus) helps pick up the occasional AICA stroke.[69] This last point is important because traditional teaching is that if hearing and dizziness coexist, the problem is peripheral (in the labyrinth). It is crucial to note, however, that the blood supply to the labyrinth is due to ischemia of branches of the AICA, so this co-involvement of hearing and dizziness can occur from a stroke.[70–72] The relative frequency of this occurring from a peripheral cause (true labyrinthitis) as opposed to stroke (AICA territory) is unknown.

A recent article with attached video clips reviews these physical examination findings.[28] Because studies of these 3 oculomotor tests have not been fully validated when done by nonspecialists, I recommend adding 2 additional components of the HINTS testing. These are the examination of the cranial nerves, cerebellar function and gait testing. The former targets cranial nerve findings that localize the pathology to the brainstem. Key elements include testing for pupillary function, facial motor and sensory symmetry, and dysarthria. Specifically, lateral medullary stroke (Wallenberg syndrome), an important cause of the AVS, merits special attention. These patients complain of dysarthria, dysphagia, or hoarseness due to lower cranial neuropathy and may have Horner syndrome with subtle ptosis and anisocoria that may only be evident in dim light (so that the normal larger pupil fully dilates, making the difference in pupil size more apparent).[73] A common physical examination finding is hemifacial decreased pain and temperature sensation. Routine testing of only light touch can miss this finding.

Finally, if all 4 initial components of the examination (nystagmus, skew deviation, HIT, and general neurologic examination) are nondiagnostic, gait testing must be performed. Ideally, have the patient walk unassisted, but for patients too symptomatic to walk, test for truncal ataxia by asking the patient to sit upright in the stretcher without holding onto the side rails. First a patient who cannot walk or sit up unassisted is unsafe for discharge. Additionally, an AVS patient who is unable to walk is more likely to have had a stroke as opposed to vestibular neuritis.[31]

Imaging is not useful in patients with the AVS. CT is a poor test for posterior circulation stroke.[56–58] MRI, even with diffusion-weighted imaging, misses 10% to 20% of strokes in spontaneous AVS during the first 24 to 48 hours.[43,59,60] In small brainstem strokes, MRI (with diffusion-weighted imaging) can still miss upward of 50% when tested within 48 hours.[60] Importantly, 50% of those small strokes were not due to small vessel disease but due to vertebral artery atherosclerosis or dissection. Therefore, in patients with the AVS, the physical examination leads to a correct diagnosis more frequently than imaging.

An Italian study in the ED (in which the emergency physicians used Frenzel lenses to test for nystagmus) exploited elements of this bedside examination and showed that it decreases both CT use and hospitalization.[63] A survey study found that American emergency physicians clearly do not understand or feel confidence in HINTS testing and overuse CT.[42] This same study showed that emergency physicians tend to overvalue the dizziness type in making a diagnosis. Although traditional vascular risk factors underperform HINTS and neurologic examination testing,[20,69] emergency physicians still value them over bedside testing.[42]

TRIGGERED EPISODIC VESTIBULAR SYNDROME

Patients with triggered EVS (t-EVS) have short-lived episodes of dizziness lasting seconds to a few minutes, depending on the underlying etiology. There is an obligate trigger, meaning that each time the specific trigger occurs, the dizziness follows. Common triggers are changes in head position or body posture, especially arising from the lying or seated position to standing. Some vestibular forms are sufficiently severe to cause vomiting, which can lead patients to overestimate episode duration. Again, clinicians must distinguish triggers (provoke new symptoms not present at baseline) from exacerbating features (worsen preexisting baseline symptoms), because episodes of acute vestibular dizziness are almost always exacerbated by head movement. The most common etiologies are BPPV and orthostatic hypotension. Dangerous causes include central (neurologic) mimics of BPPV and serious causes of orthostatic hypotension, such as internal bleeding or sepsis with relative hypovolemia. By nature of the event being triggered, the physician should be able to recreate the symptoms at the bedside.

BPPV is the most common vestibular cause of dizziness, with a lifetime prevalence of 2.4% and increasing incidence with age.[74] BPPV results from mobile crystalline debris in 1 or more semicircular canals (canaliths) in the vestibular labyrinth. Classic symptoms are repetitive brief, triggered episodes of rotational vertigo lasting more than a few seconds and less than a minute,[75,76] although nonvertiginous symptoms are frequent.[26] The diagnosis is confirmed by reproducing symptoms using canal-specific positional testing maneuvers and identifying a canal-specific nystagmus (**Table 4**).[76–78] Because the offending canal(s) are generally not known in advance, a sequence of multiple diagnostic maneuvers is typically performed starting with the Dix-Hallpike maneuver because this tests the posterior canal, which is by far the most common involved.[64] A detailed recent review of these examination maneuvers includes instructive video clips.[28] Despite that BPPV is common, a majority of emergency physicians report that they do not use the Dix-Hallpike (diagnostic) or Epley (therapeutic) maneuvers in practice.[42] Once the correct canal is identified by these maneuvers, bedside treatment with canal repositioning maneuvers can follow.[76]

Table 4
Positional nystagmus findings in triggered episodic vestibular syndrome

Positional Tests in Triggered Episodic Vestibular Syndrome	Benign Paroxysmal Positional Vertigo (Posterior Canal)	Benign Paroxysmal Positional Vertigo (Horizontal Canal)	Central
Dix-Hallpike test (diagnostic test)	Upbeat-torsional[a] 5–30 s No spontaneous reversal	None[b]	Variable direction (down-beat or horizontal; almost never up-beat) Variable duration (often >90 s) No spontaneous reversal
Supine roll test (diagnostic test)	None[b]	Pure horizontal[c] 30–90 s Spontaneous reversal typical	Variable direction (down-beat or horizontal; almost never up-beat) Variable duration (often >90 s) No spontaneous reversal

[a] The nystagmus of posterior canal BPPV has a prominent torsional component, and the 12-o'clock pole of the eye beats toward the down-facing (tested) ear. Although the nystagmus reverse on arising from the Dix-Hallpike position, there is no spontaneous reversal.
[b] Although the Dix-Hallpike test is fairly specific to posterior canal BPPV and the supine roll test to horizontal canal BPPV, the maneuvers may sometimes stimulate the other canal. If so, the nystagmus direction depends on the affected canal, not on the type of maneuver eliciting the nystagmus. The nystagmus may be considerably weaker and less evident than when using the 'correct' maneuver.
[c] The nystagmus of horizontal canal BPPV may beat toward the down ear or away from it. The nystagmus often crescendo, then slow down and reverse spontaneously, even without moving the head. When the opposite side is tested, the nystagmus usually beats in the opposite direction (eg, if right-beating initially with right ear down, then left-beating initially with left ear down).

CNS mimics of BPPV are called CPPV. This is usually caused by posterior fossa lesions, including neoplasm, infarction, hemorrhage, demyelination, cerebellar degeneration, and Chiari malformation. There are several factors to be considered in distinguishing BPPV from CPPV that are summarized in **Box 2**.[79]

Orthostatic hypotension affects 16% of adults[80] and accounts for 24% of acute syncopal presentations.[81] Classic symptoms are brief presyncope on arising, but vertigo is common[25] and underappreciated.[47] Orthostatic hypotension is a sustained decline in blood pressure of at least 20 mm Hg systolic or 10 mm Hg diastolic within 3 minutes of standing.[82] Recent work suggests optimal cutoffs should be adjusted based on baseline blood pressure.[83] The orthostasis can be delayed (onset >10 minutes), however, and the duration of monitoring remains controversial.[84–86] Measurement technique matters,[87–89] but proper bedside methods are not consistently applied in practice.[90]

Emergency physicians are familiar with the most common identifiable causes of acute orthostatic hypotension, such as medications and hypovolemia, which in turn may be caused by obvious fluid losses (bleeding, vomiting, diarrhea, and excessive urination/sweating) or by occult internal bleeding. Strong bedside predictors of moderate blood loss are postural dizziness so severe as to prevent standing or a postural pulse increment greater than 30 beats per minute, but the sensitivity of these findings is only 22%.[89] Furthermore, the benign postural orthostatic tachycardia syndrome produces similar clinical findings.[91] Absence of tachycardia or even relative bradycardia can occur with intraperitoneal blood, such as ruptured ectopic pregnancy.[92] Associated symptoms, such as fever, severe chest, back, abdominal, or pelvic pain, are clues to serious causes of orthostatic hypotension. Dangerous diseases presenting with orthostatic hypotension but sometimes lacking overt clues to the underlying cause include myocardial infarction, occult sepsis, adrenal insufficiency, and diabetic ketoacidosis.[93]

BPPV can be confused for orthostatic hypotension. BPPV produces dizziness on arising in 58%,[74] can mimic the postural lightheadedness of orthostatic hypotension,[94] and often is undiagnosed in the elderly.[26,95] Also, orthostatic hypotension

---

Box 2
Characteristics of patients with triggered episodic vestibular syndrome that suggest a central mimic rather than typical benign paroxysmal positional vertigo

1. Presence of symptoms or signs that are NOT seen in BPPV
   a. Headache
   b. Diplopia
   c. Abnormal cranial nerve or cerebellar function

2. Presence of nystagmus without dizziness

3. Atypical nystagmus characteristics
   a. Down-beating nystagmus[a]
   b. Nystagmus that beats in different directions on repeat testing

4. Poor response to therapeutic maneuvers
   a. Unable to cure patient with typical canalith repositioning maneuver
   b. Frequent recurrent symptoms

[a] Down-beating nystagmus can be seen with anterior canal BPPV. Because BPPV of this canal is rare and because down-beating nystagmus is also seen with central causes, however, it is safer for emergency physicians to consider this finding always worrisome prompting imaging and/or referral.

may be incidental and misleading, especially in older patients taking antihypertensive medications.[96] In patients with postural dizziness, BPPV and orthostatic hypotension can usually be differentiated by considering other positional triggers, such as rolling over in bed or reclining, both of which are common in BPPV but should not occur with orthostatic hypotension.

BPPV notwithstanding, orthostatic dizziness and orthostatic hypotension are not always related.[80,97] Orthostatic dizziness without systemic orthostatic hypotension has been reported with hemodynamic TIA due to vascular stenosis[98] and in patients with intracranial hypotension.[99] Neurologic evaluation is probably indicated for patients with reproducible and sustained orthostatic dizziness but no demonstrable hypotension.

SPONTANEOUS EPISODIC VESTIBULAR SYNDROME

The spontaneous EVS (s-EVS) is marked by recurrent, spontaneous episodic dizziness that ranges in duration from seconds to days, but a majority last minutes to hours. Most patients are, therefore, asymptomatic at the time of clinical assessment, and if they are, an episode cannot be provoked at the bedside (because it is not triggerable, so the evaluation relies almost entirely on history). Spells sometimes occur up to several times a day but are usually more infrequent and can be separated by months or even years, depending on the cause. The most common benign cause by far is vestibular migraine.[100–102] The most common dangerous cause is vertebrobasilar TIA.[103] This temporal pattern is also seen Meniere disease.[101] Other causes of the s-EVS include reflex (eg, vasovagal) syncope[104] and panic attacks.[105] Uncommon dangerous causes of s-EVS are cardiovascular (cardiac arrhythmia, unstable angina pectoris, and pulmonary embolus), endocrine (hypoglycemia and neurohumoral neoplasms), or toxic (intermittent carbon monoxide exposure). Diagnosis is not difficult when cases are typical. Unfortunately, classic features, such as frank loss of consciousness in reflex syncope,[106] headache in vestibular migraine,[107] and fear in panic attacks,[108] are absent in approximately 25% to 35% of cases. Atypical case presentations probably contribute to diagnostic confusion in patients with transient neurologic attacks.[109]

Some cases of vasovagal syncope may be triggered (eg, by phlebotomy) but there is often no obvious trigger. With carbon monoxide exposure, the trigger is an environmental one that is not immediately apparent. These situations differ from BPPV, however, in which there is an obligate, immediate trigger.

Definite vestibular migraine diagnosis requires recurrent attacks with vestibular symptoms, a history of migraine according to the International Classification of Headache Disorders, and migraine symptoms during at least half of the attacks.[101] Attack duration in vestibular migraine ranges from seconds to days.[101] When nystagmus is present in patients with vestibular migraine, it can be of a peripheral, central, or mixed type.[110] Headache is often absent with the attack; when headache does occur, it may begin before, during, or after the dizziness and may differ from the patient's other typical migraine headaches.[101,110] Nausea, vomiting, photophobia, phonophobia, and visual auras may accompany vestibular migraine. Hearing loss or tinnitus sometimes occur,[111] creating some overlap between vestibular migraine and Meniere disease.[112] Because there are no pathognomonic signs or biomarkers, the diagnosis is made based purely on clinical history and the exclusion of alternative causes.[101]

Although Meniere disease often features prominently in discussions of dizziness, it is probably an uncommon cause of dizziness in the ED. Patients classically present with episodic vertigo accompanied by unilateral tinnitus and aural fullness, often with reversible sensorineural hearing loss. Episodes typically last minutes to hours. Only 1 in 4 initially presents with the complete symptom triad,[113] and nonvertiginous dizziness is common.[114] Definite Meniere disease requires at least 2 spontaneous episodes of vertigo lasting at least 20 minutes, audiometrically documented hearing loss (at least once, whether transient or persistent), and tinnitus or aural fullness in the affected ear, with other causes excluded.[101]

Reflex syncope (also called neurocardiogenic or neurally mediated syncope) includes vasovagal syncope, carotid sinus hypersensitivity, and situational syncope (eg, micturition, defecation, or cough).[115] Those who faint usually experience prodromal symptoms; presyncopal spells without loss of consciousness substantially outnumber spells with syncope.[104] Dizziness is the most common presyncopal symptom and it may be of any type, including vertigo.[116] Presyncopal symptoms usually last 3 to 30 minutes.[117] Diagnosis is based on clinical history, excluding dangerous mimics (especially arrhythmia), and can be confirmed by formal head-up tilt table testing.[91]

Episodic dizziness also accompanies panic attacks, with or without hyperventilation. Dizziness begins rapidly, peaks within 10 minutes and, by definition, is accompanied by at least 3 other symptoms.[118] Although a situational precipitant (eg, claustrophobia) may be present, spells often occur without obvious incitement. Fear of dying or going crazy are classic symptoms but are absent in 30% of cases.[108] Ictal panic attacks from temporal lobe epilepsy generally last only seconds, and altered mental status is frequent.[105] Panic attacks presenting with dizziness are most closely mimicked by hypoglycemia, cardiac arrhythmias, pheochromocytoma, and basilar TIA. Each may produce a multisymptom complex with neurologic and autonomic features similar to idiopathic panic.

The principal dangerous diagnoses for s-EVS is TIA.[103] Although for years, isolated vertigo was considered to not be due to TIA, more recent evidence is strong that dizziness, even isolated attacks of vertigo, can cause TIAs.[119] TIAs can present with isolated episodes of dizziness weeks to months or even years prior to a completed infarction.[120,121] Dizziness is the most common symptom in basilar artery occlusion[122] and occurs without other neurologic symptoms in 20% of cases.[123] Dizziness is the most common presenting symptom of vertebral artery dissection,[124] which affects younger patients, mimics migraine, and is easily misdiagnosed.[5] Because 5% of TIA patients suffer a stroke within 48 hours, prompt diagnosis is critical.[125] Patients with posterior circulation TIA may have an even higher stroke risk than those with anterior circulation spells.[126,127] Rapid treatment lowers stroke risk after TIA by approximately 80%.[128,129]

Cardiac arrhythmias should also be considered in any patient with s-EVS, particularly when syncope occurs.[25] Although some clinical features may increase or decrease the odds of a cardiac cause,[115] additional testing (eg, cardiac loop recording) is often required to confirm the final diagnosis.[91]

PUTTING IT ALL TOGETHER — AN OVERARCHING ALGORITHM

Taking a history of a dizzy patient should be no different from taking a history in nearly any other patient. The timing, triggers of the dizziness (and not the descriptor used), and evolution of the symptoms, associated symptoms, and epidemiologic context inform the differential diagnosis, and bedside physical examination can frequently establish a specific diagnosis. Using this newer paradigm has not yet been validated in large numbers of ED patients treated by emergency physicians, but current evidence and experience suggest that this is possible. An overarching algorithm is suggested (**Fig. 1**).

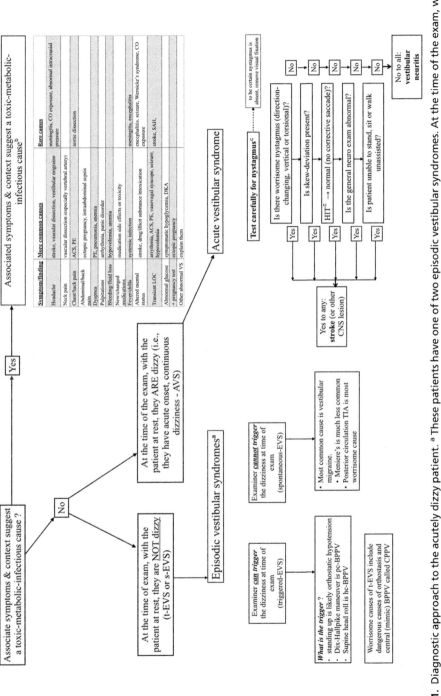

Fig. 1. Diagnostic approach to the acutely dizzy patient. [a] These patients have one of two episodic vestibular syndromes. At the time of the exam, when the patient is not moving, they are NOT dizzy. [b] This group accounts for ~ 50% of acutely dizzy patients in an ED population. [c] IMPORTANT CAVEAT: if nystagmus is absent, do not do the HIT. It is not useful and potentially misleading in these patients. CO, carbon monoxide; DKA, diabetic ketoacidosis; LOC, loss of consciousness; PE, pulmonary embolism; SAH, subarachnoid hemorrhage; VS, vital signs.

SUMMARY

Dizziness, vertigo, and unsteadiness are common complaints caused by numerous diseases that span organ systems. Diagnosis can, therefore, be difficult, leading to overutilization of resources and misdiagnosis. The current paradigm used by most physicians is based on symptom quality, a paradigm created 40 years ago; a newer paradigm, based on timing and triggers, is more consistent with current evidence. History and physical examination are more accurate, more efficient, and more likely to result in a specific diagnosis than the traditional paradigm.

REFERENCES

1. Cheung CS, Mak PS, Manley KV, et al. Predictors of important neurological causes of dizziness among patients presenting to the emergency department. Emerg Med J 2010;27:517–21.
2. Newman-Toker DE, Hsieh YH, Camargo CA Jr, et al. Spectrum of dizziness visits to US emergency departments: cross-sectional analysis from a nationally representative sample. Mayo Clin Proc 2008;83:765–75.
3. Saber Tehrani AS, Coughlan D, Hsieh YH, et al. Rising annual costs of dizziness presentations to U.S. emergency departments. Acad Emerg Med 2013;20: 689–96.
4. Improving diagnosis in health care. Washington, DC: National Academies Press; 2015.
5. Savitz SI, Caplan LR, Edlow JA. Pitfalls in the diagnosis of cerebellar infarction. Acad Emerg Med 2007;14:63–8.
6. Newman-Toker DE, Edlow JA. TiTrATE: a novel, evidence-based approach to diagnosing acute dizziness and vertigo. Neurol Clin 2015;33:577–99.
7. Newman-Toker DE, Camargo CA Jr, Hsieh YH, et al. Disconnect between charted vestibular diagnoses and emergency department management decisions: a cross-sectional analysis from a nationally representative sample. Acad Emerg Med 2009;16:970–7.
8. Cooper H, Bhattacharya B, Verma V, et al. Liquorice and soy sauce, a life-saving concoction in a patient with Addison's disease. Ann Clin Biochem 2007;44: 397–9.
9. Demiryoguran NS, Karcioglu O, Topacoglu H, et al. Painless aortic dissection with bilateral carotid involvement presenting with vertigo as the chief complaint. Emerg Med J 2006;23:e15.
10. Heckerling PS, Leikin JB, Maturen A, et al. Predictors of occult carbon monoxide poisoning in patients with headache and dizziness. Ann Intern Med 1987;107: 174–6.
11. Wolfe TR, Allen TL. Syncope as an emergency department presentation of pulmonary embolism. J Emerg Med 1998;16:27–31.
12. Choi KD, Oh SY, Kim HJ, et al. The vestibulo-ocular reflexes during head impulse in Wernicke's encephalopathy. J Neurol Neurosurg Psychiatry 2007;78: 1161–2.
13. Herr RD, Zun L, Mathews JJ. A directed approach to the dizzy patient. Ann Emerg Med 1989;18:664–72.
14. Royl G, Ploner CJ, Leithner C. Dizziness in the emergency room: diagnoses and misdiagnoses. Eur Neurol 2011;66:256–63.
15. Navi BB, Kamel H, Shah MP, et al. Rate and predictors of serious neurologic causes of dizziness in the emergency department. Mayo Clin Proc 2012;87: 1080–8.

16. Geser R, Straumann D. Referral and final diagnoses of patients assessed in an academic vertigo center. Front Neurol 2012;3:169.
17. Chase M, Joyce NR, Carney E, et al. ED patients with vertigo: can we identify clinical factors associated with acute stroke? Am J Emerg Med 2012;30:587–91.
18. Moubayed SP, Saliba I. Vertebrobasilar insufficiency presenting as isolated positional vertigo or dizziness: a double-blind retrospective cohort study. Laryngoscope 2009;119:2071–6.
19. Navi BB, Kamel H, Shah MP, et al. Application of the ABCD2 score to identify cerebrovascular causes of dizziness in the emergency department. Stroke 2012;43:1484–9.
20. Kerber KA, Meurer WJ, Brown DL, et al. Stroke risk stratification in acute dizziness presentations: a prospective imaging-based study. Neurology 2015; 85(21):1869–78.
21. Drachman DA, Hart CW. An approach to the dizzy patient. Neurology 1972;22: 323–34.
22. Edlow JA. Diagnosing dizziness: we are teaching the wrong paradigm! Acad Emerg Med 2013;20:1064–6.
23. Newman-Toker DE, Cannon LM, Stofferahn ME, et al. Imprecision in patient reports of dizziness symptom quality: a cross-sectional study conducted in an acute care setting. Mayo Clin Proc 2007;82:1329–40.
24. Kerber KA, Brown DL, Lisabeth LD, et al. Stroke among patients with dizziness, vertigo, and imbalance in the emergency department: a population-based study. Stroke 2006;37:2484–7.
25. Newman-Toker DE, Dy FJ, Stanton VA, et al. How often is dizziness from primary cardiovascular disease true vertigo? A systematic review. J Gen Intern Med 2008;23:2087–94.
26. Lawson J, Bamiou DE, Cohen HS, et al. Positional vertigo in a falls service. Age Ageing 2008;37:585–9.
27. Kerber KA, Morgenstern LB, Meurer WJ, et al. Nystagmus assessments documented by emergency physicians in acute dizziness presentations: a target for decision support? Acad Emerg Med 2011;18:619–26.
28. Edlow J, Newman-Toker D. Using the physical examination to diagnose patients with acute dizziness and vertigo. J Emerg Med 2016;50(4):617–28.
29. Braun EM, Tomazic PV, Ropposch T, et al. Misdiagnosis of acute peripheral vestibulopathy in central nervous ischemic infarction. Otol Neurotol 2011;32: 1518–21.
30. Casani AP, Dallan I, Cerchiai N, et al. Cerebellar infarctions mimicking acute peripheral vertigo: how to avoid misdiagnosis? Otolaryngol Head Neck Surg 2013; 148:475–81.
31. Lee H, Sohn SI, Cho YW, et al. Cerebellar infarction presenting isolated vertigo: frequency and vascular topographical patterns. Neurology 2006;67:1178–83.
32. Martin-Schild S, Albright KC, Tanksley J, et al. Zero on the NIHSS does not equal the absence of stroke. Ann Emerg Med 2011;57:42–5.
33. Masuda Y, Tei H, Shimizu S, et al. Factors associated with the misdiagnosis of cerebellar infarction. J Stroke Cerebrovasc Dis 2013;22:1125–30.
34. Honda S, Inatomi Y, Yonehara T, et al. Discrimination of acute ischemic stroke from nonischemic vertigo in patients presenting with only imbalance. J Stroke Cerebrovasc Dis 2014;23:888–95.
35. Kuruvilla A, Bhattacharya P, Rajamani K, et al. Factors associated with misdiagnosis of acute stroke in young adults. J Stroke Cerebrovasc Dis 2011;20:523–7.

36. Nakajima M, Hirano T, Uchino M. Patients with acute stroke admitted on the second visit. J Stroke Cerebrovasc Dis 2008;17:382–7.
37. Atzema CL, Grewal K, Lu H, et al. Outcomes among patients discharged from the emergency department with a diagnosis of peripheral vertigo. Ann Neurol 2016;79(1):32–41.
38. Kerber KA, Zahuranec DB, Brown DL, et al. Stroke risk after nonstroke emergency department dizziness presentations: a population-based cohort study. Ann Neurol 2014;75:899–907.
39. Kim AS, Fullerton HJ, Johnston SC. Risk of vascular events in emergency department patients discharged home with diagnosis of dizziness or vertigo. Ann Emerg Med 2011;57:34–41.
40. Kerber KA, Newman-Toker DE. Misdiagnosing Dizzy Patients: common pitfalls in clinical practice. Neurol Clin 2015;33:565–75.
41. Grewal K, Austin PC, Kapral MK, et al. Missed strokes using computed tomography imaging in patients with vertigo: population-based cohort study. Stroke 2015;46:108–13.
42. Kene MV, Ballard DW, Vinson DR, et al. Emergency Physician attitudes, preferences, and risk tolerance for stroke as a potential cause of Dizziness symptoms. West J Emerg Med 2015;16:768–76.
43. Tarnutzer AA, Berkowitz AL, Robinson KA, et al. Does my dizzy patient have a stroke? A systematic review of bedside diagnosis in acute vestibular syndrome. CMAJ 2011;183(9):E571–92.
44. Edlow JA, Newman-Toker DE. Medical and nonstroke neurologic causes of acute, continuous vestibular symptoms. Neurol Clin 2015;33:699–716.
45. Pula JH, Newman-Toker DE, Kattah JC. Multiple sclerosis as a cause of the acute vestibular syndrome. J Neurol 2013;260:1649–54.
46. Kerber KA, Burke JF, Brown DL, et al. Does intracerebral haemorrhage mimic benign dizziness presentations? A population based study. Emerg Med J 2012;29(1):43–6.
47. Stanton VA, Hsieh YH, Camargo CA Jr, et al. Overreliance on symptom quality in diagnosing dizziness: results of a multicenter survey of emergency physicians. Mayo Clin Proc 2007;82:1319–28.
48. Cutfield NJ, Seemungal BM, Millington H, et al. Diagnosis of acute vertigo in the emergency department. Emerg Med J 2011;28(6):538–9.
49. Arbusow V, Theil D, Strupp M, et al. HSV-1 not only in human vestibular ganglia but also in the vestibular labyrinth. Audiol Neurootol 2001;6:259–62.
50. Bergenius J, Perols O. Vestibular neuritis: a follow-up study. Acta Otolaryngol 1999;119:895–9.
51. Lee H, Kim BK, Park HJ, et al. Prodromal dizziness in vestibular neuritis: frequency and clinical implication. J Neurol Neurosurg Psychiatry 2009;80:355–6.
52. Karlberg M, Annertz M, Magnusson M. Acute vestibular neuritis visualized by 3-T magnetic resonance imaging with high-dose gadolinium. Arch Otolaryngol Head Neck Surg 2004;130:229–32.
53. Strupp M, Jager L, Muller-Lisse U, et al. High resolution Gd-DTPA MR imaging of the inner ear in 60 patients with idiopathic vestibular neuritis: no evidence for contrast enhancement of the labyrinth or vestibular nerve. J Vestib Res 1998; 8:427–33.
54. Lu YC, Young YH. Vertigo from herpes zoster oticus: superior or inferior vestibular nerve origin? Laryngoscope 2003;113:307–11.
55. Baloh RW. Clinical practice. Vestibular neuritis. N Engl J Med 2003;348: 1027–32.

56. Chalela JA, Kidwell CS, Nentwich LM, et al. Magnetic resonance imaging and computed tomography in emergency assessment of patients with suspected acute stroke: a prospective comparison. Lancet 2007;369:293–8.
57. Hwang DY, Silva GS, Furie KL, et al. Comparative sensitivity of computed tomography vs. magnetic resonance imaging for detecting acute posterior fossa infarct. J Emerg Med 2012;42:559–65.
58. Simmons Z, Biller J, Adams HP Jr, et al. Cerebellar infarction: comparison of computed tomography and magnetic resonance imaging. Ann Neurol 1986; 19:291–3.
59. Kattah JC, Talkad AV, Wang DZ, et al. HINTS to diagnose stroke in the acute vestibular syndrome: three-step bedside oculomotor examination more sensitive than early MRI diffusion-weighted imaging. Stroke 2009;40:3504–10.
60. Saber Tehrani AS, Kattah JC, Mantokoudis G, et al. Small strokes causing severe vertigo: frequency of false-negative MRIs and nonlacunar mechanisms. Neurology 2014;83:169–73.
61. Chen L, Lee W, Chambers BR, et al. Diagnostic accuracy of acute vestibular syndrome at the bedside in a stroke unit. J Neurol 2011;258(5):855–61.
62. Vanni S, Nazerian P, Casati C, et al. Can emergency physicians accurately and reliably assess acute vertigo in the emergency department? Emerg Med Australas 2015;27:126–31.
63. Vanni S, Pecci R, Casati C, et al. STANDING, a four-step bedside algorithm for differential diagnosis of acute vertigo in the Emergency Department. Acta Otorhinolaryngol Ital 2014;34:419–26.
64. Welgampola MS, Bradshaw AP, Lechner C, et al. Bedside assessment of acute Dizziness and Vertigo. Neurol Clin 2015;33:551–64, vii.
65. Strupp M, Fischer C, Hanss L, et al. The takeaway Frenzel goggles: a Fresnel-based device. Neurology 2014;83:1241–5.
66. Newman-Toker DE, Sharma P, Chowdhury M, et al. Penlight-cover test: a new bedside method to unmask nystagmus. J Neurol Neurosurg Psychiatry 2009; 80:900–3.
67. Halmagyi GM, Curthoys IS. A clinical sign of canal paresis. Arch Neurol 1988; 45:737–9.
68. Newman-Toker DE, Kattah JC, Alvernia JE, et al. Normal head impulse test differentiates acute cerebellar strokes from vestibular neuritis. Neurology 2008;70: 2378–85.
69. Newman-Toker DE, Kerber KA, Hsieh YH, et al. HINTS outperforms ABCD2 to screen for stroke in acute continuous vertigo and dizziness. Acad Emerg Med 2013;20:986–96.
70. Lee H. Neuro-otological aspects of cerebellar stroke syndrome. J Clin Neurol 2009;5:65–73.
71. Lee H, Kim JS, Chung EJ, et al. Infarction in the territory of anterior inferior cerebellar artery: spectrum of audiovestibular loss. Stroke 2009;40:3745–51.
72. Lee SH, Kim JS. Acute diagnosis and management of stroke presenting Dizziness or Vertigo. Neurol Clin 2015;33:687–98, xi.
73. Kim JS. Pure lateral medullary infarction: clinical-radiological correlation of 130 acute, consecutive patients. Brain 2003;126:1864–72.
74. von Brevern M, Radtke A, Lezius F, et al. Epidemiology of benign paroxysmal positional vertigo: a population based study. J Neurol Neurosurg Psychiatry 2007;78:710–5.
75. Baloh RW, Honrubia V, Jacobson K. Benign positional vertigo: clinical and oculographic features in 240 cases. Neurology 1987;37:371–8.

76. Fife TD, von Brevern M. Benign paroxysmal positional vertigo in the acute care setting. Neurol Clin 2015;33:601–17, viii-ix.
77. Bhattacharyya N, Baugh RF, Orvidas L, et al. Clinical practice guideline: benign paroxysmal positional vertigo. Otolaryngol Head Neck Surg 2008;139:S47–81.
78. Fife TD, Iverson DJ, Lempert T, et al. Practice parameter: therapies for benign paroxysmal positional vertigo (an evidence-based review): report of the Quality Standards Subcommittee of the American Academy of Neurology. Neurology 2008;70:2067–74.
79. Soto-Varela A, Rossi-Izquierdo M, Sanchez-Sellero I, et al. Revised criteria for suspicion of non-benign positional vertigo. QJM 2013;106:317–21.
80. Wu JS, Yang YC, Lu FH, et al. Population-based study on the prevalence and correlates of orthostatic hypotension/hypertension and orthostatic dizziness. Hypertens Res 2008;31:897–904.
81. Sarasin FP, Louis-Simonet M, Carballo D, et al. Prevalence of orthostatic hypotension among patients presenting with syncope in the ED. Am J Emerg Med 2002;20:497–501.
82. Freeman R, Wieling W, Axelrod FB, et al. Consensus statement on the definition of orthostatic hypotension, neurally mediated syncope and the postural tachycardia syndrome. Clin Auton Res 2011;21:69–72.
83. Fedorowski A, Burri P, Melander O. Orthostatic hypotension in genetically related hypertensive and normotensive individuals. J Hypertens 2009;27: 976–82.
84. Cheshire WP Jr, Phillips LH 2nd. Delayed orthostatic hypotension: is it worth the wait? Neurology 2006;67:8–9.
85. Cohen E, Grossman E, Sapoznikov B, et al. Assessment of orthostatic hypotension in the emergency room. Blood Press 2006;15:263–7.
86. Gibbons CH, Freeman R. Delayed orthostatic hypotension: a frequent cause of orthostatic intolerance. Neurology 2006;67:28–32.
87. Guss DA, Abdelnur D, Hemingway TJ. The impact of arm position on the measurement of orthostatic blood pressure. J Emerg Med 2008;34:377–82.
88. McAlister FA, Straus SE. Evidence based treatment of hypertension. Measurement of blood pressure: an evidence based review. BMJ 2001;322:908–11.
89. McGee S, Abernethy WB 3rd, Simel DL. The rational clinical examination. Is this patient hypovolemic? JAMA 1999;281:1022–9.
90. Vloet LC, Smits R, Frederiks CM, et al. Evaluation of skills and knowledge on orthostatic blood pressure measurements in elderly patients. Age Ageing 2002;31:211–6.
91. Moya A, Sutton R, Ammirati F, et al. Guidelines for the diagnosis and management of syncope (version 2009). Eur Heart J 2009;30:2631–71.
92. Birkhahn RH, Gaeta TJ, Van Deusen SK, et al. The ability of traditional vital signs and shock index to identify ruptured ectopic pregnancy. Am J Obstet Gynecol 2003;189:1293–6.
93. Gilbert VE. Immediate orthostatic hypotension: diagnostic value in acutely ill patients. South Med J 1993;86:1028–32.
94. Lawson J, Johnson I, Bamiou DE, et al. Benign paroxysmal positional vertigo: clinical characteristics of dizzy patients referred to a falls and syncope unit. QJM 2005;98:357–64.
95. Oghalai JS, Manolidis S, Barth JL, et al. Unrecognized benign paroxysmal positional vertigo in elderly patients. Otolaryngol Head Neck Surg 2000;122:630–4.

96. Poon IO, Braun U. High prevalence of orthostatic hypotension and its correlation with potentially causative medications among elderly veterans. J Clin Pharm Ther 2005;30:173–8.

97. Radtke A, Lempert T, von Brevern M, et al. Prevalence and complications of orthostatic dizziness in the general population. Clin Auton Res 2011;21(3): 161–8.

98. Stark RJ, Wodak J. Primary orthostatic cerebral ischaemia. J Neurol Neurosurg Psychiatry 1983;46:883–91.

99. Blank SC, Shakir RA, Bindoff LA, et al. Spontaneous intracranial hypotension: clinical and magnetic resonance imaging characteristics. Clin Neurol Neurosurg 1997;99:199–204.

100. Neuhauser HK, Radtke A, von Brevern M, et al. Migrainous vertigo: prevalence and impact on quality of life. Neurology 2006;67:1028–33.

101. Seemungal B, Kaski D, Lopez-Escamez JA. Early diagnosis and management of acute vertigo from Vestibular Migraine and Meniere's Disease. Neurol Clin 2015;33:619–28, ix.

102. Strupp M, Versino M, Brandt T. Vestibular migraine. Handb Clin Neurol 2010;97: 755–71.

103. Blum CA, Kasner SE. Transient ischemic attacks presenting with Dizziness or Vertigo. Neurol Clin 2015;33:629–42, ix.

104. Romme JJ, van Dijk N, Boer KR, et al. Influence of age and gender on the occurrence and presentation of reflex syncope. Clin Auton Res 2008;18:127–33.

105. Kanner AM. Ictal panic and interictal panic attacks: diagnostic and therapeutic principles. Neurol Clin 2011;29:163–75, ix.

106. Mathias CJ, Deguchi K, Schatz I. Observations on recurrent syncope and presyncope in 641 patients. Lancet 2001;357:348–53.

107. Dieterich M, Brandt T. Episodic vertigo related to migraine (90 cases): vestibular migraine? J Neurol 1999;246:883–92.

108. Chen J, Tsuchiya M, Kawakami N, et al. Non-fearful vs. fearful panic attacks: a general population study from the National Comorbidity Survey. J Affect Disord 2009;112:273–8.

109. Fonseca AC, Canhao P. Diagnostic difficulties in the classification of transient neurological attacks. Eur J Neurol 2011;18(4):644–8.

110. Lempert T, Neuhauser H, Daroff RB. Vertigo as a symptom of migraine. Ann N Y Acad Sci 2009;1164:242–51.

111. Kayan A, Hood JD. Neuro-otological manifestations of migraine. Brain 1984; 107(Pt 4):1123–42.

112. Millen SJ, Schnurr CM, Schnurr BB. Vestibular migraine: perspectives of otology versus neurology. Otol Neurotol 2011;32:330–7.

113. Mancini F, Catalani M, Carru M, et al. History of Meniere's disease and its clinical presentation. Otolaryngol Clin North Am 2002;35:565–80.

114. Faag C, Bergenius J, Forsberg C, et al. Symptoms experienced by patients with peripheral vestibular disorders: evaluation of the Vertigo Symptom Scale for clinical application. Clin Otolaryngol 2007;32:440–6.

115. van Dijk JG, Thijs RD, Benditt DG, et al. A guide to disorders causing transient loss of consciousness: focus on syncope. Nat Rev Neurol 2009;5:438–48.

116. Sloane PD, Linzer M, Pontinen M, et al. Clinical significance of a dizziness history in medical patients with syncope. Arch Intern Med 1991;151:1625–8.

117. Sheldon R, Hersi A, Ritchie D, et al. Syncope and structural heart disease: historical criteria for vasovagal syncope and ventricular tachycardia. J Cardiovasc Electrophysiol 2010;21:1358–64.

118. Katon WJ. Clinical practice. Panic disorder. N Engl J Med 2006;354:2360–7.
119. Paul NL, Simoni M, Rothwell PM, et al. Transient isolated brainstem symptoms preceding posterior circulation stroke: a population-based study. Lancet Neurol 2013;12:65–71.
120. Gomez CR, Cruz-Flores S, Malkoff MD, et al. Isolated vertigo as a manifestation of vertebrobasilar ischemia. Neurology 1996;47:94–7.
121. Grad A, Baloh RW. Vertigo of vascular origin. Clinical and electronystagmographic features in 84 cases. Arch Neurol 1989;46:281–4.
122. von Campe G, Regli F, Bogousslavsky J. Heralding manifestations of basilar artery occlusion with lethal or severe stroke. J Neurol Neurosurg Psychiatry 2003;74:1621–6.
123. Fisher CM. Vertigo in cerebrovascular disease. Arch Otolaryngol 1967;85: 529–34.
124. Gottesman RF, Sharma P, Robinson KA, et al. Clinical characteristics of symptomatic vertebral artery dissection: a systematic review. Neurologist 2012;18: 245–54.
125. Shah KH, Kleckner K, Edlow JA. Short-term prognosis of stroke among patients diagnosed in the emergency department with a transient ischemic attack. Ann Emerg Med 2008;51:316–23.
126. Flossmann E, Rothwell PM. Prognosis of vertebrobasilar transient ischaemic attack and minor stroke. Brain 2003;126:1940–54.
127. Gulli G, Khan S, Markus HS. Vertebrobasilar stenosis predicts high early recurrent stroke risk in posterior circulation stroke and TIA. Stroke 2009;40:2732–7.
128. Lavallee PC, Meseguer E, Abboud H, et al. A transient ischaemic attack clinic with round-the-clock access (SOS-TIA): feasibility and effects. Lancet Neurol 2007;6:953–60.
129. Rothwell PM, Giles MF, Chandratheva A, et al. Effect of urgent treatment of transient ischaemic attack and minor stroke on early recurrent stroke (EXPRESS study): a prospective population-based sequential comparison. Lancet 2007; 370:1432–42.

Acute Nontraumatic Back Pain

Risk Stratification, Emergency Department Management, and Review of Serious Pathologies

Jennifer Singleton, MD, Jonathan A. Edlow, MD*

KEYWORDS

- Back pain • Spinal cord compression • Cauda equine • Spinal epidural abscess
- Metastatic epidural tumor

KEY POINTS

- Of emergency department patients with acute nontraumatic back pain, physicians must understand how to diagnose the minority with serious causes while simultaneously treating the large majority with conservative measures.
- Distinguishing patients with simple back pain versus those with serious causes is based on careful history, physical examination, and in some cases inflammatory markers.
- In patients with acute back pain and new abnormalities in the neurologic examination of the lower extremities, rapid MRI to diagnose the specific lesion is critical to improving outcomes in this group of patients.

INTRODUCTION
Scope of the Problem

Back pain is common and costly, with a lifetime prevalence of 80% to 90% and rapidly increasing health-related expenditures.[1,2] Adults with acute nontraumatic back pain account for 2% to 3% of emergency department (ED) visits.[3,4] Although most have benign, self-limited causes, around 5% of patients have serious pathology that, if not rapidly diagnosed and treated, can result in poor outcomes because of neurologic damage.[5] The role of the emergency physician is to identify this subset from among a large majority of patients who often require no more than a history and physical examination. Overall, the quality of evidence on this subject as it specifically relates to ED patients is weak and recommendations in the article are mostly based on guidelines, expert opinion, and clinical experience. This article reviews the most recent literature

Department of Emergency Medicine, Beth Israel Deaconess Medical Center, Harvard Medical School, 1 Deaconess Place, Boston, MA 02115, USA
* Corresponding author.
E-mail address: jedlow@bidmc.harvard.edu

Emerg Med Clin N Am 34 (2016) 743–757
http://dx.doi.org/10.1016/j.emc.2016.06.015
0733-8627/16/© 2016 Elsevier Inc. All rights reserved.

and guideline revisions in the ED evaluation and management of atraumatic back pain, and is an updated and expanded version of a 2015 review published in the *Annals of Emergency Medicine*.[6]

Differential Diagnosis

Patients with acute, nontraumatic low back pain are broadly divided into three categories: (1) benign, self-limited musculoskeletal causes; (2) spinal pathologies that can cause severe neurologic disability because of spinal cord or cauda equina damage; and (3) other abdominal or retroperitoneal processes that can present with back pain. We refer to these groups as simple, serious, and nonspine causes of back pain, respectively.

Simple musculoskeletal causes include degenerative spine disease, muscular or ligamentous injury, and most acute disk herniations. Sciatica, the presenting symptom of lumbosacral radiculopathy, is characterized by pain in the back radiating to the leg. This specific entity carries an estimated lifetime prevalence of 3% to 5% in adults.[7] These patients may have severe pain but have normal neurologic examinations, except for some patients with a monoradiculopathy. Making a specific anatomic diagnosis (eg, ligamentous strain vs disk herniation) is neither helpful nor necessary because the initial management is identical and the outcomes are almost always excellent.

Although self-limited musculoskeletal causes of back pain cause the most presentations for this complaint in the primary care setting, one must consider more serious potential spinal pathologies in patients presenting to the ED with back pain. Among the serious causes of back pain, the most common include metastatic epidural tumor, spinal epidural abscess (SEA), epidural hematoma, and central disk herniation (**Box 1**).

It is crucial to remember that although new neurologic physical findings strongly suggest serious disease, the converse is not true. Patients with any of the common serious causes can present with normal neurologic examinations. Not surprisingly, these patients are more likely to be misdiagnosed.[8] Failure to consider a serious diagnosis is the most common cause of misdiagnosis of patients with back pain with serious causes.[9]

Finally, in the diagnostic work-up of back pain, one must consider the life-threatening nonspinal etiologies (eg, aortic aneurysm, cholangitis, retroperitoneal hematoma; see **Box 1**). This article does not focus on the subset of patients with nonspinal etiologies of back pain; however, it is incumbent on the emergency physician to keep a broad differential and appropriately tailor diagnostic strategy in patients without a convincing musculoskeletal cause of back pain. For example, it is well known that a significant minority of patients with acutely symptomatic abdominal aortic aneurysms present with isolated back pain and that ED ultrasound is a fast and sensitive diagnostic test. Each of the conditions in **Box 1** needs to be considered.

RISK STRATIFICATION

In evaluating a patient with back pain, the major decision point often comes down to whether a patient requires advanced imaging as part of a diagnostic work-up for serious causes of back pain. This decision should not be made lightly: routine imaging has not been shown to change outcomes in patients with back pain.[10–12] Additionally, the choice to pursue advanced imaging may have downstream effects on ED resource use and throughput. In most cases, this decision can be made solely with a thorough history and physical examination, after which those with simple back pain may be safely discharged from the ED.[13–15]

Box 1
Differential diagnosis of adult patients with acute atraumatic low back pain[a]

Benign Causes

Muscular and ligamentous strains and sprains

Isolated sciatica (posterolateral disk herniation)

Spinal stenosis

Serious Causes

Cancer related
   Epidural metastatic disease
   Intradural metastatic disease
   Intramedullary tumor

Infection related
   Spinal epidural abscess
   Vertebral osteomyelitis
   Infectious diskitis

Spinal epidural hematoma

Giant (central) disk herniation causing cauda equina syndrome

Nonspine-related causes[a]

Aortic disease: dissection, aneurysm, ulceration, and aortitis

Genitourinary disease: ureteral colic, renal infarction and tumor, prostatitis

Gastrointestinal causes: pancreatitis and pancreatic cancer, penetrating peptic ulcer, cholecystitis, and cholangitis

Retroperitoneal hemorrhage

Systemic infections including endocarditis, psoas abscess, and other localized abscess

   [a] These lists include the more common or more dangerous causes in each category; they are not meant to be encyclopedic.

Choosing who requires advanced imaging is usually based on the assessment of red flags or risk factors for serious causes of back pain (**Fig. 1**). The evidence for many of these red flags is weak.[4,5,16,17] The best validated red flags for fracture include older age, prolonged corticosteroid use, severe trauma, and presence of an abrasion/contusion. The probability of fracture is higher when multiple red flags are present. In 2013, Downie and colleagues[16] performed a systemic review of 14 studies to identify evidence-based red flags associated with malignancy and fracture. The authors found that the only well-supported red flag for spinal malignancy was a history of malignancy. The posttest probability of a malignant cause was much higher in the ED compared with the primary care setting, further highlighting the skewed acuity of patients presenting to the ED. Red flags classified as "minor risk" by the American College of Physicians guideline, including old age, unexplained weight loss, and failure to improve after 1 month, had posttest probability point estimates less than 3% in this review for various spinal pathology including fractures. Other frequently cited red flags, including thoracic pain, nonmechanical pain, and weight loss, were considered uninformative for serious spinal cause of back pain based on the included studies.[16]

Well-validated red flags for serious causes of back pain include abnormal neurologic physical examination findings (ie, new ataxia and saddle anesthesia). A 2014 retrospective study of 206 patients presenting to a UK teaching hospital with the chief

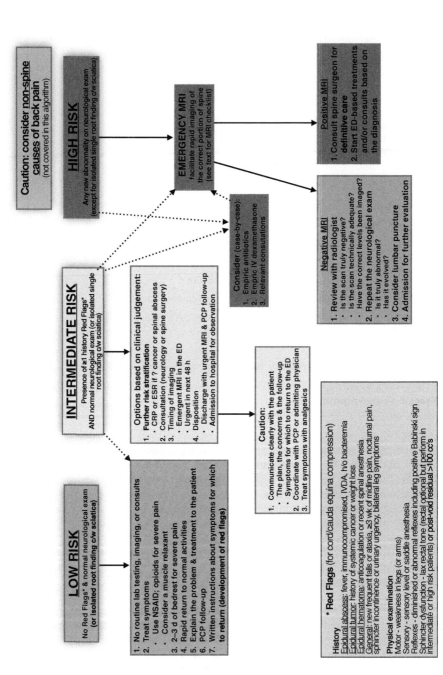

Fig. 1. Algorithm for management of nontraumatic back pain (based on expert consensus and national non-emergency-medicine-based guidelines). *Solid lines* indicate usual care; *dotted lines* indicate options based on case-by-case clinical judgment. IV, intravenous; IVDA; intravenous drug addict; NSAID, nonsteroidal anti-inflammatory drugs; PCP, primary care physician.

Caution: consider non-spine causes of back pain (not covered in this algorithm)

HIGH RISK
Any new abnormality on neurological exam (except for isolated single root finding c/w sciatica)

EMERGENCY MRI
facilitate rapid imaging of the correct portion of spine (see text for MRI checklist)

Positive MRI
1. Consult spine surgeon for definitive care
2. Start ED-based treatments and/or consults based on the diagnosis

Negative MRI
1. Review with radiologist
   • Is the scan truly negative?
   • Is the scan technically adequate?
   • Have the correct levels been imaged?
2. Repeat the neurological exam
   • Is it truly abnormal?
   • Has it evolved?
3. Consider lumbar puncture
4. Admission for further evaluation

Consider (case-by-case):
1. Empiric antibiotics
2. Empiric IV dexamethasone
3. Relevant consultations

INTERMEDIATE RISK
Presence of ≥1 history Red Flags* AND normal neurological exam (or isolated single root finding c/w sciatica)

Options based on clinical judgement:
1. Further risk stratification
   • CRP or ESR if ? cancer or spinal abscess
2. Consultation (neurology or spine surgery)
3. Timing of imaging
   • Emergent MRI in the ED
   • Urgent in next 48 h
4. Disposition
   • Discharge with urgent MRI & PCP follow-up
   • Admission to hospital for observation

Caution:
1. Communicate clearly with the patient
   • The plan, the concerns & the follow-up
   • Symptoms for which to return to the ED
2. Coordinate with PCP or admitting physician
3. Treat symptoms with analgesics

LOW RISK
No Red Flags* & normal neurological exam (or isolated root finding c/w sciatica)

1. No routine lab testing, imaging, or consults
2. Treat symptoms
   • Use NSAID; opioids for severe pain
   • Consider a muscle relaxant
3. 2–3 d of bedrest for severe pain
4. Rapid return to normal activities
5. Explain the problem & treatment to the patient
6. PCP follow-up
7. Written instructions about symptoms for which to return (development of red flags)

* Red Flags (for cord/cauda equina compression)

History
Epidural abscess: fever, immunocompromised, IVDA, h/o bacteremia
Epidural tumor: history of systemic cancer or weight loss
Epidural hematoma: anticoagulation or recent spinal anesthesia
General: new frequent falls or ataxia, ≥3 wk of midline pain, nocturnal pain, sphincter incontinence or urinary urgency, bilateral leg symptoms

Physical examination
Motor - weakness in legs (or arms)
Sensory - sensory level or saddle anesthesia
Reflexes - diminished or abnormal reflexes including positive Babinski sign
Sphincter dysfunction - lax rectal tone (rectal optional but perform in intermediate or high risk patients) or post-void residual >100 cc's

complaint of atraumatic back pain demonstrated that bowel/bladder dysfunction and saddle anesthesia had likelihood ratios greater than 2.45 and 2.11, respectively, for spinal cord compression. Taken together, the two had a likelihood ratio of 3.46.[5]

It is possible that combinations of red flags and interpreting them in the context of an individual patient could improve their utility. Patients with no red flags and normal neurologic examinations are at extremely low risk for serious causes of back pain. Patients with new hard neurologic findings (including a sensory level and saddle anesthesia) are at high risk for serious causes. Patients with the presence of historic red flags but normal neurologic examinations are at intermediate risk for cord compression or cauda equina syndrome. This group is more difficult to identify, and often requires a more diligent, careful history. To highlight the importance of historical context, primary (intradural) tumors can present with symptoms suggestive of an uncomplicated lumbosacral radiculopathy, but with the subtle element of gradually increased pain over time and with recumbency, which should lead one to consider the possibility of a neoplastic cause.

DIAGNOSTIC EVALUATION
Biomarkers

Routine laboratory testing is not useful. For example, elevated white blood cell counts are only found in two-thirds of patients with SEA.[18] Neither the percentage of neutrophils nor presence of immature forms (bands) are sensitive enough to make the diagnosis of SEA. Inflammatory markers, such as erythrocyte sedimentation rate (ESR) or C-reactive protein (CRP), are highly sensitive, although nonspecific markers, for epidural abscess and to a lesser extent for cancer.[18–20] Timing is variable between the two markers: CRP levels increase faster at the onset of inflammation and return to normal before ESR. From a sensitivity standpoint, inflammatory biomarkers may lend themselves to increased posttest probability for SEA. An ESR of greater than 20 mm has a sensitivity approaching 100% for epidural abscess but with poor specificity. As would be expected, when one increases the threshold definition of a positive ESR, the specificity improves but at the price of lowered sensitivity.[19]

A single institution study of patients with suspected SEA compared clinical outcomes before and after implementation of a guideline using ESR (cutoff of 20 mm) and CRP. Diagnostic delays dropped from 84% to 10% and the proportion of patients with motor abnormalities at time of diagnosis fell from 82% to 19%.[19] ESR performed better than CRP in this small study. Using ESR for patients with possible metastatic cancer to the spine has a lower sensitivity (78% using a cutoff of 20 mm).[20] Because of poor specificity, ESR and CRP are not recommended in patients without red flags and because of poor sensitivity, they are not useful in patients where disk herniation or epidural hematoma are the main diagnostic considerations.

Imaging

Better quality evidence underlies the recommendations against routine imaging of patients with simple back pain, although the source is mostly from primary care populations.[1,13,15] In actual ED practice, more than 30% of patients with nontraumatic back pain are imaged, possibly reflecting the skewed acuity. Over time, there has been a strong trend toward computed tomography (CT) or MRI.[4] A meta-analysis of 1804 patients from six studies comparing clinical outcomes in patients who received no imaging with those with any imaging (spine plain films or MRI) found no difference in outcomes between imaged and nonimaged patients.[21] Another study randomized 380 patients with back pain (whose physicians had ordered plain films) to plain films versus MRI.[22] Use of MRI did not improve outcomes, but costs trended higher in the MRI group, in part because of increased numbers of procedures based on abnormal MRI findings that are often incidental; fully 52% of asymptomatic individuals with no history of back pain have disk bulges and 27% have disk protrusions.[23] Similar data exist for lumbar disk herniations.[24]

Neurologic dysfunction does not always follow a linear progression of "compression" caused by increasing mass effect. Patients with SEA can abruptly decompensate because of cord infarction from vascular thrombosis.[18] Patients with metastatic spine disease can also deteriorate abruptly because of vertebral collapse with acute compression or acute vascular ischemia caused by compression on a feeding spinal artery.[25] Therefore, even in neurologically intact patients, there is urgency for the MRI if SEA is the target diagnosis and also if cancer is the major concern. The key point that bears emphasis is that neurologic dysfunction can occur abruptly in neurologically normal patients with abscess or tumor.

In patients with red flags, plain radiographs should not be used to distinguish simple from serious back pain because negative plain film are insufficient to exclude serious pathology and positive studies require follow-up MRI.

MANAGEMENT OF SIMPLE BACK PAIN

Application of heat is weakly recommended.[1,13] Rapid resumption of ordinary activity leads to faster, better outcomes than bed rest.[26] If the patient gets relief from bed rest, very short duration (2 days) results in faster recovery than longer courses.[13,14,27] Acutely, exercise is not recommended.[1,13]

Guidelines and expert opinion recommend nonnarcotic analgesics.[1,13,14] It is important to acknowledge that despite numerous studies and recommendations, there are few data about what works for ED patients with acute back pain in the first days. It is not known if overall, ED patients have more severe pain than the primary care patients for which these guidelines were developed. In practice, emergency physicians commonly (61% in a large national sample) use opioids.[4] Recently, Friedman and colleagues[28] compared functional outcomes and pain control among patients randomized to 10-day treatment of (1) naproxen and placebo, (2) naproxen and cyclobenzaprine, or (3) naproxen and oxycodone/acetaminophen. The authors found no improvement in functional outcome with the addition of either a muscle relaxant or opiate analgesic in the short-term management of back pain (1-week follow-up). Oral steroids do not help unselected patients with acute back pain, but the subset of patients with an acute radiculopathy may benefit.[29,30]

One of the most important aspects of treating the patient with simple musculoskeletal back pain is adequate counseling. Our current practice is to recommend follow-up with a primary care physician within 1 to 2 weeks and give careful instructions about symptoms for which to return sooner (red flags).

Patient satisfaction seems to be more related to the perception that a careful history and physical examination have been done and that the provider has clearly explained the diagnosis and care plan rather than to being imaged.[31]

DIAGNOSIS AND EMERGENCY DEPARTMENT MANAGEMENT OF HIGH-RISK PATIENTS
Diagnosis of Serious Causes

Classic presentations are frequently absent in patients with serious causes of back pain. Symptoms and signs may be partial and can evolve with time, even over the course of a multihour ED encounter. Many patients with cauda equina syndrome do not have rectal or urinary sphincter dysfunction or saddle anesthesia on presentation.[32,33] In a meta-analysis of 613 patients with spinal epidural hematoma (SEH), 30% of patients had no identifiable reason for the bleeding.[34]

Because some patients may not have history red flags, careful examination of the lower extremities and perineum is extremely important including testing sensation in the feet and the Babinski sign. Other than a monoradiculopathy from sciatica, new hard physical findings should drive rapid evaluation (see **Fig. 1**). Although a rectal examination is not required in all patients with back pain, testing for saddle anesthesia, which is a sensitive finding in cauda equina syndrome, should be done routinely.[32] In patients with urinary symptoms, a postvoid residual of greater than 100 mL by catheter, ultrasound, or bladder scanning is abnormal.

Although most patients without red flags and with normal neurologic examinations have simple back pain, occasional patients have one of the serious causes. These patients are extremely difficult to diagnose at initial presentation. For this reason, among others, patients being discharged with back pain should be given well-articulated discharge instructions that outline symptoms for which to return (red flags) and instructions to follow-up with another physician in 1 to 2 weeks, or sooner if any red flag symptoms develop.

Management

Patients with back pain and new neurologic findings (other than a monoradiculopathy consistent with sciatica) should undergo emergent MRI. Attention to details of the MRI expedites the procedure (**Box 2**). Communication with the radiologist is useful to determine if contrast should be used. Imaging the correct part of the spine is of obvious importance. The differential diagnosis, location of pain, and physical findings inform which levels of spine should be imaged. When evaluating for epidural abscess or metastases, the entire spine should be included because multiple foci of infection or cancer are common. A lumbosacral MRI images the cauda equina. Physicians should be aware, however, that a positive Babinski sign (an upper motor neuron finding),

---

Box 2
MRI checklist

1. Ensure that MRI safety checklist has been filled out and sent to the appropriate place
   a. If there are absolute contraindications, do not send to MRI
   b. Discuss alternative options (computed tomography or conventional myelogram) with the radiologist

2. Ensure that pain and anxiety are controlled and that the patient can lie flat for the likely duration of the scan
   a. Consider procedural sedation if there are adequate medical staff to safely monitor patient factoring in the logistics of proximity of MRI department to the ED
   b. Endotracheal intubation and sedation may be necessary

3. Decide what part of the spine needs imaging
   a. In patients with back pain and up-going toes, isolated lumbosacral imaging is insufficient
   b. If spinal epidural abscess or metastatic cancer is an important concern, the entire spine should be imaged because skip areas with abscess (that may affect surgical planning) and multiple metastases (that can affect radiation therapy planning) are common

4. Speak to radiologist
   a. Discuss the urgency of the case to prioritize based on other cases in the queue
   b. Ensure that the scan is properly protocolized for the specific diagnostic concern regarding use of contrast (note that contrast is recommended for diagnosis of epidural abscess and epidural cancer)

indicates a lesion in the thoracic and/or cervical spine, which would be missed if only the lumbosacral MRI is done. Intravenous contrast facilitates diagnosis of epidural abscess and metastatic disease.

Some of the major drawbacks to spine MRI are the significant time requirements and that patients must be able to lie flat to obtain adequate images. After sufficient analgesics and/or sedation have been administered, some patients who cannot lie flat may need to be intubated or given procedural sedation if the local human resources and logistics make this option safe. In general, patients who require emergent scanning should be transferred if MRI is not available at a given hospital. However, if a qualified local spine surgeon were willing to operate based on results of CT scanning, this would be a reasonable alternative. If the CT were normal, an MRI would still be needed. These decisions should be individualized based on institutional capabilities.

For high-risk patients with negative MRIs, physicians should re-evaluate the situation. Discussing the clinical findings with the radiologist may heighten their focus to the clinically important area of spine, re-examining the patient to confirm the examination (and evaluate for evolution), and considering lumbar puncture (to help diagnose transverse myelitis or Guillain-Barré syndrome) and neurology consultation may help clarify a diagnosis. Definitive treatment of patients with diagnostic MRI requires spine surgical consultation and is beyond the purview of emergency medicine, although some issues should be addressed in the ED (**Table 1**).

REVIEW OF SERIOUS ETIOLOGIES
Spinal Epidural Abscess

In recent decades, the prevalence of SEA ranged from 0.2 to 1.2 cases per 10,000 hospital admissions. This condition has seen an increasing prevalence, now comprising a rate of 12.5 per 10,000 hospital admissions in the tertiary referral setting, likely caused by a combination of factors including increasing prevalence of diabetes, intravenous drug abuse, the use of immunosuppressive medications, and increased rate of invasive spinal procedures.[35] The diagnosis is notoriously difficult to make: approximately half of patients are misdiagnosed at initial presentation (range, 11%–75%).[36,37] This is probably caused by the relative rarity of the condition on the overall

Table 1
Initial management steps to be considered in the ED for patients diagnosed with common serious cause of back pain

Condition Diagnosed	Definitive Treatment	Steps to Be Initiated or Considered in the Emergency Department
Metastatic epidural tumor	Steroids, radiotherapy, surgery, and chemotherapy	Consider early consultation with oncology, radiation oncology Empiric dexamethasone should also be considered early
Spinal epidural abscess or vertebral osteomyelitis	Antibiotics and surgery	Always obtain two blood cultures before antibiotics
Spinal epidural hematoma	Anticoagulation reversal and surgery	Reversal of anticoagulation
Giant (central) disk herniation	Surgery	

Spine surgical consultation should occur for all cases.

spectrum of back pain disorders, and a lack of classic findings. Only about 10% of SEA patients present with the classic triad of fever, back pain, and neurologic deficits.[36] Moreover, only 66% have fever at presentation.[38] Back pain is the most common presenting complaint, seen in 70% to 90% of patients and described as severe and unremitting. When the diagnosis is considered, one must perform an MRI of the whole spine with and without gadolinium.

Historically, the management of SEA has consisted of a combined approach of parenteral antibiotics and surgical decompression. Neurologic function at time of presentation is a key predictor of outcome; however, patients with SEA can have abrupt neurologic decompensation, leading many spine specialists to advocate for a combination of medical and surgical management regardless of neurologic examination findings. Recently, a pattern of antibiotic-only management with close observation has emerged because of encouraging early results of this management strategy.[39–41] In 2005, a single-center retrospective review demonstrated an 83% success rate of medical management in carefully selected patients with a normal neurologic examination and without evidence of systemic inflammatory response syndrome or sepsis.[42] However, in 2014 a separate group published a retrospective review of 128 cases of SEA managed with either antibiotics plus surgical decompression or antibiotics plus observation alone. The investigators found that the antibiotic approach failed in 21 out of 51 patients (41%), requiring surgical decompression because of either worsening neurologic function or pain. Both groups had similar posttreatment motor scores.[43] Four factors that predicted failure of medical management included a history of diabetes mellitus, white blood cell count greater than 12,500, positive blood cultures, and CRP greater than 115 mg/L. Other groups have shown similarly high failure rates of medical management alone, leading to a current state of controversy over the optimal management of SEA.[44,45]

Based on previous research and the known success of surgical decompression, a combined approach remains the standard of care for patients with SEA. Although medical management may be an attractive option in specific patient groups, such as those with minimal neurologic deficit and high operative risk, this decision must be made carefully in consultation with a spine specialist.

Metastatic Epidural Tumor

Spinal fracture and malignancy are the two most common serious pathologic conditions affecting the spine.[46] Having a high index of suspicion for serious pathology in a patient with ongoing back pain may shorten time to treatment and preservation of neurologic function, particularly given that in about 20% of patients, a vertebral metastasis is the first symptom of cancer.[25]

According to a recent population-based study of more than 15,000 hospitalizations for neoplastic extradural spinal cord compression (ESCC), the three most common underlying primary sources are lung cancer, breast cancer, and multiple myeloma.[47] However, in patients without a previously known malignancy, lung cancer, multiple myeloma, and non-Hodgkin lymphoma were responsible for 78% of cases of ESCC.[48] By location, approximately 60% of cases of ESCC occur in the thoracic spine, 30% in the lumbosacral spine, and 10% in the cervical spine.[25]

The pathophysiology of epidural spinal metastases is thought to stem from one of four pathways: (1) arterial embolization to bone, (2) shunting of venous blood from the abdomen and pelvis to Batson epidural venous plexus during Valsalva maneuver, (3) contiguous spread from a paraspinal mass through the intervertebral foramen (particularly common in lymphoma), and (4) new tumor growth without a bony or paraspinal component. Neurologic symptoms typically result from obstruction of the epidural venous plexus related to mass effect, followed by vasogenic edema in the white matter and gray matter eventually leading to neurologic symptoms.[49]

Pain is typically the first symptom encountered with ESCC, affecting at least 83% of patients at time of diagnosis, and can precede neurologic symptoms by 7 weeks on average.[50] Weakness is detectable in 60% to 85% of patients at time of diagnosis.[51,52] When compression occurs at or above the level of the conus medullaris, this manifests as an upper motor neuron pattern, with hyperreflexia below the level of compression, extensor plantar response, and preferential involvement of the lower extremity flexor and upper extremity extensor muscle groups. Bowel and bladder dysfunction is generally a late finding and is confounded by high-dose opiate use in patients with advanced malignancy.[52]

Treatment of ESCC is divided broadly into three main categories: (1) chemotherapy, (2) radiation, and (3) surgery. The early use of steroids in metastatic spinal disease with neurologic involvement has seen mainstream adoption in recent years. In 1994, Sorensen and colleagues[53] randomized 57 patients with newly diagnosed ESCC secondary to solid tumor to radiotherapy with either high-dose dexamethasone (96 mg intravenous bolus, followed by 96 mg orally for 3 days and gradual taper) or no steroidal treatment. The authors found a significant difference in functional deficit, with 59% of patients in the dexamethasone group maintaining ability to ambulate compared with 33% in the control group. Median survival was equivalent between the two groups.[53] A Cochrane review published in 2015 found only three small trials addressing the role of steroids in acute management of ESCC. The authors concluded that there was no difference in survival, pain, or neurologic outcome with the use of high-dose versus moderate-dose steroids, and an association with drug-related adverse events in patients who received high-dose dexamethasone. British and Canadian guidelines recommend moderate-dose dexamethasone (16 mg/day), and based on both the suspected benefit and widespread use of steroids in ESCC it is unlikely that a placebo-controlled trial would ever be undertaken to investigate the therapeutic effects of this intervention.[54]

Although long-term treatment of ESCC is beyond the scope of this article, the appropriate acute management is based largely on examination and prognostic factors. In general, radiotherapy is considered the primary treatment of neurologically stable patients with ESCC and can significantly improve pain and preservation of neurologic function. Decompressive surgery should be considered in patients younger than 65 years old, those who have lost motor function within 48 hours, have localized cord compression, and estimated survival greater than 3 months. Surgery should also be considered in ambulatory patients with poor prognostic factors for radiotherapy, such as bony instability or compression, rapidly progressive neurologic deficits, or radiation-insensitive malignancy.[54]

Spinal Epidural Hematoma

SEH is a rare and elusive cause of back pain. The precise incidence of SEH is unknown; the best estimate is from a Swedish retrospective survey that reported a 1:200,000 occurrence of SEH in obstetric patients undergoing epidural anesthesia.[55] In 2013, the Multicenter Perioperative Outcomes Group published a retrospective chart review of complications in patients undergoing either spinal or epidural anesthesia. The authors found that approximately 1 in 8920 patients undergoing epidural catheterization developed hematoma requiring surgical evacuation; interestingly, none of the 79,837 obstetric patients included in this study developed an epidural hematoma.[56] Neuraxial analgesia and diagnostic procedures, such as lumbar puncture, constitute major risk factors for SEH, and this diagnosis should be strongly considered in anyone presenting to the ED with back pain or new neurologic deficit following a spinal procedure.

Spontaneous SEH (SSEH) is considerably less common with a reported incidence of 0.1 per 100,000, but gaining recognition in light of increasing oral anticoagulant use in the general population.[57] SSEH is thought to result from venous hemorrhage. This hypothesis is widely supported based on the valveless anatomic makeup of spinal epidural veins, which are thus more vulnerable to injury from abrupt changes in abdominal or thoracic pressure.[58] Most spinal hematomas are located in the dorsal aspect of the spinal column at the cervicothoracic or thoracolumbar junctions. The main risk factors for SSEH include clotting disorders (congenital or acquired), which account for up to one-third of cases; vascular malformations; and tumors.[59]

Patients with SEH tend to present with severe back or neck pain, frequently with a radicular component, followed by loss of sensory, motor, bladder, and bowel function. In an extensive review of 613 case studies spanning the past two centuries, one group found a common pattern of presentation with patients describing "intense, knife-like pain at the location of the hemorrhage, a 'coup de poignard' " followed in some cases by a symptom-free interval up to several days, leading to progressive paralysis below the affected vertebral level.[34]

In the ED, if the patient is on an anticoagulant, strong consideration should be given to reversing that drug, although this depends on many factors including the indication for the anticoagulation, the availability of a reversal agent, time since last dose of the anticoagulant, and the ability to measure its effect (eg, international normalized ratio vs antithrombin X levels). Most patients with SEH require decompressive laminectomy. As would be expected, prognosis is closely tied to the time from symptom onset and degree of neurologic deficit at diagnosis. In 2004, Liao and colleagues[60] published a retrospective study of 35 patients presenting with SSEH. The authors found that 88.9% of patients with incomplete neurologic deficits at presentation experienced full recovery following surgical decompression, compared with only 37.5% of those presenting with complete neurologic deficits. A symptom duration of less than 48 hours and duration of complete neurologic deficit less than 12 hours, if present, were both correlated with better neurologic recovery.[60]

Giant Disk Herniation

Giant lumbar disk herniation (GLDH) (sometimes called central disk herniation) has a reported incidence of 8% to 22% among all types of disk herniation. This entity has been variably defined as occupying anywhere from 33% to 75% of the anterior-posterior diameter of the spinal canal, or resulting in a complete block on CT myelogram. As one would expect, the threat to neurologic function is disproportionately increased with GLDH, with studies estimating GLDH to underlie between 45% and 60% of all cases of cauda equina syndrome.[61,62]

Although the etiologic mechanism of GLDH is not fully known, predisposition to large disk herniation has been documented in patients with unusual movements, that is, heavy labor, traction, spinal manipulation, and hypermobility. Importantly, as with any acute disk herniation, the inciting trauma can be minimal or absent. The mean age at time of diagnosis was 42 years in a series of patients undergoing decompressive surgery for GLDH.

A 2014 retrospective study by Akhaddar and colleagues[63] reviewed the patient characteristics and outcomes following surgical management of GLDH, which was defined as occupying more than half of the sagittal diameter of the lumbar spinal canal. The indications for surgery included cauda equina syndrome, progressive motor deficits, or intolerable symptoms. Compared with patients who underwent surgical decompression for simple posterolateral disk herniation, those with giant disk herniation had statistically significantly shorter duration of symptoms (7.8 months vs 11.1 months), hyperalgesic radicular pain (21.4% vs 14.2%), bilateral symptoms (11% vs 4.4%), preoperative motor deficits (18.8% vs 10.4%), and clinical picture consistent with cauda equina syndrome (7.1% vs 1.3%). The location was more likely central in patients with giant disk herniation (21.4% vs 7.3%), and more frequently required decompressive laminectomy (33.1% vs 20.9%).[63]

Treatment of symptomatic GLDH is with decompressive surgery, whether in the form of discectomy alone or with additional laminectomy. Although large central disk herniations were previously thought to represent a high-risk category for spinal instability necessitating spinal fusion, recent studies have shown equivalent outcomes in patients undergoing decompression alone compared with decompression and spinal fusion.[62,64,65]

SUMMARY

Acute nontraumatic back pain comprises a steady proportion of ED visits and affects most patients over time. Simple musculoskeletal back pain is effectively managed with a short course of nonsteroidal anti-inflammatory drugs with or without the addition of opioid analgesic and muscle relaxant medications, and encouraging the patient to achieve a quick return to previous level of physical activity. Neuroimaging is rarely necessary or likely to change long-term management when a reassuring history and physical examination are obtained in the emergency setting.

Among the many possible causes of back pain, a small portion of dangerous entities may harbor devastating neurologic and functional consequences if not considered and appropriately ruled out with the use of a compressive history, examination, and neuroimaging. In particular, the incidence of SEA and SSEH may be on the rise because of the increased use of intravenous drugs of abuse and prophylactic oral anticoagulants, respectively. Although many patients with high-risk back pain present with telltale neurologic signs or historical findings, this is not always the case. It is important for the emergency physician to remain vigilant in the evaluation of a patient presenting with nontraumatic back pain.

REFERENCES

1. Balague F, Mannion AF, Pellise F, et al. Non-specific low back pain. Lancet 2012; 379:482–91.
2. Martin BI, Deyo RA, Mirza SK, et al. Expenditures and health status among adults with back and neck problems. JAMA 2008;299(6):656–64.
3. Pitts SR, Niska RW, Xu J, et al. National Hospital Ambulatory Medical Care Survey: 2006 emergency department summary. Natl Health Stat Rep 2008;6(7):1–38.
4. Friedman BW, Chilstrom M, Bijur PE, et al. Diagnostic testing and treatment of low back pain in United States emergency departments: a national perspective. Spine 2010;35:E1406–11.
5. Raison NT, Alwan W, Abbot A, et al. The reliability of red flags in spinal cord compression. Arch Trauma Res 2014;3:e17850 (was 10).
6. Edlow JA. Managing nontraumatic acute back pain. Ann Emerg Med 2015;66: 148–53.
7. Tarulli AW, Raynor EM. Lumbosacral radiculopathy. Neurol Clin 2007;25(2):387.
8. Dugas AF, Lucas JM, Edlow JA. Diagnosis of spinal cord compression in nontrauma patients in the emergency department. Acad Emerg Med 2011;18: 719–25.

9. Pope JV, Edlow JA. Avoiding misdiagnosis in patients with neurological emergencies. Emerg Med Int 2012;2012:949275.

10. Anderson JC. Is immediate imaging important in managing low back pain? J Athl Train 2011;46(1):99–102.

11. Gilbert FJ, Grant AM, Gillan MG, et al. Low back pain: influence of early MR imaging or CT on treatment and outcome – multicenter randomized trial. Radiology 2004;231(2):343–51.

12. Lurie JD, Birkmeyer NJ, Weinstein JN. Rates of advanced spinal imaging and spine surgery. Spine 2003;28(6):616–20.

13. Chou R, Qaseem A, Snow V, et al. Diagnosis and treatment of low back pain: a joint clinical practice guideline from the American College of Physicians and the American Pain Society. Ann Intern Med 2007;147:478–91.

14. Deyo RA, Weinstein JN. Low back pain. N Engl J Med 2001;344:363–70.

15. Goertz M, Thorson D, Bonsell B, et al. ARHQ guideline: adult acute and subacute low back pain. National Guideine Clearinghouse, Guideline summary NGC-9520. 2012.

16. Downie A, Williams CM, Henschke N, et al. Red flags to screen for malignancy and fracture in patients with low back pain: systematic review. BMJ 2013;347: f7095.

17. Thiruganasambandamoorthy V, Turko E, Ansell D, et al. Risk factors for serious underlying pathology in adult emergency department nontraumatic low back pain patients. J Emerg Med 2014;47:1–11.

18. Darouiche RO. Spinal epidural abscess. N Engl J Med 2006;355:2012–20.

19. Davis DP, Salazar A, Chan TC, et al. Prospective evaluation of a clinical decision guideline to diagnose spinal epidural abscess in patients who present to the emergency department with spine pain. J Neurosurg Spine 2011;14:765–70.

20. Deyo RA, Diehl AK. Cancer as a cause of back pain: frequency, clinical presentation, and diagnostic strategies. J Gen Intern Med 1988;3:230–8.

21. Chou R, Fu R, Carrino JA, et al. Imaging strategies for low-back pain: systematic review and meta-analysis. Lancet 2009;373:463–72.

22. Jarvik JG, Hollingworth W, Martin B, et al. Rapid magnetic resonance imaging vs radiographs for patients with low back pain: a randomized controlled trial. JAMA 2003;289:2810–8.

23. Jensen MC, Brant-Zawadzki MN, Obuchowski N, et al. Magnetic resonance imaging of the lumbar spine in people without back pain. N Engl J Med 1994; 331:69–73.

24. Frymoyer JW, Moskowitz RW. Spinal degeneration. Pathogenesis and medical management. In: Frymoyer JW, editor. The adult spine: principles and practice. New York: Raven; 1991. p. 611–34.

25. Cole JS, Patchell RA. Metastatic epidural spinal cord compression. Lancet Neurol 2008;7:459–66.

26. Malmivaara A, Hakkinen U, Aro T, et al. The treatment of acute low back pain: bed rest, exercises, or ordinary activity? N Engl J Med 1995;332:351–5.

27. Deyo RA, Diehl AK, Rosenthal M. How many days of bed rest for acute low back pain? A randomized clinical trial. N Engl J Med 1986;315:1064–70.

28. Friedman BW, Dym AA, Davitt M, et al. Naproxen with cyclobenzaprine, oxycodone/acetaminophen, or placebo for treating acute low back pain: a randomized clinical trial. JAMA 2015;314(15):1572–80.

29. Balakrishnamoorthy R, Horgan I, Perez S, et al. Does a single dose of intravenous dexamethasone reduce Symptoms in Emergency department patients with low

Back pain and RAdiculopathy (SEBRA)? A double-blind randomised controlled trial. Emerg Med J 2014;32(7):525–30.

30. Eskin B, Shih RD, Fiesseler FW, et al. Prednisone for emergency department low back pain: a randomized controlled trial. J Emerg Med 2014;47:65–70.

31. Carey TS, Garrett J, Jackman A, et al. The outcomes and costs of care for acute low back pain among patients seen by primary care practitioners, chiropractors, and orthopedic surgeons. The North Carolina Back Pain Project. N Engl J Med 1995;333:913–7.

32. Balasubramanian K, Kalsi P, Greenough CG, et al. Reliability of clinical assessment in diagnosing cauda equina syndrome. Br J Neurosurg 2010;24:383–6.

33. Domen PM, Hofman PA, van Santbrink H, et al. Predictive value of clinical characteristics in patients with suspected cauda equina syndrome. Eur J Neurol 2009;16:416–9.

34. Kreppel D, Antoniadis G, Seeling W. Spinal hematoma: a literature survey with meta-analysis of 613 patients. Neurosurg Rev 2003;26(1):1–49.

35. Rigamonti D, Liem L, Sampath P, et al. Spinal epidural abscess: contemporary trends in etiology, evaluation and management. Surg Neurol 1999;52:189–96.

36. Davis DP, Wold RM, Patel RJ, et al. The clinical presentation and impact of diagnostic delays on emergency department patients with spinal epidural abscess. J Emerg Med 2004;26:285–91.

37. Tang HJ, Lin HJ, Liu YC, et al. Spinal epidural abscess: experience with 46 patients and evaluation of prognostic factors. J Infect 2002;45:76–81.

38. Reihsaus E, Waldbaur H, Seeling W. Spinal epidural abscess: a meta-analysis of 915 patients. Neurosurg Rev 2000;23:175–204 [discussion: 5].

39. Butler JS, Shelly MJ, Timlin M, et al. Nontuberculous pyogenic spinal infection in adults: a 12-year experience from a tertiary referral center. Spine 2006;31: 2695–700.

40. Karikari IO, Powers CJ, Reynolds RM, et al. Management of a spontaneous spinal epidural abscess: a single-center 10-year experience. Neurosurgery 2009;65: 919–24.

41. Siddiq F, Chowfin A, Tight R, et al. Medical vs surgical management of spinal epidural abscess. Arch Intern Med 2004;164:2409–12.

42. Savage K, Holtom PD, Zalavras CG. Spinal epidural abscess: early clinical outcome in patients treated medically. Clin Orthop Relat Res 2005;439:56–60.

43. Patel AR, Alton TB, Bransford RJ, et al. Spinal epidural abscesses: risk factors, medical versus surgical management, a retrospective review of 128 cases. J Spine 2014;14(2):326–30.

44. Connor DE Jr, Chittiboina P, Caldito G, et al. Comparison of operative and nonoperative management of spinal epidural abscess: a retrospective review of clinical and laboratory predictors of neurological outcome. J Neurosurg Spine 2013;19: 119–27.

45. Pereira CE, Lynch JC. Spinal epidural abscess: an analysis of 24 cases. Surg Neurol 2005;63(Suppl 1):S26–9.

46. Williams CM, Henschke N, Maher CG, et al. Red flags to screen for vertebral fracture in patients presenting with low back pain. Cochrane Database Syst Rev 2013;(1):CD008643.

47. Mak KS, Lee LK, Mak RH, et al. Incidence and treatment patterns in hospitalizations for malignant spinal cord compression in the United States, 1998-2006. Int J Radiat Oncol Biol Phys 2011;80(3):824.

48. Schiff D, O'Neill BP, Suman VJ. Spinal epidural metastasis as the initial manifestation of malignancy: clinical features and diagnostic approach. Neurology 1997; 49(2):452.
49. Siegal T. Spinal cord compression: from laboratory to clinic. Eur J Cancer 1995; 31A(11):1748.
50. Bach F, Larsen BH, Rohde K, et al. Metastatic spinal cord compression. Occurrence, symptoms, clinical presentations and prognosis in 398 patients with spinal cord compression. Acta Neurochir 1990;107(1–2):37.
51. Greenberg HS, Kim JH, Posner JB. Epidural spinal cord compression from metastatic tumor: results with a new treatment protocol. Ann Neurol 1980;8(4):361.
52. Helweg-Larsen S, Sorensen PS. Symptoms and signs in metastatic spinal cord compression: a study of progression from first symptom until diagnosis in 153 patients. Eur J Cancer 1994;30A(3):396.
53. Sorensen S, Helweg-Larsen S, Mouridsen H, et al. Effect of high-dose dexamethasone in carcinomatous metastatic spinal cord compression treated with radiotherapy: a randomized trial. Eur J Cancer 1994;30A(1):22–7.
54. George R, Jeba J, Ramkumar G, et al. Interventions for the treatment of metastatic extradural spinal cord compression in adults. Cochrane Database Syst Rev 2015;(9):CD006716.
55. Moen V, Dahlgren N, Irestedt L. Severe neurological complications after central neuraxial blockades in Sweden 1990-1999. Anesthesiology 2004;101(4):950.
56. Bateman BT, Mhyre JM, Ehrenfeld J, et al. The risk and outcomes of epidural hematomas after perioperative and obstetric epidural catheterization: a report from the Multicenter Perioperative Outcomes Group Research Consortium. Anesth Analg 2013;116(6):1380–5.
57. Holtas S, Heiling M, Lonntoft M. Spontaneous spinal epidural hematoma: findings at MR imaging and clinical correlation. Radiology 1996;199(2):409–13.
58. Marmey G, Doyon D, David P, et al. D'un hematome epidural cervical. J Radiol 1990;71(10):549–53.
59. Harik SI, Raichle ME, Reis DJ. Spontaneously remitting spinal epidural hematoma in a patient on anticoagulants. N Engl J Med 1971;284:1355–7.
60. Liao CC, Lee ST, Hsu WC, et al. Experience in the surgical management of spontaneous spinal epidural hematoma. J Neurosurg 2004;100:38–45.
61. Qureshi A, Sell P. Cauda equina syndrome treated by surgical decompression: the influence of timing on surgical outcome. Eur Spine J 2007;16:2143–51.
62. Koh YD, Rhee SJ, Kim DJ. Radiological and clinical outcome after simple discectomy of central massive lumbar disc herniation. J Korean Soc Spine Surg 2010; 17:169–76.
63. Akhaddar A, Belfquih H, Salami M, et al. Surgical management of giant lumbar disc herniation: analysis of 154 patients over a decade. Neurochirurgie 2014; 60(5):244–8.
64. Barr JS, Kubik GS, Molloy MK, et al. Evaluation of end results in treatment of ruptured lumbar intervertebral discs with protrusion of nucleus pulposus. Surg Gynecol Obstet 1967;125:250–6.
65. LaMont RL, Morawa LG, Pederson HE. Comparison of disc excision with combined disc excision and spinal fusion for lumbar disc ruptures. Clin Orthop 1976;121:212–6.

Status Epilepticus
What's New?

Danya Khoujah, MBBS, Michael K. Abraham, MD, MS*

KEYWORDS

- Status epilepticus • Seizures • Epilepsy

KEY POINTS

- Status epilepticus (SE) is diagnosed at 5 minutes of continuous seizure activity, and has the potential for high morbidity and mortality if not diagnosed promptly and treated accurately and effectively.
- Devising specific protocols for management of SE improves outcomes.
- The first line for management of SE is benzodiazepines, followed by phenytoin, fosphenytoin, or valproic acid.
- Second line adjuncts for management of SE are levetiracetam, lacosamide, phenobarbital and ketamine, followed by intravenous anesthetics.
- Subtle SE occurs frequently after convulsive SE and should be treated in the same manner.
- Underlying causes leading to provoked seizures should be considered early on in the disease, especially in patients not responding to first line agents.

INTRODUCTION

Seizures are commonly encountered in the emergency department (ED) because approximately 5% to 10% of people who live to the age of 80 years experience a seizure.[1] The spectrum of disease, from a partial complex seizure to refractory status epilepticus (SE), can present a daunting treatment task to emergency physicians. Epilepsy is defined as 2 or more unprovoked seizures occurring at least 24 hours apart, a heightened tendency toward unprovoked seizures (as shown by electroencephalographic or neuroimaging testing), or an epilepsy syndrome.[2] The determination of a provoked versus an unprovoked seizure is paramount because the underlying treatment options can be very different. At the far end of the spectrum of disease, generalized convulsive SE (GCSE) can be defined in a variety of ways, but

Disclosures: None.
Department of Emergency Medicine, University of Maryland School of Medicine, 110 South Paca Street, 6th Floor, Suite 200, Baltimore, MD 21201, USA
* Corresponding author. Department of Emergency Medicine, University of Maryland School of Medicine, 110 South Paca Street, 6th Floor, Suite 200, Baltimore, MD 21201.
E-mail address: mabraham@em.umaryland.edu

the most common is an active seizure lasting greater than 5 minutes or 2 seizures without return to baseline. There are also subclassifications of subclinical or nonconvulsive, refractory, and super-refractory SE as well. SE is associated with increased morbidity and mortality, with the reported mortality after the first episode of GCSE approaching 20%.[3] The mortality is partly a function of the underlying cause, refractoriness of the seizure, age, and medical comorbidities, with the last 2 factors playing the greatest role. Reported mortality is from 4% to 40%, depending on the definition of SE used in the study and the underlying cause, with hypoxic ischemic brain injury producing the worst outcomes.[4–6]

The patient's hospital course from the prehospital setting, continuing through the ED, and ultimately the time spent in an intensive care unit (ICU) can be greatly affected by the choices the emergency physician makes. This article reviews the current diagnosis and treatment recommendations for GCSE, including refractory and other forms of SE.

PATHOPHYSIOLOGY

The common pathway for all seizures is an abnormal electrical discharge of cortical neurons, in which a hyperexcitable neuron group fires in a coordinated manner, recruiting adjacent neurons in a synchronized manner. The most common excitatory neurotransmitter is glutamate, which works via the N-methyl-D-aspartate (NMDA) receptor. In contrast, the most common inhibitory neurotransmitter is gamma-aminobutyric acid (GABA), which works via the $GABA_A$ receptors. In normal circumstances, the neuronal membrane only allows a single action potential to pass from one neuron to another in a given time interval. Seizures can occur once this stability is altered, which could either be caused by sensitized inhibitory $GABA_A$ receptors (eg, in the setting of alcohol or benzodiazepine withdrawal), an altered ion concentration (eg, hyponatremia), or altered cellular metabolism (eg, hypoglycemia). If these mechanisms are involved, these seizures are considered provoked (**Box 1**).

Unprovoked seizures, which by definition are epileptic, are mostly caused by abnormalities of sodium channels, but other mechanisms can be involved, such as self-excitation, abnormal calcium channel stimulation, or a mutation in acetylcholine receptors.[7]

The imbalance of excess excitation and decreased inhibition is what ultimately manifests as a seizure. Many abortive medications, such as benzodiazepines, barbiturates, propofol, and some anesthetics, work via enhancing GABA inhibition. There are many endogenous seizure-terminating processes, which is why most seizures last for only 1 or 2 minutes before spontaneously aborting, but, when they fail, a single seizure is transformed into SE. A seizure that has lasted 30 minutes or more will not spontaneously stop, because at this point the seizure has become self-sustaining even if the inciting factor was removed.[8]

Physiologic Changes in Generalized Convulsive Status Epilepticus

Multiple systemic physiologic changes accompany GCSE, mostly caused by the catecholamine surge. These changes can include hyperthermia, leukocytosis, cerebrospinal fluid (CSF) pleocytosis, increased blood pressure, pupillary dilatation, and other cardiovascular and respiratory abnormalities. Attributing hyperthermia, leukocytosis, and CSF pleocytosis to the seizure is a diagnosis of exclusion, because a true infectious cause needs to be excluded first. As the seizure progresses there can also be resultant lactic acidosis caused by the conversion to anaerobic metabolism as the

---

Box 1
Underlying medical conditions leading to provoked seizures

- Tumor/structural brain lesion
- Vascular:
  - Ischemic stroke
  - Subarachnoid hemorrhage
  - Subdural/epidural hematoma
  - Vasculitis
- Toxic:
  - Cocaine
  - Tricyclics
  - Anticholinergics
  - Lithium
  - Isoniazid (INH)
  - Alcohol intoxication/withdrawal
  - Benzodiazepine withdrawal
- Pregnancy (eclampsia)
- Metabolic:
  - Hyponatremia
  - Hypernatremia
  - Hypoglycemia
  - Hyperglycemia
  - Hypocalcemia
  - Hypomagnesemia
- Infectious:
  - Meningitis/encephalitis
  - Brain abscess
- Hypertensive encephalopathy
- Heat stroke

---

seizure progresses. The lactic acidosis should clear spontaneously once the clonic nature of the seizures is terminated and normal metabolism returns.

Early during the course of a seizure, brain metabolism is increased, but cerebral blood flow and substrate supply are adequate for demands. Eventually, at some point between 30 and 60 minutes, excitotoxic cell injury occurs, leading to irreversible neuronal damage. In this second phase of SE, brain metabolism remains high, but cerebral blood flow and substrate supply decline, and cerebral autoregulation mechanisms fail, leading to mismatch and decompensation. This detrimental effect on neurons is compounded by systemic hypoxia, hypercarbia, hypotension, and hypothermia, which occur frequently during this second phase. Bradycardia and other arrhythmias can occur as well.

Excitotoxic cell injury is thought to occur when glutamate binds to the NMDA receptors. In normal circumstances, the channel is blocked by a magnesium ion. However, in GCSE the cells are severely depolarized and the magnesium ions are not available, leaving the channel open. This situation allows calcium and other ions to flow into the cell, causing intracellular accumulation of calcium, with resulting acute necrosis, delayed cell death, or both. The length of the early phase depends on an intact airway, oxygenation and circulation, and the ability of the brain to compensate for this increased metabolism, which is decreased in patients with underlying illness.

Pharmacoresistance in Prolonged Seizures

Multiple mechanisms contribute to time-dependent pharmacoresistance in patients with GCSE. Benzodiazepines become less effective because of downregulation and alteration of $GABA_A$ receptors, decreasing their availability and affinity for binding.[9] After 20 to 30 minutes of SE, inflammatory changes of molecular transporters decrease transport across the blood-brain barrier, decreasing the affinity of phenytoin and phenobarbital.[10] This process explains why these medications are less effective in controlling a seizure when given later than when given early in the disease process.[11,12] In addition, the upregulation of NMDA receptors leads to increased excitotoxicity, which is why pharmacoresistance is not thought to occur as much with NMDA antagonists, such as ketamine, making it a potentially attractive option for the treatment of super-refractory SE.[13,14]

Evaluation and Management

As with all critically ill patients, the focus of evaluation should be on the primary survey, including evaluation of airway, breathing, and circulation. When dealing with neurologic emergencies, and seizures in particular, is important to always obtain a bedside glucose level at the outset of the resuscitation. If possible, the seizing patient should be placed in the lateral decubitus position and protected from harm with padded guardrails.

Airway management

In generalized seizures, the gag reflex is suppressed and vomiting may occur, leading to aspiration of gastric contents. If an airway adjunct is needed, then a nasopharyngeal airway should be used, because oropharyngeal airways and bite blocks are not recommended because of the risk of injury to the provider. The decision to control the airway in a seizing patient is difficult and often anxiety provoking for the emergency provider. If the patient is aspirating or apneic, then immediate intubation is necessary. A patient may need to be intubated after multiple antiepileptic medications are administered. Otherwise, not all patients in SE have to be emergently intubated, because intubation may complicate matters. If the decision is made to intubate the patient on arrival, rapid sequence intubation is recommended, and the recommended agents for this are discussed later in the article.

After assessment of the airway, breathing, and circulatory support, the next step should be to focus efforts on termination of the seizures because this is the most important step in returning the patient to normal physiology. For the reasons listed earlier it becomes exponentially more difficult to manage patients with GCSE as time elapses, so many of the interventions must happen using parallel processing, including obtaining a history and diagnostic testing while concurrently managing the patient. An important consideration is that paralytics eliminate the outwards signs of seizure activity but not the electrical discharges underlying it; therefore, patients intubated for GCSE who are receiving long-acting paralytics should have electroencephalogram (EEG) monitoring.

History

As discussed earlier, seizures can be provoked or unprovoked and obtaining history from emergency medical services (EMS), family members, bystanders, and medical records can be crucial in this determination. Some of the relevant aspects of the history are shown in **Box 2**. The relevant history should help determine whether the seizure is provoked and whether there is a reversible or treatable cause to terminate the seizure (see **Box 1**).

Box 2
Relevant and important clinical history

- Description of episodes:
  - Duration
  - Loss of consciousness
  - Urinary or stool incontinence
  - Tongue biting
  - Apnea
  - Preceding aura

- Medications (and compliance/possibility of overdose)
  - Anticonvulsants
  - Tramadol
  - Tricyclics
  - Lithium
  - Isoniazid (INH)

- Past medical history:
  - Seizure disorder
  - Diabetes mellitus
  - Chronic kidney disease
  - Cancer

- Alcohol consumption and recent changes in pattern

- Illicit drug use, specifically synthetic cannabinoids, cocaine

- Recent illness, fever

- Trauma

- Pregnancy

Diagnostic testing

Diagnostic tests should be focused on investigating and verifying the relevant history to identify the cause of the seizure and looking for complications from prolonged seizing. Immediate point-of-care glucose level should be measured, if it has not already been by EMS. Serum electrolyte levels (specifically sodium), renal function, and liver function tests should be obtained. A pregnancy test in all women of child-bearing age is necessary. In addition, blood levels of any anticonvulsant medication the patient is on should be done. Even if the results will not be available in a timely fashion, they may help the inpatient team make later decisions. Depending on the history, a toxicology screen for ethanol, aspirin, tricyclic antidepressants, lithium, and drugs of abuse can be obtained, but rarely influences the acute management of SE. If clinically indicated, creatine kinase testing can be ordered to screen for rhabdomyolysis. A lumbar puncture (LP) for suspected meningitis/encephalitis should be done after the patient is stable and the seizure is terminated, but if a strong clinical suspicion exists then empiric antibiotics should be given within 1 hour of arrival and not delayed to perform the LP. Unless there is a clear reason for the seizure (eg, hypoglycemia), noncontrast head computed tomography should be done in all patients with refractory SE once they have been stabilized. There is no role for MRI in acute diagnosis and management of SE. EEG monitoring is not necessary in the initial diagnosis and management of SE, but is recommended (if available) in patients who remain unresponsive after the apparent termination of convulsive SE, those who are pharmacologically paralyzed, and when a patient has been placed in a pharmacologically induced coma in refractory SE. This testing is important to diagnose and appropriately manage subtle SE.

Management

As discussed earlier, there are a few important concepts that govern the successful management of SE. The first is that decreased time to administering abortive medications increases their success rate. Another is that in order to successfully terminate provoked seizures, treatment of the underlying cause must occur. In addition, health care providers need to be vigilant about preventing and treating potential complications of seizures.

The only widely accepted first-line treatment of GCSE is benzodiazepines. There are no nationally accepted treatment protocols for refractory SE, mostly because of a paucity of large randomized controlled studies in humans that show the superiority of one agent to another. Therefore the guidelines, specifically for medications that are second, third, or fourth line, are based on consensus rather than evidence.[15–18] However, guidelines and protocols are important to provide prompt treatment and improve outcome, and the use of a treatment protocol within an institution results in better and faster seizure control, and decreased hospital and ICU length of stay.[19,20] The protocol depends on availability of certain medications and familiarity with administration, because rapidity of administration is essential to successfully terminating SE. **Fig. 1** shows a tiered approach to the management of SE.

Treatment of underlying conditions

Some seizures are provoked by an underlying cause (see **Box 1**), and the treatment of the causative disorder needs to occur in order to terminate the seizure and improve outcome. The history and/or physical may enable the provider to suspect such conditions, but the refractoriness of the seizure should itself prompt the provider to

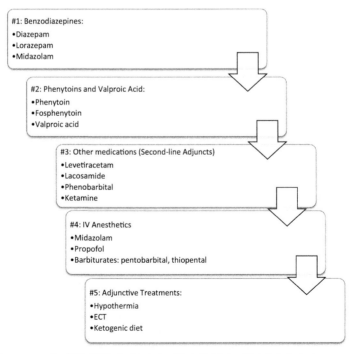

Fig. 1. Management of SE. ECT, electroconvulsive therapy; IV, intravenous.

reconsider such causes. Some of the underlying conditions and specific treatments are listed in **Table 1**.

First-line Agents

Benzodiazepines

Benzodiazepines are the mainstay of abortive treatment of seizures, and the first line in the management of SE.[21] They are the only class 1a level A recommendation in the management of SE,[15,18] which was supported by a randomized controlled study that found lorazepam more efficacious than phenytoin in controlling SE, and just as efficacious as phenobarbital, or a combination of diazepam and phenytoin, but less cumbersome to use.[20] The most commonly used benzodiazepines in the treatment of SE are diazepam, lorazepam, and midazolam, which are often administered before the patient's presentation to the hospital by family members or EMS.

Although benzodiazepines are the mainstay of first-line treatment, there are some aspects of each medication that should be considered when approaching a patient with GCSE, because some may be more appropriate than others. Benzodiazepines differ in their time to onset and duration of action, but the most clinically significant difference is the mode of administration and ease of storage (**Table 2**).

Diazepam has a longer half-life than lorazepam, but lorazepam has a smaller volume of distribution and active metabolites, leading to a longer duration of action than diazepam, with no significant difference in effectiveness.[18] In contrast, midazolam has the shortest duration of action of the 3.[22] All of these medications can be given through the intravenous (IV) route, and also by the intraosseous route. Obtaining IV access on a patient who is actively seizing can be a difficult, time-consuming, and hazardous

Table 1
Cause-specific management of seizures

Cause	Treatment	Notes
Eclampsia	Magnesium sulfate 4–6 g IV over 15–20 min followed by an infusion of 1–3 g/h Blood pressure control with labetalol (20 mg IV every 10 min) or hydralazine 5–10 mg IV every 20 min	Must monitor magnesium levels
Isoniazid	Pyridoxine (B₆) 5 g IV at the rate of 0.5–1 mg/min	May repeat every 5–10 min as needed
Hypoglycemia	Dextrose 50% 50 mL IV or glucagon 1 mg IM (if no IV access)	—
Hyponatremia	3% hypertonic saline 100 mL IV over 10 min	May be repeated
Hypocalcemia	Calcium gluconate or calcium chloride 1–2 g over 10 min	Calcium gluconate is preferred
Meningitis	Ceftriaxone 2 g IV q 12 h Plus Vancomycin 15–20 mg/kg IV q 8–12 h	Add ampicillin 1.5–3 g IV q 4–6 h in elderly patients and alcoholics
Aspirin, tricyclics, or lithium overdose	Hemodialysis	—
Subdural or epidural hematoma	Neurosurgical evaluation for evacuation of hematoma	—

Abbreviations: IM, intramuscular; IV, intravenous; q, every.

Table 2
Benzodiazepines: time to onset, duration of action, mode of administration, and weight-based dosing

Drug	Time to Onset	Duration of Action	Mode of Administration	Incremental Dosage	Weight-based Dosage
Diazepam	Longest	Intermediate	IV	5 mg q 10–15 min	0.2 mg/kg
Lorazepam	Intermediate	Longest	IV, IM	2 mg q 5–10 min	0.1 mg/kg
Midazolam	Shortest	Shortest	IV, IM, IN	2 mg q 5–10 min	0.15–0.3 mg/kg for IM

procedure, necessitating a faster and safer route of administration. Intramuscular (IM) administration is an attractive alternative, but can only be used for lorazepam and midazolam. IM midazolam is preferable because it is more water soluble, and thus has a faster onset.[23] Diazepam should not be used intramuscularly because it is not water soluble and this leads to erratic absorption, and can take as long as 90 minutes to take effect.[24]

Many studies have compared different benzodiazepines in the prehospital setting and have shown little differences.[21] However, one of the more recent trials was the 2012 study, the Rapid Anticonvulsant Medication Prior to Arrival Trial (RAMPArT), which was a randomized controlled trial that compared IM midazolam with IV lorazepam in SE in the prehospital setting. IM midazolam was superior to IV lorazepam, with a shorter time for active treatment and similar rates for intubation and seizure recurrence. This superiority was attributed to shorter time to administration rather than innate properties of the medications, so the choice depends on the presence of vascular access.[25] A significant concern regarding the use of lorazepam solution in the ambulatory setting is the instability of the drug at room temperature, because the manufacturer recommends that it be refrigerated. Studies show that it can be stored at room temperature for up to 60 days, and has to be discarded afterward.[26,27] It is worth noting that rectal diazepam has been shown to be effective in seizure termination, but logistics hinder its common use by EMS and in the ED.[24]

Another option is using intranasal (IN) midazolam. Using a nasal spray is more convenient than rectal diazepam, and may be more effective.[28] The rapid uptake and high bioavailability are comparable with IV midazolam, and it is therefore dosed similarly.[29]

In the absence of clear evidence on optimal dosing of benzodiazepines in SE, most investigators recommend setting a weight-based target dose, and administer the chosen benzodiazepine in increments to effect (**Tables 2** and **3**). This recommendation does not apply to patients who are seizing because of alcohol withdrawal, because they usually require very large amounts of benzodiazepines and possibly phenobarbital.

Benzodiazepines can cause sedation and muscle relaxation resulting in upper airway obstruction, and in large doses hypotension. These side effects should not deter providers from using the appropriate dosages of benzodiazepines because uncontrolled SE is more likely than benzodiazepines to cause hypoxemia or airway compromise.[21] Proper dosing and intubation is preferred to underdosing and continued seizure activity.

Second-line Agents

Between 33% and 66% of patients in SE continue to seize despite appropriate benzodiazepine administration, necessitating a second-line agent.[30,31] Phenytoin has been

Table 3 Anticonvulsant dosages			
Medication	**Dosage**	**Infusion Rate**	**Notes**
Diazepam	0.2 mg/kg	5 mg/min	—
Lorazepam	0.1 mg/kg	2 mg/min	—
Midazolam	10 mg[a]	100–300 µg/min[b]	—
Phenytoin	20–25 mg/kg	50 mg/min	Slower in geriatric and known cardiac disease
Fosphenytoin	20–25 mg PE/kg	150 mg PE/min	—
Valproic acid	20–40 mg/kg	60 mg/min or 10 mg/kg/min	Dose can be repeated to a maximum of 60 mg/kg
Levetiracetam	2000–4000 mg	Up to 500 mg/min	—
Lacosamide	200–400 mg IV	30–40 mg/min	
Phenobarbital	20 mg/kg	60 mg/min	
Ketamine	Bolus: 1.5–4.5 mg/kg Infusion: 2–10 mg/kg/h		—
Midazolam infusion	Bolus: 0.2 mg/kg, repeated every 3–5 min to a maximum of 2 mg/kg Infusion: 0.05–2 mg/kg/h		Can result in hypotension requiring vasopressors
Propofol infusion	Bolus: 1–5 mg/kg, repeated in 3–5 min Infusion: 1–15 mg/kg/h		
Pentobarbital infusion	Bolus: 5 mg/kg, repeated q3–5 min to a max of 15 mg/kg over 1 h Infusion: 0.5–10 mg/kg/h		
Thiopental infusion	Bolus: 1–2 mg/kg Infusion: 5 mg/h		

Abbreviation: PE, phenytoin equivalent.
[a] Dosage used in the adult arm of the RAMPArT trial.[25]
[b] Off-label usage for refractory SE.

a long-standing choice, but valproic acid has recently become more favorable. A much needed study is underway; the Established Status Epilepticus Treatment Trial (ESETT), which is a randomized, double-blind, comparative study of levetiracetam, fosphenytoin, and valproic acid in subjects with refractory SE who have already received benzodiazepines. Some investigators recommend that patients be given a second-line treatment even if benzodiazepines abort the seizure, to prevent recurrence.[17]

Phenytoins

Phenytoins work on sodium channels, slowing their rate of reactivation after depolarization (**Table 4**). Fosphenytoin is a phenytoin prodrug, metabolized to phenytoin in the body. It is more water soluble, and does not require the propylene glycol and ethanol diluents that are necessary for phenytoin, allowing a faster infusion and fewer side effects. Increased cost associated with fosphenytoin was an initial concern on introduction to the market, but may be lower than those of phenytoin, now that it is available in generic forms. With the lower rate of adverse effects,[32] it is preferred to phenytoin.[18]

Phenytoin is dosed at 20 to 25 mg/kg and infused at a maximum of 50 mg/min, and even slower (25 mg/min) in geriatric patients and patients with known cardiovascular disease.[15] It is important to deliver weight-based amounts and the common practice

Table 4
Anticonvulsants by site of action

Na Channel	GABA$_A$	Ca Channel	NMDA Antagonist
Phenytoin	Benzodiazepines:	Propofol	Ketamine
Valproic acid	• Diazepam	Lacosamide	Propofol
	• Lorazepam		
	• Midazolam		
	Barbiturates:		
	• Phenobarbital		
	• Pentobarbital		
	• Thiopental		
	Valproic acid		
	Propofol		

of giving a gram of phenytoin underdoses many patients. Fosphenytoin dosage is calculated in phenytoin equivalents (PE) because it is a prodrug, and dosed at 20 to 25 mg PE/kg. It can be infused at a maximum rate of 150 mg PE/min, but preferably slower in the elderly and patients at high risk for arrhythmias. Phenytoin cannot be administered intramuscularly, but fosphenytoin can. However, given the long absorption time and delayed onset of action, this method should not be used in SE (see **Table 3**).

Phenytoin directly affects the myocardium, prolonging the QT interval. If not administered appropriately, hypotension and cardiac arrhythmias can occur, which happens in approximately 3.5% of patients. This condition usually resolves with slowing or temporarily stopping the infusion, and may necessitate the administration of a fluid bolus. Local irritation from diluents in IV phenytoin can result in phlebitis, and in the event of extravasation there can be localized tissue necrosis with possible resulting limb loss, named purple glove syndrome.[33]

Valproic acid
Valproic acid works by prolonging the recovery of voltage-gated sodium channels from inactivation, similar to phenytoin. In addition, valproic acid increases the availability of GABA by stimulating its synthesis and inhibiting its degradation (see **Table 4**). It has been used in Europe for the treatment of SE since 2004, and since then more than 300 cases have been documented.[34] Valproic acid is at least as effective as phenytoin in terminating SE with a more favorable side effect profile, especially in cardiorespiratory patients.[35,36] A 2014 systematic review showed that IV valproate was effective in 68.5% of adult patients, which is comparable with, if not superior to, published data for phenytoin and phenobarbital.[20,37,38] Valproic acid is dosed at 20 to 40 mg/kg, and can be infused over 10 minutes, or even faster, at a rate of 10 mg/kg/min. A repeat dose of another 20 mg/kg can be used, to a maximum of 60 mg/kg (see **Table 3**). The incidence of serious side effects with valproate is low, mostly consistent with mild hypotension, with good cardiorespiratory tolerability. The most serious side effect is idiosyncratic encephalopathy, which is rare and may be associated with hepatic abnormality or hyperammonemia, and is reversible with discontinuation of the drug.[37]

Intubation
At this point in the management, if the patient's airway has not been controlled, the patient should be intubated. The patient may not need a separate induction agent depending on the mental status that is present because of the combined results of the seizure and the medications used to abort it. Multiple induction agents exist,

including benzodiazepines, propofol, etomidate, and ketamine. Propofol is regarded by many experts as the induction agent of choice in SE given its anticonvulsant properties. However, because it can cause hypotension, it should be avoided in hypotensive patients. Ketamine, which has antiepileptic properties (discussed later), is another induction agent that can be safely used for intubation, especially in patients who are hypotensive. Etomidate has long been regarded as a less favorable agent for induction, because of concerns for its lowering of seizure threshold, making it a counterintuitive choice for patients in SE. However, this fear is extrapolated from EEG data from patients undergoing electroconvulsive therapy (ECT) for psychiatric diagnoses,[39] and has not been truly studied in seizing patients.

Two classes of paralytic medications exist: depolarizing short-acting agents, such as succinylcholine; and nondepolarizing agents, which are longer acting, such as rocuronium and vecuronium. Nondepolarizing agents are considered safer because they do not carry the concomitant risk of hyperkalemia, which could be significant in patients who have been seizing and may have developed rhabdomyolysis. However, another consideration is the duration of their paralytic effect (30 minutes for rocuronium, 45 to 65 minutes for vecuronium) compared with 4 to 6 minutes for succinylcholine. The paralytic stops the motor activity of the seizure despite ongoing neuronal firing, which can lead to false reassurance regarding seizure control despite continuous neuronal damage. Therefore, if a nondepolarizing paralytic is used, EEG monitoring is indicated to guide management.[16] However, given that an EEG is not immediately available in most settings, a short-acting agent is recommended.[40] Although there is a reversal agent for the nondepolarizing agents, sugammadex, its use is not widespread outside of anesthesia, and most emergency providers are not comfortable with its use.

Third-line Agents (Second-line Adjuncts)

Three percent of patients continue to seize despite the use of a second-line agent, necessitating the use of another anticonvulsant.[31] Previous convention has been that, if a second-line medication fails, then a second-line adjunct or third-line anticonvulsant should be used before using IV anesthetics. However, experts are now moving toward early escalation to IV anesthetics for seizure termination while adding a second-line adjunct concomitantly. This aggressive method of management may not be suitable in elderly patients, patients with multiple comorbidities, or patients with subtle seizures.

Levetiracetam

Levetiracetam's exact mechanism of action is unknown, but it has been an increasingly popular agent since its introduction to the US market. It is unclear how effective levetiracetam is in controlling refractory SE. A retrospective study suggested that levetiracetam is less effective than valproic acid as a second-line agent in controlling benzodiazepine-refractory SE, but it seems to be an acceptable third-line treatment of refractory SE, after benzodiazepines and phenytoin, making it a level C recommendation.[36,41,42] As mentioned previously, ESETT is underway to compare fosphenytoin, levetiracetam, and valproic acid, and should provide evidence on the true efficacy of levetiracetam. Despite the lack of strong evidence regarding the efficacy of levetiracetam, it is the most commonly used antiepileptic for SE after benzodiazepines and phenytoin.[15] Levetiracetam is not hepatically metabolized, resulting in practically no drug interactions and a favorable safety profile, because it has no effect on respiratory drive or blood pressure either. However, it is renally excreted and therefore should be avoided in patients with renal disease.

It is administered as an IV loading dose of 2000 to 4000 mg at the rate of 500 mg/min (see **Table 3**).

Lacosamide

Intravenous lacosamide was approved in the United States in 2009, and the data on its use in SE are limited. It seems to enhance the slow inactivation of voltage-dependent sodium channels.

A review article in 2013 included all patients given IV lacosamide in SE (a total of 314 patients), all in retrospective studies or case series. The overall success rate was 56%, with 4.4% having a serious side effect, which included angioedema, hypotension, or third-degree heart block with paroxysmal asystole.[43] One study specifically compared lacosamide with phenytoin as a third-line agent (after benzodiazepines and levetiracetam), with similar success rates for seizure control but with a significantly safer side effect profile.[44] Since then, a small Spanish prospective study was done (N = 34 patients), which showed that IV lacosamide was effective in 64.7% of patients when used as a third or later agent; however, there was no control group.[45] Another multicenter retrospective observational study in Spain studied the use of IV lacosamide in SE and acute repetitive seizures, with a total of 98 patients and a 76.5% success rate.[46] A consistent trend among all these studies is that there is decreased response to lacosamide with a longer time lag before administration, which is not surprising. Large randomized trials are still needed. The dose is 200 to 400 mg, with a greater trend for success with 400 mg, at the rate of 30 to 40 mg/min. The infusion is generally well tolerated with minimal side effects and low drug interaction potential.[47]

Phenobarbital

Phenobarbital, a barbiturate, is a $GABA_A$ agonist. It is the oldest anticonvulsant drug still in use and used to be a first-line treatment of SE, but has been replaced by benzodiazepines because of its numerous side effects, which include hypotension caused by vasodilatation, and respiratory depression, and which are compounded when used with a benzodiazepine. In addition, the very long half-life (2–6 days) makes complications difficult to manage. It is dosed at 20 mg/kg, and infused at a rate of 60 mg/min (see **Table 3**).

Ketamine

Ketamine is a dissociative agent that inhibits the NMDA receptors, making it a logical option for management of seizures, because it functions via a mechanism that is different from all other currently used anticonvulsants, particularly one that does not display pharmacoresistance. In addition, its sympathomimetic properties decrease the need for the vasopressors that are usually needed with IV anesthetics in refractory SE.

Ketamine has been investigated for refractory SE over the past 25 years, mostly in small retrospective series, with only 3 prospective cohort studies, totaling 23 studies, and a total of 162 patients (110 adults and 52 children).[48] Variable results were recorded, from complete response in all study patients to complete treatment failure, with a total of 56.5% of the adult patients having electrographic response. This great variability in results is probably caused by heterogeneity in timing of ketamine (from 16 hours after start of SE to 140 days), and variability of anticonvulsant drugs used in conjunction with ketamine.[49]

The side effects of treatment and functional outcomes were sparingly documented, raising concerns about the safety of ketamine in this setting. Previous concerns about the negative effects of ketamine on the intracranial pressure (ICP) that stemmed from older studies in the 1960s has been challenged, because ketamine does not seem to increase the ICP, especially in patients who are premedicated with benzodiazepines or are already on a sedative, as is the case in SE.[50]

In conclusion, data are lacking to prove the efficacy of ketamine in refractory SE, but it looks promising, and a large study (preferably randomized and controlled) is needed. In the meantime, it is reasonable to use ketamine in patients who are in refractory SE, after IV anesthetics have failed. The optimal bolus dose seems to be 1.5 to 4.5 mg/kg, with an infusion of up to 10 mg/kg/h.

Fourth-line Treatment

At this point, the patient should have been intubated and placed on a continuous EEG monitor. Most of the fourth-line agents, which are IV anesthetics, cause hypotension, sometimes severe enough to require vasopressors, especially barbiturates. This hypotension is compounded by the previous treatments the patient has received. Two recent retrospective studies suggest increased mortality with the use of IV anesthetics, heightening awareness of complications, such as increased infection and mechanical ventilation. This increased mortality might be caused by variable seizure causes in the patients included in these studies, and perhaps a uniform SE protocol irrespective of the underlying cause is not appropriate. Also, the retrospective nature of these studies introduces bias, necessitating prospective studies to further clarify this concern.[51,52] Infusions are frequently used in combination to achieve EEG burst suppression. If EEG is not available, the current recommendation is to titrate until convulsions cease and EEG becomes available.[17] Infusions should be maintained for 24 hours after seizure cessation, followed by controlled withdrawal of anesthesia.

Midazolam infusion
Midazolam is the preferred benzodiazepine for continuous infusion, given its short duration of action and ability to be titrated. Lorazepam is not used as an infusion, given its longer half-life, which makes weaning from the infusion more difficult. A bolus of 0.2 mg/kg is used, and repeated every 3 to 5 minutes to a maximum of 2 mg/kg until seizure control is achieved. The patient is then started on an infusion of 0.05 to 2 mg/kg/h. Of note, prolonged administration of midazolam is complicated by tachyphylaxis, an acute decrease in response, necessitating increasing the dose to maintain seizure control.[53]

Propofol infusion
Propofol can be used as an induction agent for intubation or as an IV infusion to control seizures. Propofol is a sedative and anesthetic that has antiepileptic properties. It works on $GABA_A$ receptors, and is a sodium channel blocker, NMDA inhibitor, and calcium channel modulator. It has a short duration of action, which makes it easily titrated. There is evidence that propofol efficiently suppresses seizures. A retrospective study in 2004 showed a 67% success rate in terminating refractory SE in patients on a propofol infusion. The caveat of that study is that the patients also received thiopental, clonazepam, or another anticonvulsant.[54] However, most of the evidence comes from an underpowered study that compared propofol with barbiturates, resulting in comparable seizure control and complications, with a marked increase in mechanical ventilation days in patients on thiopental.[55] A bolus of 3 to 5 mg/kg is used, and is repeated until seizure control is achieved. The patient is then started on an infusion of 1 to 15 mg/kg/h. Some limitations to prolonged use of high-dose propofol infusion are hypotension and propofol infusion syndrome; a combination of lactic acidosis, bradycardia, heart failure, lipemia, rhabdomyolysis, and renal failure, which

can be fatal.[56] Note that propofol has been reported to cause jerking movements and induce seizures as well.[57]

Barbiturate infusion

Pentobarbital and thiopental are much shorter acting than phenobarbital, and are therefore used as infusions. As with all barbiturates, they are highly lipid soluble, accumulating in fat stores and prolonged elimination. Pentobarbital is started as a bolus of 5 mg/kg, which is repeated every few minutes to a maximum of 15 mg/kg until seizure control is achieved. The patient is then maintained on an infusion of 0.5 to 10 mg/kg/h. Given that one-third of patients on pentobarbital have severe hypotension requiring a vasopressor or inotrope, it is recommended that these agents be readily available when initiating the infusion.[58] A systematic review in 2002 comparing pentobarbital with propofol and midazolam infusions found pentobarbital to be superior in effectively controlling refractory SE with fewer breakthrough seizures but also with an increased incidence of hypotension.[59] Therefore, the convention has been to reserve pentobarbital for patients refractory to propofol and midazolam. Another cohort in 2012 found that pentobarbital effectively controlled super-refractory SE in almost 90% of patients, with infrequent complications.[58]

Thiopental is metabolized into pentobarbital. It is more lipid soluble than pentobarbital, and therefore requires longer to be eliminated. The dose is 1 to 2 mg/kg, repeated every 3 to 5 minutes, and then infused at 5 mg/h. High-dose thiopental is effective in clinical and electrophysiologic seizure control, but requires inotropes or vasopressors in approximately 40% of cases.[60]

Adjunctive therapies

In addition to pharmacologic therapies there are multiple adjunctive therapies that may help terminate seizures. Therapeutic hypothermia has been tested for a variety of intracranial pathologies since the 1960s, and has been proposed to treat super-refractory SE because it slows nerve conduction in vitro and decreases excitatory neurotransmission. Its minimal evidence in super-refractory SE comes from a case report and case series, in addition to multiple animal studies. It is also extrapolated from neurosurgical data in which local cooling is applied directly to the brain. Hypothermia can either be generalized, with a goal core temperature of 31°C to 35°C, or local, applied to the head and neck area to achieve a surface temperature of 30°C to 31°C.[61]

Ketogenic diets have been investigated for the management of super-refractory SE that has failed pentobarbital in addition to multiple antiepileptic drugs and has been ongoing for at least 24 hours. Achieving ketogenesis requires a mean of 2.8 days, making this a nonemergent intervention, albeit a fairly successful one in carefully chosen candidates.[62]

MANAGEMENT OF SUBTLE STATUS EPILEPTICUS

Treatment options depend on impairment of consciousness. If severely impaired, then the patient should be treated the same as in convulsive SE. If consciousness is partially preserved, then it might be reasonable to wait longer before initiation of IV anesthetics, and perhaps start a third-line anticonvulsant (also referred to as a second-line adjunct) first, because treatment may be more harmful than continued seizures.[17,63,64]

FAILURES IN THE MANAGEMENT OF STATUS EPILEPTICUS

There are many causes for failure of management of SE, the major one being delay to treatment. Poor drug selection and inappropriate dosing are others. Failure to identify

---

Box 3
Metabolic derangements worsening neuronal damage

- Hypoxia
- Hypoglycemia
- Hyperglycemia
- Hypercarbia
- Hypotension
- Fever

---

the underlying cause is important as well, because some toxin-induced seizures are less responsive to certain medications, such as phenytoin.[17]

COMPLICATIONS

Because prolonged seizures are a major physiologic stress to the human body, several derangements in certain parameters are expected. As the body continues to use anaerobic metabolism during the seizure, lactic acid can accumulate and the patient can have a wide anion gap acidosis. If the seizures are not terminated in a timely fashion, an increase in the serum creatinine kinase levels is also expected, indicating rhabdomyolysis and all of the resultant complications, including renal failure. These patients should receive supportive care and proper IV hydration during their ED course. It is prudent to optimize the patient's metabolic status to prevent further neuronal damage, because that would increase the metabolic demand and/or decrease substrate delivery and worsen neurologic outcome (**Box 3**). Most metabolic abnormalities resolve promptly after the resolution of the convulsive episodes. In addition, there are reports of reversible cerebral edema caused by GCSE that is also self-resolving, but may complicate the clinical picture.[65]

SUMMARY

The emergent evaluation and treatment of GCSE presents challenges for emergency physicians. This disease is one of the few in which minutes can mean the difference between life and significant morbidity and mortality. It is imperative to use parallel processing and have multiple treatment options planned in advance, in case the current treatment is not successful. There is also benefit to exploring, or initiating, treatment algorithms to standardize the care for these critically ill patients.

REFERENCES

1. Angus-Leppan H. First seizures in adults. BMJ 2014;348:g2470.
2. Fisher RS, Acevedo C, Arzimanoglou A, et al. ILAE official report: a practical clinical definition of epilepsy. Epilepsia 2014;55(4):475–82.
3. Logroscino G, Hesdorffer DC, Cascino G, et al. Mortality after a first episode of status epilepticus in the United States and Europe. Epilepsia 2005;46(Suppl 11):46–8.
4. Hocker SE, Britton JW, Mandrekar JN, et al. Predictors of outcome in refractory status epilepticus. JAMA Neurol 2013;70(1):72–7.
5. Koubeissi M, Alshekhlee A. In-hospital mortality of generalized convulsive status epilepticus: a large US sample. Neurol 2007;69(9):886–93.

6. Chen JW, Wasterlain CG. Status epilepticus: pathophysiology and management in adults. Lancet Neurol 2006;5(3):246–56.
7. Huff JS, Fountain NB. Pathophysiology and definitions of seizures and status epilepticus. Emerg Med Clin North Am 2011;29(1):1–13.
8. Chen JWY, Naylor DE, Wasterlain CG. Advances in the pathophysiology of status epilepticus. Acta Neurol Scand 2007;115:7–15.
9. Deeb TZ, Maguire J, Moss SJ. Possible alterations in GABAA receptor signaling that underlie benzodiazepine-resistant seizures. Epilepsia 2012;53(s9):79–88.
10. Löscher W, Potschka H. Drug resistance in brain diseases and the role of drug efflux transporters. Nat Rev Neurosci 2005;6(8):591–602.
11. Mazarati AM, Baldwin RA, Sankar R, et al. Time-dependent decrease in the effectiveness of antiepileptic drugs during the course of self-sustaining status epilepticus. Brain Res 1998;814(1):179–85.
12. Kapur J, Macdonald RL. Rapid seizure-induced reduction of benzodiazepine and Zn2+ sensitivity of hippocampal dentate granule cell GABAA receptors. J Neurosci 1997;17(19):7532–40.
13. Naylor DE, Liu H, Niquet J, et al. Rapid surface accumulation of NMDA receptors increases glutamatergic excitation during status epilepticus. Neurobiol Dis 2013; 54:225–38.
14. Mazarati AM, Wasterlain CG. N-methyl-D-asparate receptor antagonists abolish the maintenance phase of self-sustaining status epilepticus in rat. Neurosci Lett 1999;265(3):187–90.
15. Brophy GM, Bell R, Claassen J, et al. Guidelines for the evaluation and management of status epilepticus. Neurocrit Care 2012;17(1):3–23.
16. Shearer P, Riviello J. Generalized convulsive status epilepticus in adults and children: treatment guidelines and protocols. Emerg Med Clin North Am 2011;29(1): 51–64.
17. Hocker SE. Status epilepticus. Continuum (Minneap Minn) 2015;21(5 Neurocritical Care):1362–83.
18. Glauser T, Shinnar S, Gloss D, et al. Evidence-based guideline: treatment of convulsive status epilepticus in children and adults: report of the guideline committee of the American epilepsy society. Epilepsy Curr 2016;16(1):48–61.
19. Aranda A, Foucart G, Ducassé JL, et al. Generalized convulsive status epilepticus management in adults: a cohort study with evaluation of professional practice. Epilepsia 2010;51(10):2159–67.
20. Treiman DM, Meyers PD, Walton NY, et al. A comparison of four treatments for generalized convulsive status epilepticus. N Engl J Med 1998;339(12):792–8.
21. Alldredge BK, Gelb AM, Isaacs SM, et al. A comparison of lorazepam, diazepam, and placebo for the treatment of out-of-hospital status epilepticus. N Engl J Med 2001;345(9):631–7.
22. Reves JG, Fragen RJ, Vinik HR, et al. Midazolam: pharmacology and uses. Anesthesiology 1985;62(3):310–24.
23. Towne AR, DeLorenzo RJ. Use of intramuscular midazolam for status epilepticus. J Emerg Med 1999;17(2):323–8.
24. Gamble J, Dundee J, Assaf R. Plasma diazepam levels after single dose oral and intramuscular administration. Anaesthesia 1975;30(2):164–9.
25. Silbergleit R, Durkalski V, Lowenstein D, et al. Intramuscular versus intravenous therapy for prehospital status epilepticus. N Engl J Med 2012;366(7):591–600.
26. Gottwald MD, Akers LC, Liu P, et al. Prehospital stability of diazepam and lorazepam. Am J Emerg Med 1999;17(4):333–7.

27. Jahns BE, Bakst CM. Extension of expiration time for lorazepam injection at room temperature. Am J Hosp Pharm 1993;50(6):1134.
28. Wolfe TR, Macfarlane TC. Intranasal midazolam therapy for pediatric status epilepticus. Am J Emerg Med 2006;24(3):343–6.
29. Knoester P, Jonker D, Van der Hoeven R, et al. Pharmacokinetics and pharmacodynamics of midazolam administered as a concentrated intranasal spray. a study in healthy volunteers. Br J Clin Pharmacol 2002;53(5):501–7.
30. Bleck T, Cock H, Chamberlain J, et al. The established status epilepticus trial 2013. Epilepsia 2013;54(s6):89–92.
31. Mayer SA, Claassen J, Lokin J, et al. Refractory status epilepticus: frequency, risk factors, and impact on outcome. Arch Neurol 2002;59(2):205–10.
32. Marchetti A, Magar R, Fischer J, et al. A pharmacoeconomic evaluation of intravenous fosphenytoin (Cerebyx®) versus intravenous phenytoin (Dilantin®) in hospital emergency departments. Clin Ther 1996;18(5):953–66.
33. Earnest MP, Marx JA, Drury LR. Complications of intravenous phenytoin for acute treatment of seizures: recommendations for usage. JAMA 1983;249(6):762–5.
34. Knake S, Hamer HM, Rosenow F. Status epilepticus: a critical review. Epilepsy Behav 2009;15(1):10–4.
35. Agarwal P, Kumar N, Chandra R, et al. Randomized study of intravenous valproate and phenytoin in status epilepticus. Seizure 2007;16(6):527–32.
36. Huff JS, Melnick ER, Tomaszewski CA, et al. Clinical policy: critical issues in the evaluation and management of adult patients presenting to the emergency department with seizures. Ann Emerg Med 2014;63(4):437–47.e15.
37. Trinka E, Höfler J, Zerbs A, et al. Efficacy and safety of intravenous valproate for status epilepticus: a systematic review. CNS Drugs 2014;28(7):623–39.
38. Yasiry Z, Shorvon SD. The relative effectiveness of five antiepileptic drugs in treatment of benzodiazepine-resistant convulsive status epilepticus: a meta-analysis of published studies. Seizure 2014;23(3):167–74.
39. Gábor G, Judit T, Zsolt I. Comparison of propofol and etomidate regarding impact on seizure threshold during electroconvulsive therapy in patients with schizophrenia. Neuropsychopharmacol Hung 2007;9(3):125–30.
40. Betjemann JP, Lowenstein DH. Status epilepticus in adults. Lancet Neurol 2015; 14(6):615–24.
41. Alvarez V, Januel J, Burnand B, et al. Second-line status epilepticus treatment: comparison of phenytoin, valproate, and levetiracetam. Epilepsia 2011;52(7): 1292–6.
42. Tripathi M, Vibha D, Choudhary N, et al. Management of refractory status epilepticus at a tertiary care centre in a developing country. Seizure 2010;19(2):109–11.
43. Höfler J, Trinka E. Lacosamide as a new treatment option in status epilepticus. Epilepsia 2013;54(3):393–404.
44. Kellinghaus C, Berning S, Stögbauer F. Intravenous lacosamide or phenytoin for treatment of refractory status epilepticus. Acta Neurol Scand 2014;129(5):294–9.
45. Miró J, Toledo M, Santamarina E, et al. Efficacy of intravenous lacosamide as an add-on treatment in refractory status epilepticus: a multicentric prospective study. Seizure 2013;22(1):77–9.
46. Garcés M, Villanueva V, Mauri JA, et al. Factors influencing response to intravenous lacosamide in emergency situations: LACO-IV study. Epilepsy Behav 2014; 36:144–52.
47. Legros B, Depondt C, Levy-Nogueira M, et al. Intravenous lacosamide in refractory seizure clusters and status epilepticus: comparison of 200 and 400 mg loading doses. Neurocrit Care 2014;20(3):484–8.

48. Zeiler F, Teitelbaum J, Gillman L, et al. NMDA antagonists for refractory seizures. Neurocrit Care 2014;20(3):502–13.
49. Zeiler F. Early use of the NMDA receptor antagonist ketamine in refractory and superrefractory status epilepticus. Crit Care Res Pract 2015;2015:831260.
50. Zeiler FA, Teitelbaum J, West M, et al. The ketamine effect on intracranial pressure in nontraumatic neurological illness. J Crit Care 2014;29(6):1096–106.
51. Kowalski RG, Ziai WC, Rees RN, et al. Third-line antiepileptic therapy and outcome in status epilepticus: the impact of vasopressor use and prolonged mechanical ventilation. Crit Care Med 2012;40(9):2677–84.
52. Sutter R, Marsch S, Fuhr P, et al. Anesthetic drugs in status epilepticus: risk or rescue? A 6-year cohort study. Neurology 2014;82(8):656–64.
53. Kumar A, Bleck TP. Intravenous midazolam for the treatment of refractory status epilepticus. Crit Care Med 1992;20(4):483–8.
54. Rossetti AO, Reichhart MD, Schaller M, et al. Propofol treatment of refractory status epilepticus: a study of 31 episodes. Epilepsia 2004;45(7):757–63.
55. Prabhakar H, Bindra A, Singh GP, et al. Propofol versus thiopental sodium for the treatment of refractory status epilepticus (Review). Evid Based Child Health 2013; 8(4):1488–508.
56. Iyer VN, Hoel R, Rabinstein AA. Propofol infusion syndrome in patients with refractory status epilepticus: an 11-year clinical experience. Crit Care Med 2009; 37(12):3024–30.
57. Mäkelä J, Iivanainen M, Pieninkeroinen I, et al. Seizures associated with propofol anesthesia. Epilepsia 1993;34(5):832–5.
58. Pugin D, Foreman B, De Marchis GM, et al. Is pentobarbital safe and efficacious in the treatment of super-refractory status epilepticus: a cohort study. Crit Care 2014;18(3):R103.
59. Claassen J, Hirsch LJ, Emerson RG, et al. Treatment of refractory status epilepticus with pentobarbital, propofol, or midazolam: a systematic review. Epilepsia 2002;43(2):146–53.
60. Parviainen I, Uusaro A, Kalviainen R, et al. High-dose thiopental in the treatment of refractory status epilepticus in intensive care unit. Neurology 2002;59(8): 1249–51.
61. Bennett AE, Hoesch RE, DeWitt LD, et al. Therapeutic hypothermia for status epilepticus: a report, historical perspective, and review. Clin Neurol Neurosurg 2014; 126:103–9.
62. Kossoff EH, Nabbout R. Use of dietary therapy for status epilepticus. J Child Neurol 2013;28(8):1049–51.
63. Ferguson M, Bianchi MT, Sutter R, et al. Calculating the risk benefit equation for aggressive treatment of non-convulsive status epilepticus. Neurocrit Care 2013; 18(2):216–27.
64. Meierkord H, Boon P, Engelsen B, et al. EFNS guideline on the management of status epilepticus in adults. Eur J Neurol 2010;17(3):348–55.
65. Nandhagopal R. Generalised convulsive status epilepticus: an overview. Postgrad Med J 2006;82(973):723–32. Available at: http://www.ncbi.nlm.nih.gov/pmc/articles/PMC2660499/.

Initial Diagnosis and Management of Coma

Stephen J. Traub, MD[a],*, Eelco F. Wijdicks, MD[b]

KEYWORDS

- Coma • Coma mimics • Pathophysiology

KEY POINTS

- Coma is a life-threatening process that requires immediate stabilization and a structured approach to diagnosis and management.
- The differential diagnosis for coma is long, but is often divided into structural vs. diffuse neuronal dysfunction; the latter is subdivided into toxic vs. metabolic.
- When available, historical information may be of great use in determining the etiology of coma; in all cases, a focused physical examination can help greatly refine the differential diagnosis.
- The definitive treatment of patients with coma is ultimately disease-specific.

INTRODUCTION

Many patients present to the emergency department with an alteration in mental status simply as a complication of many serious illnesses. A subset of these patients will present comatose, a clinical state that is a true medical emergency. Although coma is a relatively rare presenting condition in the emergency department, patients who present with coma are often in extremis and necessitate immediate evaluation and stabilization.

The approach to coma by the emergency physician is described, beginning with a discussion of pathophysiology and cause. Then, the practical clinical aspects of coma are addressed, including initial stabilization, obtaining the correct historical information, performing a thorough physical examination, ordering appropriate testing and imaging studies, and providing appropriate treatment.

PATHOPHYSIOLOGY

A neuronal network in the dorsal pons and midbrain give rise to the ascending reticular activing system (ARAS), which is responsible for arousal.[1] Neurons from these centers

[a] Department of Emergency Medicine, Mayo Clinic Arizona, 1-738, 5777 East Mayo Boulevard, Phoenix, AZ 85054, USA; [b] Department of Neurology, Mayo Clinic, Rochester, MN, USA
* Corresponding author.
E-mail address: traub.stephen@mayo.edu

Emerg Med Clin N Am 34 (2016) 777–793
http://dx.doi.org/10.1016/j.emc.2016.06.017
0733-8627/16/© 2016 Elsevier Inc. All rights reserved.
emed.theclinics.com

run together through the thalamus and then to the bilateral cerebral cortex; the cortex controls sensory processing and understanding, which generates awareness.[2,3] Coma results from an impairment of this axis by a process that affects the brain's arousal center, consciousness center, the tracts that connect them, or some combination thereof. Patients are, therefore, not aware and not awake. Importantly, coma from cortical impairment can only result from a bilateral insult; unilateral cortical deficits do not cause coma. Prolonged coma may result in awakening cycles (eyes open coma) without awareness. Because the comatose state is difficult to quantify, some patients diagnosed as comatose may be minimally aware (minimally conscious state) and others may be more aware than can be assumed or tested.

Although the final common physiologic pathway of coma is neuronal dysfunction in the ARAS-thalamic-cortical pathway, it is useful to subdivide the pathophysiology into structural versus diffuse neuronal dysfunction. Structural causes of coma are defined as those that precipitate cellular dysfunction through a mechanical force, such as pressure on key area or a blockade of delivery of critical cellular substrate. Diffuse neuronal dysfunction precipitates coma by abnormalities only at the cellular level and may be further divided into two general categories: toxic and metabolic. In a toxin-induced coma, an exogenous substance is responsible for the clinical findings; in a metabolic coma, a perturbation of an endogenous process, such as temperature or sodium regulation, has gone awry.

This classification, although useful, does have limitations. A metabolic process, such as hypoglycemia or hypoxia, may initially produce coma through diffuse neuronal dysfunction; however, if the process is uncorrected and cell death occurs, the cause of coma becomes structural. Similarly, a diffuse neuronal process, such as cerebral edema, may become a structural problem if the edema occludes vessels in the posterior circulation and produces brainstem ischemia.

CAUSES

A causal overview of coma is presented in **Table 1**, categorized based on this logic, and includes coma mimics, which are several disorders that may be easily mistaken

Table 1
Causal overview of coma and coma mimics

	Coma		
	Diffuse Neuronal Dysfunction		
Structural	**Toxic**	**Metabolic**	**Coma Mimics**
Neoplasia	Sedative-hypnotics	Respiratory	Locked-in syndrome
Hydrocephalus	agents	insufficiency	Neuromuscular paralysis
Intracranial	Opioids	Dysthermia	Akinetic mutism
hemorrhage	Dissociative agents	Dysglycemia	Psychogenic unresponsiveness
Vascular	Carbon monoxide	Electrolyte disorders	
occlusion	Toxic alcohols	Infection	
	Antidepressants	Hypothyroidism	
	Antiepileptics	Thiamine deficiency	
	Agents of	Nonconvulsive status	
	histotoxic hypoxia	epilepticus	
	Simple asphyxiants		
	Serotonin syndrome		
	Neuroleptic malignant		
	syndrome		
	Clonidine		

for coma but do not involve interruption of the ARAS-thalamic-cortical pathway. For the purposes of this article, the focus is on relatively common entities that may present with coma, rather than those that are uncommon or in which coma is a late finding.

STRUCTURAL CAUSES OF COMA
Tumors

Tumors may cause coma by exerting pressure on either a key area (eg, the brainstem) or by causing a diffuse increase in intracranial pressure. More commonly, however, patients with tumors have a slow progression of neurologic findings. Abrupt onset of coma in such patients often results from hemorrhage into an expanding mass. Even small tumors, however, may cause obstructive hydrocephalus or focal infarctions, each of which may in turn lead to the relatively abrupt onset of coma.

Acute Hydrocephalus

There is approximately 100 to 150 mL of cerebrospinal fluid (CSF) in the adult brain. CSF is produced predominantly in the choroid plexus, circulates through the ventricular system, and empties into the subarachnoid space where it is absorbed predominantly into the venous system through the arachnoid villi.[4] Occlusion of this flow via tumor, clotting of intraventricular blood, or dysfunction of the arachnoid villi may lead to an increase in intraventricular CSF, with a concurrent increase in intracranial pressure and resultant coma.

Intracranial Hemorrhage

Central nervous system (CNS) hemorrhage resulting in coma may have 1 of 4 causes.

Spontaneous subarachnoid hemorrhage
Spontaneous subarachnoid hemorrhage (SAH) usually results from the rupture of an aneurysm in the Circle of Willis (often referred to as a berry aneurysm). Thunderclap headache on presentation is present in more than 95% of patients.[5] Coma in the setting of SAH may be due to acute hydrocephalus or anoxic-ischemic injury.

Subdural hemorrhage
Subdural hemorrhage (SDH) is an accumulation of blood between the dura and the arachnoid membrane. SDH is often associated with a trauma but may also be associated with low intracranial pressure, as occurs after lumbar puncture.[6] SDH may occur because of either shearing of bridging veins[7] or arterial interruption.[8] The use of both antiplatelet agents and anticoagulants increase the risk of SDH.[9] SDH may produce a rapid shift of brain parenchyma, resulting in compression of the thalamus and pressure on the brainstem. Seizures, including nonconvulsive status epilepticus (NCSE), may mimic structural injury and are more often seen after hematoma evacuation.

Epidural hemorrhage
Epidural hemorrhage (EDH) is most often due to blunt force trauma that disrupts an epidural artery, with blood collecting in the potential space between the dura and the skull. Patients may present with initial confusion or loss of consciousness from which they recover, only to subsequently "talk and deteriorate." This lucid interval occurs in approximately half of all EDH patients.[10] Coagulopathy is associated with a poorer outcome in patients with EDH.[11] Similar to SDH, brain parenchymal shift, brainstem pressure, and seizures may result.

Intraparenchymal hemorrhage

Intraparenchymal hemorrhage (IPH) is usually due to longstanding hypertension and associated vascular changes, although amyloid angiopathy and coagulopathy are other possible causes.[12] Coma from an IPH may be caused by the disruption of key tracts or a general increase in intracranial pressure, depending on the location of the lesion.

Vascular Occlusion

Arterial vascular occlusion may be either thrombotic or embolic; both may produce coma if critical structures are affected. Of note, arterial vascular occlusion causing coma is usually a posterior circulation event, with occlusion in the vertebrobasilar system leading to hypoperfusion of crucial structures within the ARAS. Arterial occlusion in the anterior circulation is an uncommon cause of coma because bilateral cortical disruption is required to produce the requisite depression of consciousness. This may occur, however, in patients who have suffered a stroke on one side of the brain and subsequently suffer an acute arterial vascular occlusion on the other.

DIFFUSE NEURONAL DYSFUNCTION CAUSES OF COMA: METABOLIC
Respiratory Insufficiency

Respiratory insufficiency may produce coma in two ways. First, the brain is particularly sensitive to the effects of hypoxia, with coma possible within minutes of acute oxygen deprivation. Second, hypercarbia may cause coma; the exact mechanism is unclear, but may involve an alteration in neurotransmitter levels or changes in intracranial pressure as increases in carbon dioxide levels are associated with increases in cerebral blood flow.

Dysthermia

Extremes of body temperature may accompany other primary causes of coma or be a primary cause. Although the exact temperature at which coma occurs will vary by individual, loss of consciousness in hypothermic patients generally occurs around 28°C[13] and hyperthermia-induced coma generally does not occur below a temperature of 40°C.[14]

Hypertension

Rarely, severe hypertension may result in a loss of vascular epithelial integrity in small vessels of the brain, resulting in a patchwork pattern of vascular narrowing and vasodilation, resulting in cerebral edema.[15] This condition, called posterior reversible encephalopathy syndrome, may present with significant alterations in consciousness.

Dysglycemia

Hypoglycemia may produce virtually any neurologic sign, symptom, or syndrome, including coma. Hypoglycemia is most common in diabetic patients who are taking hypoglycemic agents, such as insulin or sulfonylureas, and the rate of coma in such patients is about 1% to 2% per year.[16,17] Hyperglycemia may also cause coma, most commonly in the setting of a hyperosmolar hyperglycemic state (HHS) in which glucose levels are greater than 600 mg/dL and osmolality greater than 320 mOsm/kg.[18] Coma is more common in HHS than diabetic ketoacidosis (DKA). Serum osmolality is the driver of mental status changes in hyperglycemic states and HHS is associated with higher serum osmolality levels than DKA.[19]

Electrolyte Disorders

Disorders of sodium hemostasis, particularly when they are acute, may produce coma. Hyponatremia produces an imbalance of intracellular versus extracellular osmolality, the flow of free water into the brain parenchyma, and the development of cerebral edema.[20] Hypernatremia may also cause coma, and overly-rapid correction (particularly when the hypernatremia develops acutely) may lead to either demyelination or intracranial hemorrhage due to abrupt changes in intraparenchymal volume.[21]

Hypercalcemia is common in patients with advanced malignancy, occurring in 10% to 20% of such patients.[22] Although the most common neurologic presentations of hypercalcemia are confusion, delirium, or lethargy, coma is reported.[23]

Infection

Coma in the setting of infection may be due to one of several CNS infections. Profound coma is a rare presentation of meningitis[24] but is more commonly seen in fulminant cases. In one series, approximately 10% of subjects with encephalitis presented with coma (defined by the investigators as Glasgow Coma Scale [GCS] ≤ 8) and these subjects had poorer outcomes.[25]

Systemic non-CNS infections, such as sepsis, may also produce coma. The myriad biochemical and microcirculatory changes involved in sepsis-induced coma are incompletely understood but seem to activate neuroinflammatory and ischemic pathways culminating in dysfunction of the brain parenchyma.[26]

Thyroid Disorders

Myxedema coma is a severe form of hypothyroidism in which alterations in cerebral blood flow and glucose metabolism may lead to significant changes in mental status[27] and coma.[28] The alterations in mental status that accompany hyperthyroidism classically include nervousness and anxiety,[29] but decreases in mental status (which may include coma) may occur and are more common in the elderly.[30,31]

Renal Failure

Renal failure produces neurologic findings that include uremic encephalopathy, which in severe cases may manifest as coma.[32] The molecular basis of uremic encephalopathy is not fully elucidated but it is likely a multifactorial process that includes the accumulation of false neurotransmitters.

Hepatic Failure

Hepatic failure may lead to an encephalopathic state caused by either an accumulation of endogenous toxins (including ammonia) or cerebral edema.[33]

Hyperammonemia

Although hyperammonemia is a common finding in hepatic failure, nonhepatic hyperammonemia may cause coma as well. Valproic acid therapy in the setting of carnitine deficiency, infection with urease-producing bacteria, recent surgery (particularly lung transplantation, bariatric surgery or ureterosigmoidostomy), hyperalimentation, and errors of metabolism are also potential causes.[34]

Thiamine Deficiency

Thiamine deficiency is a common problem in malnourished patients. In the emergency department, thiamine deficiency is of particular concern in patients with alcohol-related presentations, not only in alcoholics but in binge drinkers as well.[35] Severe thiamine deficiency, usually seen in the context of alcoholism, may lead to Wernicke encephalopathy (characterized by encephalopathy, oculomotor dysfunction, and gait ataxia) or Korsakoff psychosis (a chronic amnestic condition). Coma as a presenting symptom of thiamine deficiency, however, is very uncommon.[36,37]

Nonconvulsive Status Epilepticus

NCSE is an epileptogenic condition in which the classic manifestations of seizure (eg, focal or general motor activity) are absent. NCSE may be mistaken for coma or unresponsiveness, and is an under-recognized cause of altered mental status in the emergency department.[38]

DIFFUSE NEURONAL DYSFUNCTION CAUSES OF COMA: TOXINS
Sedative-Hypnotic Agents

Sedative-hypnotic agents are a broad class of drugs that include ethanol, benzodiazepines, barbiturates, baclofen, gamma-hydroxybutyrate, and others. Most sedative-hypnotic agents act by facilitating the effect of the neurotransmitter gamma-aminobutyric acid (GABA), hyperpolarizing neurons either through an increase in chloride conductance (GABA$_A$)[39] or through an increase in potassium conductance (GABA$_B$).[40] Ethanol, in addition to interacting with the GABA system,[41] also produces some effects via interference with the excitatory neurotransmitter N-methyl-D-asparate (NMDA).[42]

Opioids

Opioids (ie, heroin, morphine, oxycodone, hydrocodone, and others) may produce profound decreases in mental status, including coma, in addition to other clinical findings such as respiratory depression. Opioid receptors are coupled to G proteins, which may exert their effects via adenylate cyclase, calcium channels, or potassium channels.[43] Opioids have multiple receptor subtypes, with the mu receptor responsible for coma.

Dissociative Agents

Phencyclidine and ketamine depress (and therefore interrupt) thalamic-cortical tracts,[44] producing a temporary state in which cardiorespiratory functions are preserved but in which the patient is dissociated from his or her higher functions. Dissociative agents likely exert most of their effects via NMDA antagonism but also have effects on opiate receptors and sympathetic neurotransmission.[45]

Carbon Monoxide

Carbon monoxide (CO) poisoning is alarmingly prevalent, accounting for approximately 50,000 visits per year to US emergency departments[46] and, in severe cases, presenting with coma.[47] CO is a complex toxin that affects oxyhemoglobin dissociation, increases oxidative stress, interrupts cellular respiration, and leads to the generation of reactive oxygen species. All of these may contribute to the development of neurologic impairment.[48]

Serotonin Syndrome and Neuroleptic Malignant Syndrome

Serotonin syndrome (SS) and neuroleptic malignant syndrome (NMS) are distinct entities with overlapping presentations that, when severe, include profound alterations in mental status, muscular rigidity, and hyperthermia. SS results from an excess of central and peripheral serotonin activity, often when two or more serotonergic agents are used together[49] NMS (although less well understood) likely results from central dopaminergic blockade.[50]

Miscellaneous Toxins

Several other toxins may produce coma. Toxic alcohols, such as methanol and ethylene glycol, are CNS depressants that produce coma in a manner similar to ethanol. Psychiatric medications, such as tricyclic antidepressants and serotonin selective reuptake inhibitors, may produce coma as an exaggeration of their normal pharmacologic effects. Simple asphyxiants, such as nitrogen, act by displacing oxygen and producing hypoxia. Agents of histotoxic hypoxia, such as cyanide, interfere with aerobic metabolism and the generation of adenosine triphosphate. Clonidine alters central sympathomimetic neurotransmission.

Coma Mimics

Four conditions deserve mention as coma mimics. The locked-in syndrome describes paralysis of all voluntary muscles of the body save the eyes, usually as a result of ischemia or infarction to key CNS tracts often involving the pons, with preservation of consciousness and higher cortical functions.[51] Neuromuscular paralysis may be iatrogenic, after the administration of succinycholine or curare-like drugs, or may arise from varied environmental sources, such as the toxin of *Clostridium botulinum*, the venom of elapid snakes,[52] or tetrodotoxin-producing organisms such as the blue-ringed octopus.[53] Akinetic mutism usually results from injury to the frontal or prefrontal motor cortex, in which patients cannot initiate voluntary motor movements.[54] In all 3 of these diseases, consciousness is preserved. The fourth coma mimic is psychogenic unresponsiveness, a complex disorder in which there is no neurologic insult; the condition resolves spontaneously.[55]

INITIAL STABILIZATION

The initial stabilization of comatose patients is the same as that for that of all emergency department patients and consists of securing the patients airway (with attention to the cervical spine), breathing, and circulation.

Decisions regarding airway management are often very difficult, driven by gestalt rather than algorithmic decision making, and are based on several factors. Mechanism of coma is important; although a GCS of 8 or less in a trauma patient is often viewed as an indication for intubation,[56,57] poisoned patients with such GCS levels can be managed without intubation and with low levels of complications.[58,59] Monitoring concerns may also enter into the decision-making process. Patients who require significant time out of the department for diagnostic imaging, as may occur during a computerized tomography (CT) scan, may require intubation; whereas patients who remain in an acute care area might be managed expectantly, even at the same level of consciousness. Expected clinical course, particularly in poisoned patients, is also a factor. The patient with an isolated alprazolam ingestion will likely do well without intubation, whereas a patient with carbamazepine ingestion is more likely to have a complicated course and require airway intervention.

Concurrently with airway management, the cervical spine must be stabilized whenever there is a possibility that the patient's alteration in mental status has a traumatic cause. Cervical spine injuries are commonly associated with alterations mental status of traumatic cause, occurring in 5% or more of such patients.[60,61]

HISTORY

Comatose patients by definition cannot give details of their illness, so it is crucial that the provider actively seek alternative sources of information. Emergency medical service responders often provide the most valuable information. They can relay information obtained from family members or bystanders, describe the patient's initial level of consciousness and how that has changed en route, provide a description of how the patient was found, and contribute important situational information such as the presence or absence of prescription bottles or drug paraphernalia. Ideally, the belongings of comatose patients should also be examined for clues, such as pill bottles in coat pockets or a purse, a pharmacy phone number, or a medication list in a wallet. Finally, medical alert bracelets or information from the institution's medical record may shed light on an otherwise confusing presentation.

To the extent possible, the clinician should establish the rate of progression of symptoms. Coma because of subarachnoid hemorrhage, cerebellar infarction, and IPH is usually of abrupt onset, whereas coma from infection may evolve over hours to days. Coma from poisoning may occur over minutes if caused by a large dose of drug (eg, an opioid) or a rapidly acting toxin (eg, volatilized cyanide after malicious mixing with a soft drink). Alternatively, it may occur over the course of hours if the patient over-titrates a self-administered substance (eg, ethanol) or ingests a substance that may have delayed toxicity (eg, baclofen).

Importantly, when obtaining historical information, providers must avoid the errors of premature closure and diagnostic anchoring.[62] For example, alcohol is ubiquitous in many western countries and its presence may be coincident with, rather than causative of, coma. SDH and hypoglycemia are life-threatening causes of coma that may coexist with ethanol intoxication.[63,64] As with any condition, physicians evaluating patients with coma must be willing to reconsider initial impressions when additional data, such as a fever or classic physical examination findings, are inconsistent with the initial working diagnosis.

PHYSICAL EXAMINATION

A complete physical examination will provide clues to the diagnosis of coma and help streamline the patient's diagnostic evaluation. Crucial physical examination findings, and the important causes of coma associated with them, are listed below.

VITAL SIGNS
Pulse

Bradycardia may occur in the context of sympatholytic drugs, such as clonidine; in the setting of sedative hypnotic toxicity, particularly with barbiturates and gamma-hydroxybutyrate; and with increases in intracranial pressure, characteristically accompanied by systemic hypertension. Tachycardia is common with psychotropic drug poisoning, ketamine intoxication, adrenergic hyperactivity from intracranial hemorrhage, and 3,4-methylenedioxymethamphetamine (MDMA) intoxication, which produces coma via symptomatic hyponatremia.[65]

Blood Pressure

Hypotension may occur in sepsis and many poisonings, particularly tricyclic antidepressants, sedative-hypnotic agents, and clonidine. Hypertension is a prerequisite for the diagnosis of hypertensive encephalopathy and is common in ketamine or phencyclidine intoxication, MDMA intoxication, and in the setting of increased intracranial pressure. In the cases of elevated intracranial pressure, the hypertension is usually accompanied by bradycardia, a combination known as Cushing response.

Respiratory Rate

Tachypnea is common with metabolic acidosis of any cause. Bradypnea may be seen in both opioid and sedative-hypnotic toxicity but is much more pronounced in the former. Bradypnea in the setting of structural CNS disease suggests medullary involvement and is often a preterminal event.

Temperature

Hyperthermia may be due to environmental exposure, infection, NMS, SS, salicylate poisoning, and several primary CNS disorders, including subarachnoid hemorrhage and hypothalamic injury. Hypothermia is commonly due to environmental exposure but may also be seen with hypoglycemia of any cause, sedative-hypnotic toxicity, hypothyroidism, and overwhelming infection.

Physical Examination

Head, eyes, ears, nose, and throat
Head Examination of the head may show obvious signs of deformity, such as crepitus or bony step-offs in the setting of a skull fracture. Other signs suggestive of basilar skull fracture that should be specifically evaluated are bilateral orbital ecchymosis (Raccoon Eyes) and postauricular bruising (Battle's sign).

Eyes Miosis is commonly seen in opioid and clonidine toxicity, and may also be seen in the setting of pontine hemorrhage. Mydriasis is common in poisoning with compounds with anticholinergic properties (eg, tricyclic antidepressants) and MDMA. Horizontal nystagmus is common in ethanol intoxication and with toxicity from antiepileptic drugs. Vertical nystagmus is uncommon and suggests dissociative agents (eg, phencyclidine and ketamine) or brainstem dysfunction. Gaze deviation may be in response to an ipsilateral hemispheric lesion, a contralateral pontine lesion, or a seizure focus. Roving eye movements do not specifically localize a lesion but suggest that the brainstem is intact. When ice water irrigation of the ear is performed in normal patients, there is tonic deviation of the eyes toward the side of the irrigation followed by rapid nystagmus away from the side of the irrigation. Loss of the former suggests a midbrain or pontine lesion, loss of the latter suggests a cortical lesion, and loss of neither suggests psychogenic coma.

Ears Hemotympanum may be seen in approximately 50% of basilar skull fractures.[66]

Throat Dry mucous membranes are suggestive of profound dehydration or anticholinergic toxicity, whereas increased salivation may be seen with ketamine toxicity.

Skin

Excessively dry skin suggests poisoning with a drug with anticholinergic properties, such as tricyclic antidepressants. Diaphoresis may be seen in any hyperadrenergic state. Coma bullae are classically associated with barbiturate toxicity but may also be seen in other settings, such as infection.[67] Small linear areas of pinprick-size trauma over veins (track marks) suggest the ongoing abuse of intravenous drugs, particularly opioids, but cannot be used in and of themselves to diagnose the cause of a comatose state.

Bowel Sounds

Markedly decreased bowel sounds are associated with both anticholinergic toxicity and opioid toxicity.

The Toxidrome-Oriented Physical Examination

Syndromes are a constellation of signs or symptoms that together suggest a certain disease entity. In humans, certain toxins or classes of toxins produce stereotypical physical examination findings. These toxic syndromes, or toxidromes, can provide invaluable information. In comatose patients, the use of vital signs and examination of the eye, throat (mucous membranes), skin, and bowel sounds may yield a pattern that strongly suggests a given class of toxins (**Table 2**).

IMAGING AND LABORATORY TESTING

Although a thorough history and physical examination will often generate a refined differential diagnosis, imaging studies and laboratory testing play an important role in the diagnosis of coma. Such interventions, however, should serve to refine clinical impressions and should not be ordered indiscriminately as a substitute for thoughtful patient evaluation.

When coma is obviously caused by diffuse neuronal dysfunction, such as hypoglycemia or a known ingestion, CT is rarely if ever necessary. The diagnostic yield of CT in this setting is exceedingly low.[68] When a structural cause is suspected, particularly in the setting of trauma, CT of the head is essential and will often identify the lesion. In the emergency department, most patients with a structural cause of coma will have a hemorrhagic syndrome.

MRI scans allow greater definition of cortical and subcortical structures and may show cortical injury, laminar necrosis, or white matter disease that is not apparent on a CT scan. Magnetic resonance angiography allows for excellent visualization of the arterial system and is the preferred method for visualization of suspected acute basilar artery occlusion; however, this may not be possible at all institutions. In such instances, CT angiogram or conventional angiography can allow for rapid visualization of the arterial system. The major drawbacks of MRI scans include accessibility, cost, and time necessary to complete the scan.

The authors believe that basic laboratory testing should include the following at a minimum: a complete blood count, to assess for leukocytosis as corroborating evidence of infection and to assess the numerical adequacy of platelets in the event of CNS hemorrhage; an electrocardiogram, to exclude toxin-induced conduction system abnormalities; serum glucose, preferably via a rapid bedside test; serum electrolytes,

Table 2
Physical examination findings for ingestions producing coma

Finding	Opiates	Sedative-Hypnotic Agents	Dissociative Agents
Pulse	Normal vs decreased	Normal vs decreased	Increased
Blood pressure	Normal vs decreased	Normal vs decreased	Increased
Respiratory rate	Markedly decreased	Normal vs decreased	Normal
Mucous membranes	Normal	Normal	Salivation (ketamine)
Eyes	Miosis	Normal	Nystagmus
Skin	Normal	Normal	Normal
Bowel sounds	Markedly decreased	Normal	Normal

including calcium; and tests of renal and hepatic function. Additional high-yield testing in the correct clinical setting may include a serum ammonia level as a marker for hepatic encephalopathy, or as a primary hyperammonemic disorder that may occur in the setting of valproic acid treatment.[69] An arterial or venous blood gas may also be helpful, particularly when poisoning with salicylates, toxic alcohols, or CO is suspected.

The authors discourage the routine use of urine drug screen (UDS) testing, for several reasons. First, such tests do not measure intoxication or toxicity but, instead, the presence of a drug or drug metabolite, meaning that findings on a positive UDS may be coincident with, rather than causative of, coma. Second, UDS tests may show false negative results. For example, not all benzodiazepines react with commonly used commercial benzodiazepine assays.[70] In such cases, over-reliance on a UDS may cause a clinician to reject a diagnosis that is clinically apparent. Third, UDS tests may generate false-positive results; this is particularly true with the phencyclidine assay, which is often positive in the setting of commonly used medications such as the cough suppressant dextromethorphan.[71] Finally, and perhaps most importantly, studies suggest that UDS testing does not significantly affect clinical decision making.[72,73]

Electroencephalographic (EEG) testing may be useful in patients who have a history of a seizure disorder, or who have had several seizures before the development of coma, to exclude NCSE. The authors strongly recommend against emergency department EEG testing when an alternative diagnosis is clear, such as a large subdural hematoma, or strongly suspected in the case of patients with clear alcohol intoxication. When EEG is used in the ED, the authors suggest that an abbreviated protocol be used if at all possible.[74]

Lumbar puncture should be performed in any case in which meningitis or encephalitis is suspected. Historical context, such as a close contact with meningitis; symptoms, such as photophobia or neck pain; or physical signs, such as a fever or meningismus, may all suggest a CNS infection. Unfortunately, historical and physical examination findings are neither sensitive nor specific for the diagnosis of CNS infection.[75] Therefore, the decision to perform a lumbar puncture must be made on a case-by-case basis by the treating physician. Generally, the authors do not advocate for routine lumbar puncture in all comatose patients, particularly in those for whom an alternative diagnosis is established or strongly suspected.

GRADING SYSTEMS

Grading systems allow providers to quickly convey a general sense of the patient's condition. This is particularly important when one provider cannot examine the patient, as may occurs in telephone discussions between providers or during emergency medical service communications.

Two major grading systems are used to assess the depths of coma (**Table 3**). The GCS, first described in 1974,[76] is a 15-point composite score of eye, motor, and verbal responses developed to assess patients with head trauma. The Full Outline of Unresponsiveness (FOUR) score, first described in 2005, is a 16-point scale that assesses eye, motor, brainstem reflexes, and respirations.[77] Both rely on clinical findings, have high inter-rater reliability,[78] and can be performed quickly. The FOUR score has a benefit over GCS in that one of three of the GCS criteria is unreliable in intubated patients. The FOUR score is also a better predictor of mortality in critically ill patients.[79]

Table 3
Glasgow coma scale and full outline of unresponsiveness (FOUR) score

Glasgow Coma Scale	Full Outline of Unresponsiveness Score
Eye Opening Response	Eye response
Spontaneously, 4	Open and tracking or blinking to command, 4
To speech, 3	Open but not tracking, 3
To pain, 1	Closed but open to loud voice, 2
Best Verbal Response	Closed but open to pain, 1
Oriented, 5	Closed with pain, 0
Disoriented, 5	Motor response
Inappropriate words, 4	Thumbs up, fist or peace sign, 4
Incomprehensible sounds, 3	Localizes pain, 3
No response, 1	Flexion response to pain, 2
Best Motor Response	Extension response to pain, 1
Obeys commands, 6	No response to pain or myoclonic status, 0
Localizes pain, 5	Brainstem reflexes
Withdrawal from pain, 4	Pupil and corneal reflexes present, 4
Decorticate flexion, 3	1 pupil wide and fixed, 3
Decerebrate extension, 2	Pupil or corneal reflexes absent, 2
No movement, 1	Pupil and corneal reflexes absent, 1
	Absent pupil, corneal and cough reflex, 0
	Respiration
	Not intubated, regular pattern, 4
	Not intubated, Cheyne-Stokes pattern, 3
	Not intubated, irregular breathing, 2
	Breathes above ventilator rate, 1
	Breathes at ventilator rate or apnea, 0

Importantly, both systems exist as scales, meaning that coma is rarely a yes or no delineation. Although many investigators define coma as a GCS of less than 8, this cutoff represents an arbitrary choice more than a significant physiologic distinction.

TREATMENT

The ultimate treatment of coma depends on the cause. In general, there are three overarching themes regarding the treatment of coma.

First, coma from structural causes may be catastrophic and untreatable. However, when the cause is treatable, it can be treated surgically or with geographically targeted pharmacologic or mechanical intervention. The authors advocate for the early involvement of neurosurgical specialists for patients with coma from intracranial hemorrhage or hydrocephalus because early intervention can have an extraordinary effect on both mortality and long-term outcomes. Patients with ischemic cerebrovascular disease should be promptly assessed, ideally by a team that includes a neurologist, to assess their candidacy for either intravenous or intra-arterial thrombolysis.

Second, in patients whose coma is a result of a metabolically induced diffuse neuronal dysfunction, treatment involves progress toward homeostasis. In some cases, such as hypoglycemia and respiratory insufficiency, the goal is expeditious normalization of values such as serum glucose or the partial pressure of oxygen or carbon dioxide in the blood. In other cases, such as hypertensive encephalopathy and hyponatremia, the correct initial treatment involves only a partial correction, and an abrupt return to normal could be clinically devastating.[80]

Third, in patients whose coma is a result of a toxin-induced diffuse neuronal dysfunction, the most important intervention, established more than 50 years ago, is the provision of appropriate supportive care.[81] Initial supportive care includes securing the airway, assuring adequate oxygenation and ventilation, and assuring appropriate circulation with intravenous fluids and, if necessary, vasopressors. Advanced supportive care may include altering systemic or compartmental pH to reduce drug toxicity or increase drug excretion, such as administering sodium bicarbonate for tricyclic antidepressant or salicylate toxicity, or the administration of intravenous lipid emulsion to alter drug distribution.[82] Although there are specific toxins that induce coma for which specific antidotal therapy may be critical or lifesaving (eg, fomepizole for toxic alcohols, hydroxocobalamin for cyanide, or naloxone for opioids), antidotal therapy plays little or no role in treating most toxins that may produce coma.

SUMMARY

Coma represents a true medical emergency. Although drug intoxications are a leading cause of coma in patients who present to the emergency department, other metabolic disturbances and traumatic brain injury are common causes as well. The general emergency department approach to the patient with coma begins with stabilization of airway, breathing, and circulation, followed by a thorough physical examination to generate a limited differential diagnosis that is then refined by focused testing. Definitive treatment is ultimately disease-specific.

REFERENCES

1. Edlow BL, Takahashi E, Wu O, et al. Neuroanatomic connectivity of the human ascending arousal system critical to consciousness and its disorders. J Neuropathol Exp Neurol 2012;71(6):531–46.
2. Sarasso S, Rosanova M, Casali AG, et al. Quantifying cortical EEG responses to TMS in (un)consciousness. Clin EEG Neurosci 2014;45(1):40–9.
3. Widjicks EFM. The comatose patient. Oxford University Press; 2014.
4. Han CY, Backous DD. Basic principles of cerebrospinal fluid metabolism and intracranial pressure homeostasis [review]. Otolaryngol Clin North Am 2005; 38(4):569–76.
5. Gorelick PB, Hier DB, Caplan LR, et al. Headache in acute cerebrovascular disease. Neurology 1986;36(11):1445–50.
6. Gaucher DJ Jr, Perez JA Jr. Subdural hematoma following lumbar puncture. Arch Intern Med 2002;162(16):1904–5.
7. Miller JD, Nader R. Acute subdural hematoma from bridging vein rupture: a potential mechanism for growth [review]. J Neurosurg 2014;120(6):1378–84.
8. Maxeiner H, Wolff M. Pure subdural hematomas: a postmortem analysis of their form and bleeding points. Neurosurgery 2007;61(Suppl 1):267–72 [discussion: 272–3].
9. De Bonis P, Trevisi G, de Waure C, et al. Antiplatelet/anticoagulant agents and chronic subdural hematoma in the elderly. PLoS One 2013;8(7):e68732.
10. Bullock MR, Chesnut R, Ghajar J, et al, Surgical Management of Traumatic Brain Injury Author Group. Surgical management of acute epidural hematomas [review]. Neurosurgery 2006;58(Suppl 3):S7–15 [discussion: Si–Siv].
11. Mayr R, Troyer S, Kastenberger T, et al. The impact of coagulopathy on the outcome of traumatic epidural hematoma. Arch Orthop Trauma Surg 2012; 132(10):1445–50.
12. Aguilar MI, Freeman WD. Spontaneous intracerebral hemorrhage [review]. Semin Neurol 2010;30(5):555–64.

13. Brown DJ, Brugger H, Boyd J, et al. Accidental hypothermia [review]. N Engl J Med 2012;367(20):1930–8 [Erratum appears in N Engl J Med 2013;368(4):394].
14. Bouchama A, Knochel JP. Heat stroke [review]. N Engl J Med 2002;346(25): 1978–88.
15. Strandgaard S, Paulson OB. Cerebral blood flow and its pathophysiology in hypertension. Am J Hypertens 1989;2(6 Pt 1):486–92.
16. Schloot NC, Haupt A, Schütt M, et al, German/Austrian DPV Initiative. Risk of severe hypoglycemia in sulfonylurea-treated patients from diabetes centers in Germany/Austria: how big is the problem? which patients are at risk? Diabetes Metab Res Rev 2016;32(3):316–24.
17. Kurien M, Mollazadegan K, Sanders DS, et al. A nationwide population-based study on the risk of coma, ketoacidosis and hypoglycemia in patients with celiac disease and type 1 diabetes. Acta Diabetol 2015;52(6):1167–74.
18. Pasquel FJ, Umpierrez GE. Hyperosmolar hyperglycemic state: a historic review of the clinical presentation, diagnosis, and treatment [review]. Diabetes Care 2014;37(11):3124–31.
19. Lorber D. Nonketotic hypertonicity in diabetes mellitus [review]. Med Clin North Am 1995;79(1):39–52.
20. Verbalis JG, Goldsmith SR, Greenberg A, et al. Diagnosis, evaluation, and treatment of hyponatremia: expert panel recommendations. Am J Med 2013;126(10 Suppl 1):S1–42.
21. Sterns RH. Disorders of plasma sodium–causes, consequences, and correction [review]. N Engl J Med 2015;372(1):55–65.
22. Legrand SB. Modern management of malignant hypercalcemia [review]. Am J Hosp Palliat Care 2011;28(7):515–7.
23. Ben-Asuly S, Horne T, Goldschmidt Z, et al. Coma due to hypercalcemia in a patient with Paget's disease and multiple parathyroid adenomata. Am J Med Sci 1975;269(2):267–75.
24. Lucas MJ, Brouwer MC, van der Ende A, et al. Outcome in patients with bacterial meningitis presenting with a minimal Glasgow Coma Scale score. Neurol Neuroimmunol Neuroinflamm 2014;1(1):e9.
25. Singh TD, Fugate JE, Rabinstein AA. The spectrum of acute encephalitis: causes, management, and predictors of outcome. Neurology 2015;84(4):359–66.
26. Adam N, Kandelman S, Mantz J, et al. Sepsis-induced brain dysfunction [review]. Expert Rev Anti Infect Ther 2013;11(2):211–21.
27. Constant EL, de Volder AG, Ivanoiu A, et al. Cerebral blood flow and glucose metabolism in hypothyroidism: a positron emission tomography study. J Clin Endocrinol Metab 2001;86(8):3864–70.
28. Kwaku MP, Burman KD. Myxedema coma [review]. J Intensive Care Med 2007; 22(4):224–31.
29. Devereaux D, Tewelde SZ. Hyperthyroidism and thyrotoxicosis [review]. Emerg Med Clin North Am 2014;32(2):277–92.
30. Boelaert K, Torlinska B, Holder RL, et al. Older subjects with hyperthyroidism present with a paucity of symptoms and signs: a large cross-sectional study. J Clin Endocrinol Metab 2010;95(6):2715–26.
31. Ghobrial MW, Ruby EB. Coma and thyroid storm in apathetic thyrotoxicosis [review]. South Med J 2002;95(5):552–4.
32. Seifter JL, Samuels MA. Uremic encephalopathy and other brain disorders associated with renal failure [review]. Semin Neurol 2011;31(2):139–43.
33. Bernal W, Wendon J. Acute liver failure. N Engl J Med 2013;369(26):2525–34.

34. LaBuzetta JN, Yao JZ, Bourque DL, et al. Adult nonhepatic hyperammonemia: a case report and differential diagnosis [review]. Am J Med 2010;123(10):885–91.
35. Li SF, Jacob J, Feng J, et al. Vitamin deficiencies in acutely intoxicated patients in the ED. Am J Emerg Med 2008;26(7):792–5.
36. Wallis WE, Willoughby E, Baker P. Coma in the Wernicke-Korsakoff syndrome. Lancet 1978;2(8086):400–1.
37. Gibb WR, Gorsuch AN, Lees AJ, et al. Reversible coma in Wernicke's encephalopathy. Postgrad Med J 1985;61(717):607–10.
38. Zehtabchi S, Abdel Baki SG, Malhotra S, et al. Nonconvulsive seizures in patients presenting with altered mental status: an evidence-based review [review]. Epilepsy Behav 2011;22(2):139–43.
39. Olsen RW, Yang J, King RG, et al. Barbiturate and benzodiazepine modulation of GABA receptor binding and function [review]. Life Sci 1986;39(21):1969–76.
40. Emson PC. GABA(B) receptors: structure and function [review]. Prog Brain Res 2007;160:43–57.
41. Valenzuela CF, Jotty K. Mini-review: effects of ethanol on GABAA receptor-mediated neurotransmission in the cerebellar cortex–recent advances. Cerebellum 2015;14(4):438–46.
42. He Q, Titley H, Grasselli G, et al. Ethanol affects NMDA receptor signaling at climbing fiber-Purkinje cell synapses in mice and impairs cerebellar LTD. J Neurophysiol 2013;109(5):1333–42.
43. Waldhoer M, Bartlett SE, Whistler JL. Opioid receptors [review]. Annu Rev Biochem 2004;73:953–90.
44. Miyasaka M, Domino EF. Neural mechanisms of ketamine-induced anesthesia. Int J Neuropharmacol 1968;7(6):557–73.
45. Stahl SM. Mechanism of action of ketamine. CNS Spectr 2013;18(4):171–4.
46. Hampson NB, Weaver LK. Carbon monoxide poisoning: a new incidence for an old disease. Undersea Hyperb Med 2007;34(3):163–8.
47. Ku CH, Hung HM, Leong WC, et al. Outcome of patients with carbon monoxide poisoning at a far-east poison center. PLoS One 2015;10(3):e0118995.
48. Weaver LK. Clinical practice. Carbon monoxide poisoning [review]. N Engl J Med 2009;360(12):1217–25.
49. Boyer EW, Shannon M. The serotonin syndrome [review]. N Engl J Med 2005; 352(11):1112–20 [Erratum appears in N Engl J Med 2009;361(17):1714; N Engl J Med 2007;356(23):2437].
50. Caroff SN, Mann SC. Neuroleptic malignant syndrome [review]. Med Clin North Am 1993;77(1):185–202.
51. Cardwell MS. Locked-in syndrome. Tex Med 2013;109(2):e1.
52. Bawaskar HS, Bawaskar PH. Envenoming by the common krait (*Bungarus caeruleus*) and Asian cobra (*Naja naja*): clinical manifestations and their management in a rural setting. Wilderness Environ Med 2004;15(4):257–66.
53. Cavazzoni E, Lister B, Sargent P, et al. Blue-ringed octopus (*Hapalochlaena* sp.) envenomation of a 4-year-old boy: a case report. Clin Toxicol (Phila) 2008;46(8): 760–1.
54. Ackermann H, Ziegler W. Akinetic mutism–a review of the literature [review]. Fortschr Neurol Psychiatr 1995;63(2):59–67 [in German].
55. Baxter CL, White WD. Psychogenic coma: case report. Int J Psychiatry Med 2003;33(3):317–22.
56. Dunham CM, Barraco RD, Clark DE, et al, EAST Practice Management Guidelines Work Group. Guidelines for emergency tracheal intubation immediately after traumatic injury [review]. J Trauma 2003;55(1):162–79.

57. Davis DP. Prehospital intubation of brain-injured patients [review]. Curr Opin Crit Care 2008;14(2):142–8.

58. Dietze P, Horyniak D, Agius P, et al. Effect of intubation for gamma-hydroxybutyric acid overdose on emergency department length of stay and hospital admission. Acad Emerg Med 2014;21(11):1226–31.

59. Duncan R, Thakore S. Decreased Glasgow Coma Scale score does not mandate endotracheal intubation in the emergency department. J Emerg Med 2009;37(4): 451–5.

60. Schenarts PJ, Diaz J, Kaiser C, et al. Prospective comparison of admission computed tomographic scan and plain films of the upper cervical spine in trauma patients with altered mental status. J Trauma 2001;51(4):663–8 [discussion: 668–9].

61. Diaz JJ Jr, Gillman C, Morris JA Jr, et al. Are five-view plain films of the cervical spine unreliable? A prospective evaluation in blunt trauma patients with altered mental status. J Trauma 2003;55(4):658–63 [discussion: 663–4].

62. Eva KW, Link CL, Lutfey KE, et al. Swapping horses midstream: factors related to physicians' changing their minds about a diagnosis. Acad Med 2010;85(7): 1112–7.

63. Heninger M. Subdural hematoma occurrence: comparison between ethanol and cocaine use at death. Am J Forensic Med Pathol 2013;34(3):237–41.

64. Williams HE. Alcoholic hypoglycemia and ketoacidosis [review]. Med Clin North Am 1984;68(1):33–8.

65. Traub SJ, Hoffman RS, Nelson LS. The "ecstasy" hangover: hyponatremia due to 3,4-methylenedioxy-methamphetamine. J Urban Health 2002;79(4):549–55.

66. Liu-Shindo M, Hawkins DB. Basilar skull fractures in children. Int J Pediatr Otorhinolaryngol 1989;17(2):109–17.

67. Bosco L, Schena D, Colato C, et al. Coma blisters in children: case report and review of the literature [review]. J Child Neurol 2013;28(12):1677–80.

68. Forsberg S, Höjer J, Ludwigs U, et al. Metabolic vs structural coma in the ED–an observational study. Am J Emerg Med 2012;30(9):1986–90.

69. Cuturic M, Abramson RK. Acute hyperammonemic coma with chronic valproic acid therapy. Ann Pharmacother 2005;39(12):2119–23.

70. Bertol E, Vaiano F, Borsotti M, et al. Comparison of immunoassay screening tests and LC-MS-MS for urine detection of benzodiazepines and their metabolites: results of a national proficiency test. J Anal Toxicol 2013;37(9):659–64.

71. Rengarajan A, Mullins ME. How often do false-positive phencyclidine urine screens occur with use of common medications? Clin Toxicol (Phila) 2013; 51(6):493–6.

72. Brett AS. Implications of discordance between clinical impression and toxicology analysis in drug overdose. Arch Intern Med 1988;148(2):437–41.

73. Bast RP, Helmer SD, Henson SR, et al. Limited utility of routine drug screening in trauma patients. South Med J 2000;93(4):397–9.

74. Bautista RE, Godwin S, Caro D. Incorporating abbreviated EEGs in the initial workup of patients who present to the emergency room with mental status changes of unknown etiology. J Clin Neurophysiol 2007;24(1):16–21.

75. Brouwer MC, Thwaites GE, Tunkel AR, et al. Dilemmas in the diagnosis of acute community-acquired bacterial meningitis [review]. Lancet 2012;380(9854): 1684–92.

76. Teasdale G, Jennett B. Assessment of coma and impaired consciousness. A practical scale. Lancet 1974;2(7872):81–4.

77. Wijdicks EF, Bamlet WR, Maramattom BV, et al. Validation of a new coma scale: the FOUR score. Ann Neurol 2005;58(4):585–93.
78. Sadaka F, Patel D, Lakshmanan R. The FOUR score predicts outcome in patients after traumatic brain injury. Neurocrit Care 2012;16(1):95–101.
79. Wijdicks EF, Kramer AA, Rohs T Jr, et al. Comparison of the full outline of unresponsiveness score and the Glasgow Coma Scale in predicting mortality in critically ill patients. Crit Care Med 2015;43(2):439–44.
80. Rafat C, Flamant M, Gaudry S, et al. Hyponatremia in the intensive care unit: how to avoid a Zugzwang situation? Ann Intensive Care 2015;5(1):39.
81. Cemmmesen C, Nilson E. Therapeutic trends in the treatment of barbiturate poisoning. The Scandinavian method. Clin Pharmacol Ther 1961;2:220–9.
82. Ozcan MS, Weinberg G. Intravenous lipid emulsion for the treatment of drug toxicity [review]. J Intensive Care Med 2014;29(2):59–70.

Acute Generalized Weakness

Latha Ganti, MD, MS, MBA[a],*, Vaibhav Rastogi, MD[b]

KEYWORDS

- Acute weakness • Guillain-Barre syndrome • Myasthenia gravis • Periodic paralysis
- Transverse myelitis • Tick paralysis • Botulism

KEY POINTS

- True neuromuscular weakness needs to be distinguished from fatigue, asthenia, and malaise.
- Asking the patient what he or she can no longer is an excellent method of localizing weakness.
- Although many of the neuromuscular diseases discussed in this article are each relatively rare, as a combined entity they represent the largest percent of etiologies for neuromuscular weakness.
- Evaluation of acute generalized weakness in the emergency department begins with a broad differential that is systematically narrowed down with clues from the history, physical examination and diagnostic investigations.

INTRODUCTION

Weakness is a common complaint in the emergency department (ED), and a most challenging one, because before the emergency physician can proceed with an evaluation, the complaint of weakness must be fully clarified to determine about what the patient is actually complaining.

A prospective observational study from Switzerland underscores the vast differential diagnosis of the chief complaint of weakness.[1] Of 79 consecutive patients presenting to the ED with generalized weakness, the spectrum of diagnoses spanned 14 distinct international classification of disease-10 codes. The most frequent were diseases of the respiratory system (18%), followed by endocrine, nutritional, and metabolic diseases (14%), and neoplasms (10%). Infections were the most common cause of generalized weakness. The authors attributed this to the median age of 78 in their cohort; this

Disclosures: The authors have nothing to disclose.
a University of Central Florida College of Medicine, 6850 Lake Nona Blvd, Orlando, FL 32827, USA; b Department of Internal Medicine, North Florida Regional Medical Center, 6500 W Newberry Road, Gainesville, FL, USA
* Corresponding author.
E-mail addresses: lathagantimd@gmail.com; latha.ganti@ucf.edu

highlights the fact that older patients may not have fever, cough, or other specific signs of infection, but rather present with generalized weakness.

When patients complain about weakness, the first distinction that is important to make is whether it is true neuromuscular weakness, or rather feeling fatigue, malaise, or asthenia. Fatigue is the inability to continue performing a task after multiple repetitions; the muscle gets weak after sustained activity. Malaise is a general feeling of being ill or having no energy. Malaise is perhaps more properly described as asthenia, which is defined as a sense of weariness or exhaustion in the absence of muscle weakness.[2] The key difference is that with true neuromuscular weakness, the patient is unable to partially or fully perform the task in the first place.

Weakness can be unilateral or bilateral. The most common cause of unilateral weakness is acute brain infarction or ischemia (stroke or transient ischemic attack) and intracerebral hemorrhage (including subarachnoid hemorrhage). As these entities are covered elsewhere in this issue, they will not be discussed here. Poisons are also a class of other potential contributors to weakness, which have their own vast separate discussion. The focus of this article will thus be causes of acute generalized nontraumatic bilateral weakness. Evaluation begins with the history and physical examination, followed by diagnostic testing in some cases.

HISTORY
Onset

The timing of weakness can sometimes provide a clue to diagnosis. Generally, weakness that develops minutes to hours prior to presentation is due to metabolic (electrolyte) or toxic disorders or stroke. Weakness that have begun within the last 24 hours includes etiologies such as acute porphyric neuropathy, Guillian Barre syndrome (GBS), myasthenia gravis (MG), and tick paralysis. Weakness that has been going on for a week or longer is often associated with peripheral nerve problems, and neuromuscular junction (NMJ) diseases. Weakness characterized by frequent relapses is suggestive of multiple sclerosis, periodic paralysis, and myasthenia gravis. Weakness that is transient in nature is seen with peripheral nerve entrapment problems, hemiplegic migraine, and periodic paralysis.

Description of Weakness

Asking the patient what he or she can no longer do or do without difficulty is a good start to localizing the problem. For example, difficulty combing one's hair or climbing stairs suggests proximal muscle weakness, whereas difficulty buttoning one's shirt, or turning a door knob indicate distal muscle weakness. Dysphagia, a nasal voice, and dysarthria are associated with bulbar muscle weakness and raise concern for impending airway compromise. Generally, proximal muscle weakness suggests a myopathic process, while distal muscle weakness indicates a (poly)neuropathy.

Comorbidities

Underlying systemic illnesses can contribute to the presentation of weakness. For example, diabetes and some rheumatic disorders cause neuropathy.

Family History

A family history of dystrophy, periodic paralysis, porphyria, paraneoplastic syndromes, and hereditary predisposition to pressure palsies can be important in generating an appropriate differential diagnosis. Sometime patients may not know the names of diseases, so asking about specific symptoms as in the patient history may be more useful.

Medications

A number of medications can cause myopathy (muscle disease), most notably the statins that are in widespread use. **Box 1** summarizes some of the most common drugs associated with myopathies.[3,4] Myopathies can also be inherited (eg, muscular dystrophies) or acquired.

PHYSICAL EXAMINATION
Motor Nervous System

Weakness can be caused by problems affecting upper motor neurons (UMNs), lower motor neurons (LMNs), NMJ, or the muscle itself (**Fig. 1**).

The LMNs are comprised of anterior horn cells and innervate the skeletal muscle. UMNs provide impulses and regulate the activity of lower motor neurons.[5] The neuromuscular junction is a chemical synapse formed by the contact between the motor neuron and a muscle fiber.

The motor neuronal pathway originates in the primary motor cortex (precentral gyrus) of the cerebral cortex. The corticobulbar and corticospinal tracts are the 2 main pathways of motor conduction, with the majority of axons from the corticospinal tract. Corticobulbar fibers terminate in the brain stem. Corticospinal fibers pass through the internal capsule; most of them cross to the contralateral side in the brain stem (pyramidal decussations of the medulla) and continue as lateral corticospinal tract in the spinal cord. They ultimately terminate in the gray matter of the spinal cord. Peripheral

Box 1
Drugs that can cause myopathy
HMG Co-A reductase inhibitors (statins)
Gemfibrozil
Alcohol
D-penicillamine
Interferon α
Procainamide
Zidovudine
Lamivudine
Germanium
Colchicine
Vincristine
Quinine drugs
Amiodarone
Emetine
Ipecac
Corticosteroids
Hydroxyurea
Leuprolide
Sulfonamides

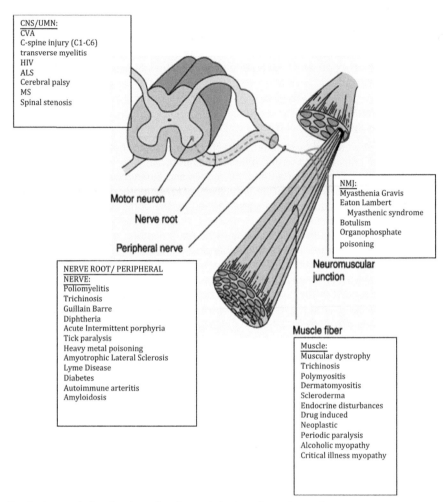

Fig. 1. Anatomic localization of various etiologies of muscle weakness.

nerves (LMNs) arising from the spinal cord supply skeletal muscle. LMN disorders affect a particular muscle that is innervated by that nerve. Signs of LMN disease include decreased muscle tone, hyporeflexia, fasciculations, and an absent Babinski sign (**Table 1**). The Babinski sign is extension, (rather than the normal flexion response)

Table 1 Comparison of the signs of upper motor neuron versus lower motor neuron		
Sign	**UMN**	**LMN**
Reflexes	↑	↓
Atrophy	−	+
Weakness	+	+
Fasciculations	−	+
Tone	↑	↓
Extensor	+	−

of the hallux (great toe) in response to stimulation of the sole of the foot with a blunt instrument.

Examples of LMN problems include: poliomyelitis, lower spinal cord injury (L4-S2) with nerve root compression, amyotrophic lateral sclerosis (ALS), progressive spinal muscular atrophy, spondylotic myelopathy, and radiation myelopathy. Problems that affect the peripheral nerves include

Trauma (including entrapment)
Toxins such as lead, alcohol, and many drugs
Infectious causes such as diphtheria, Lyme disease, and human immunodeficiency
    virus (HIV)
Inflammatory polyneuropathies such as GBS
Metabolic derangements such as diabetes and porphyria
Vascular problems such as autoimmune arteritis
Nutritional disturbances such as vitamin B1 or B12 deficit or pyridoxine toxicity
Heredity conditions such as Charcot-Marie-Tooth disease
Neoplasms
Abnormal proteins (amyloidosis).

By contrast, UMN disorders have widespread manifestations and a more complicated pathophysiology. Signs of UMN disease include increased muscle tone (spasticity), hyper-reflexia, and a positive Babinski. Examples of problems associated with UMN disease include cerebrovascular accidents, intracranial tumor, cervical spine injury (C1-C6), transverse myelitis, HIV, ALS, cerebral palsy, multiple sclerosis, and spinal stenosis.

Diseases of the NMJ are characterized by fluctuating strength based on muscle use. The classic examples of NMJ diseases are myasthenia gravis, where repeated contractions result in decreasing power, and Lambert Eaton myasthenic syndrome, in which repeated contractions result in increasing power. Botulism and organo phosphate poisoning are other examples.

Diseases that cause myopathy include

Congenital problems such as muscular dystrophy
Infection such as trichinosis
Connective tissue disease such as polymyositis, scleroderma, and mixed connec-
    tive tissue disorder
Endocrine derangements such hypo/hyperthyroidism, hyperparathyroidism, and
    hypo/hyperadrenalism
Neoplastic diseases
Drug-induced diseases

Elements of the Motor Examination

The motor component of the neurologic examination comprises of 4 main elements[6]: muscle bulk, tone, strength, and stretch reflexes. These assist in localizing the lesion responsible for the weakness.

Bulk

To ascertain muscle bulk, careful inspection of the muscles bilaterally is required. Decreased muscle bulk (atrophy) is seen in denervation disorders involving the peripheral nerves. Fasciculations (rapid twitching of the muscle) can also be noticed in the atrophic muscle. Non-neurological disorders can also result in atrophy (eg, disuse, and patient history can help in this regard.

Tone

Passive movement of the muscles can elucidate the tone, which is basically a resistance in the movements. Tone can be normal, increased, or decreased. A slight resistance is observed in normotonic muscle. Hypertonicity most commonly presents in the form of rigidity or spasticity. Rigidity is constant increase in tone over the entire range of motion, also described as lead pipe. Spasticity on the other hand is a variable increase in the tone and is dependent on velocity, also known as the clasp knife form. Rigidity is classically associated with a basal ganglia disorder, whereas spasticity is commonly observed in diseases involving corticospinal tracts. Hypotonicity (decreased muscle tone) is seen in lower motor neuron disorders.

Assessment of muscle strength

Strength (power) of the muscle can be graded per The British Research Council system (**Table 2**).[7]

Stretch reflexes

Stretch reflexes are muscle contractions occurring when the tendon is percussed over a stretched muscle. They can be normal, decreased (lower motor neuronal disorders), or increased (upper motor neuronal disorders). They are graded on the basis on intensity of contraction: 4, clonus (very brisk); 3, brisk but normal; 2, normal; 1, minimal and 0, absent.

EMERGENCY DEPARTMENT MANAGEMENT

The first priority with any patient presenting to the ED for any complaint always includes the ABCs of airway, breathing, and circulation. In this immediate assessment, a quick mental checklist of life-threatening causes of weakness (not necessarily true neuromuscular weakness) is helpful (**Box 2**) to decide which further investigations might be warranted. In general, obtaining a complete blood cell (CBC) count, chemistry, and urinalysis covers a broad scope. If there is any respiratory compromise, an arterial blood gas and an inspiratory pressure (or negative inspiratory force, NIF) should be obtained also. CPK is useful when considering rhabdomyolysis. Blood cultures and lactate are obtained when sepsis is in the differential diagnosis. For most cases of acute generalized weakness, brain imaging will be of low yield, unless an acute stroke is still in the differential (discussed elsewhere in this issue). A lumbar puncture is helpful for diagnosing encephalitis. Once initial stabilization is complete, focusing on a detailed history and physical examination can provide clues as to which specific disease entity may be present (**Table 3**).

Table 2	
Grading scale for muscle strength	
Grade	**Description**
Grade 5	Normal strength
Grade 4	Reduced strength but can still move joints against resistance
Grade 3	Movements against gravity but not against resistance
Grade 2	Movements only with the elimination of gravity
Grade 1	Only fasciculations are noticed, and no movement is observed
Grade 0	No muscle contractions.

Box 2
Acute life-threatening causes of weakness
Myasthenia gravis
GBS
Botulism
Adrenal insufficiency/hypermagnesemia
Organophosphate poisoning
Carbon monoxide poisoning
Hypokalemia
Hypoglycemia
Cerebrovascular accident
Seizure
Spinal cord compression
Encephalopathy
Sepsis

GUILLAIN-BARRÉ SYNDROME

Although GBS is an uncommon presentation in the ED, it is the most common cause of acute paralysis.[8] Also known as acute inflammatory demyelinating polyneuropathy (AIDP), GBS is an immune-mediated neuropathy that typically starts after a respiratory or gastrointestinal infection. *Campylobacter jejuni* gastroenteritis has been most commonly associated with GBS. It typically presents as numbness in the distal extremities followed by progressive ascending weakness. The weakness progresses symmetrically from the distal extremities proximally. Pain can be present in the disease, most often in the back and extremities, and can overshadow the weakness. Areflexia is typical. The weakness can progress to involve the respiratory muscles in 10% to 30% of patients, at which point the patient requires respiratory support in the form of early intubation and mechanical ventilation. Indications for intubation include: forced vital capacity less than 20 mL/kg, maximum inspiratory pressure less than 30 cmH$_2$O, and maximum expiratory pressure less than 40 cmH$_2$O (20–30–40 rule).[9,10] Softer indicators, but perhaps more useful in the ED, are the inability of the patient to lift his or her head or shoulders or to cough, and fewer days between onset of symptoms and presentation to the ED. Succinylcholine should be avoided for paralysis during intubation because of the significant risk of hyperkalemia, which is a result of upregulation of muscle acetylcholine receptors.[11]

Seventy percent of patients have autonomic dysfunction, which manifests as tachycardia, urinary retention, hypertension alternating with hypotension, ileus, and loss of sweating. The Miller Fisher variant of GBS is characterized by ophthalmoplegia with ataxia and areflexia, and comprises about 5% of GBS cases.

Cerebrospinal fluid (CSF) analysis reveals albumino-cytologic dissociation, which is an increase in protein levels without associated pleocytosis, but the elevated protein may be absent in the first week of the disease.

Plasmapheresis and intravenous immunoglobulins (IVIGs) are used to treat GBS, and are more efficacious when given during first 1 to 2 weeks.[12] A Cochrane review of 649 patients noted more improvement with plasma exchange than with supportive

Table 3
Features of various diseases that cause generalized weakness

	Symptom Onset	Pattern of Paralysis	Deep Tendon Reflexes	Sensory Exam	CSF
GBS	5–7 d after viral illness	Ascending, symmetric	Absent or diminished	Abnormal	High Protein
Botulism	12–36 h after ingestion of preformed toxin	Descending, symmetric	Normal	Normal	Normal
Organo-phoshate toxicity	24–96 h after exposure (intermediate syndrome)	Proximal muscle weakness, neck flexion weakness	Diminished	Normal	Normal
Diphtheria	Few days after high fever, oral lesions	Ascending, symmetric Cranial nerves affected first	Absent or diminished	Normal	Normal
Tick paralysis	3–7 d after tick attaches	Ascending, symmetric	Absent	Normal	Normal
Acute intermittent porphyria	Hours to days	Descending, symmetric Proximal upper extremities to lower extremities	Absent or diminished	Pain in extremities, patchy numbness, paresthesia, and dysesthesias	Normal
Myasthenia gravis	Few days	Ocular muscle, bulbar weakness, Fatigable weakness, normal pupil function	Normal	Normal	Normal
Eaton Lambert syndrome	Insidious	Progressive proximal lower limb weakness, autonomic symptoms, strength gets better with brief exercise	Absent or diminished	Normal	Normal
Transverse myelitis	Symptoms develop over hours	Flaccid paralysis below lesion level	Brisk	Sensory level below lesion level (increased or decreased, +/– parsathesias	Pleocytosis, elevated IgG
Polio	2–3 d after high fever, headache, and myalgia	Asymmetric proximal	Absent or diminished	Normal	Pleocytosis, mildly elevated protein, normal glucose
Hypokalemic Periodic paralysis	Hours to days	Fixed proximal weakness	Diminished during episode	Normal	Normal

care alone.[13] IVIG started within 2 weeks hastens recovery as much as plasma exchange. However, IVIG is more likely to be completed by the patient.[14] Adverse effects of IVIG include hypertension, headache, nausea, fever, chills, and renal failure. Adverse effects of plasmapheresis include hypotension, bleeding, and allergic reaction. There is no role for corticosteroids in the treatment of GBS.[15] Prompt treatment is associated with a good long-term prognosis, with 85% recovering fully.[16]

MYASTHENIA GRAVIS

Myasthenia gravis (MG), although rare, is the most common disease of the NMJ. It most commonly is a T-cell mediated disease in which autoantibodies are generated against the postsynaptic acetylcholine receptors. After binding to these receptors, they prevent the binding of the neurotransmitter (acetylcholine). This prevents the transmission of action potentials from nerve to muscle, ultimately resulting in weakness. Although this is a chronic process that involves the blockade, down regulation, and complement-mediated destruction of the postsynaptic receptor, it can also appear as an acute entity in the form of acute myasthenic crisis, or cholinergic crisis, both of which will be described. MG affects approximately 59,000 people in United States (2003 estimate[17]) with a predisposition toward women and people aged 20 to 30 and 60 to 70 years. Acute myasthenic crisis occurs in approximately 3% of MG patients and can be a presenting symptom in 13% to 20% of patients.

The most common initial presenting symptoms are ptosis and diplopia.[18] Dysarthria, dysphagia, fatigue, and generalized weakness (proximal > distal) can also be seen. Symptoms are less severe in the morning, with severity increasing as the day progresses, and they are worsened by exertion.

Eighty percent of general MG patients have anticholinesterase receptor immunoglobulin G (IgG), while 30% to 50% of those with the ocular variant of MG do. Another 30% to 40% of patients have the anti-Msk antibody, while 5% have no identifiable antibody.[19] Clinical features of MG include ptosis and diplopia in about half of all MG patients, and bulbar symptoms of dysarthria, dysphagia, and fatigable chewing in 15% of patients. Ocular dysfunction in MG is variable over the course of the day, and ranges from internucelar ophthalmoplegia to vertical gaze paresis. One hallmark is that pupillary function is always spared in MG.

The mainstay of treatment for MG is a cholinesterase inhibitor such as pyridostigmine. Twenty percent of patients will undergo a crisis requiring mechanical ventilation. In contrast to GBS, the best respiratory support strategy in MG is bilevel positive airway pressure (BiPAP). Thymic dysplasia is present in 65% of MG patients, and 10% of patients have a thymoma.

Patients with MG can present with acute weakness either because they have too much medication (resulting in a cholinergic crisis), or because of an exacerbation of their myasthenia, usually secondary to an acute illness or stress (myasthenic crisis), which results in not enough anticholinesterase inhibitor. It is not always possible to distinguish the 2 types of crises based on physical examination. The edrophonium test can be used to differentiate the two; a patient with a myasthenic crisis will improve, while the patient with a cholinergic crisis will worsen. Both problems can coexist. However, this puts patients with cholinergic crisis at risk for airway compromise; further, there are several false positives seen with the edrophonium test, resulting in further danger for patients with cholinergic crisis. The preferred approach to MG in crisis from either cause is to admit to a monitored setting (intensive care unit [ICU]), provide respiratory support in the form of BiPaP (preferred) or intubation (if BiPAP not adequate), take away all cholinergic medications, and slowly add pyridostigmine

(0.5 mg/kg every 3 hours) while carefully monitoring the patient.[20] Although BiPAP is the preferred mode of ventilation for respiratory failure in myasthenia gravis, if one does proceed to endotracheal intubation, it should be noted that succinylcholine will be relatively ineffective to achieve muscle relaxation. Either a higher dose (approximately 2.5 times standard dose) of succinylcholine or a half-dose of a nondepolarizing agent (eg, rocuronium 0.5–0.6 mg/kg) should be used.[21]

Plasma exchange, IVIGs, and corticosteroids can be helpful in managing crises. First-line treatment for long-term immunosuppression is with azathioprine. Alternative immunosuppressive drugs for MG include cyclosporine, cyclophosphamide, methotrexate, mycophenolate mofetil, and tacrolimus and rituximab.[19]

BOTULISM

Botulism results from ingestion of preformed toxin or infection with botulinum spores that elaborate botulinum toxin by the bacteria *Clostridium botulinum*. It is a rare disease in adults, with most outbreaks related to ingesting contaminated foods (foodborne botulism). Less common modes of contracting it include via open wounds, and more recently, from direct inoculation for cosmetic purposes.[22] It presents with acute onset of bilateral cranial neuropathies approximately 12 to 36 hours after ingesting the toxin and symmetric descending weakness. Patients are afebrile, and have intact mental status. Reflexes are normal, and there are generally no sensory deficits. Cranial nerve involvement is manifested by blurred vision, diplopia, nystagmus, ptosis, dysphagia, dysarthria, and facial weakness. Pupils are often involved in botulism, distinguishing it from MG. Smooth muscle paralysis results in urinary retention and constipation. Paralysis of the diaphragm results in respiratory compromise that requires mechanical ventilation.[23] The disease spectrum can range from mild cranial nerve palsies to rapid death. Treatment of foodborne and wound botulism consists of

- Antitoxin therapy with equine serum heptavalent botulism antitoxin[24] in an attempt to prevent neurologic progression of a moderate, slowly progressive illness, or to shorten the duration of ventilatory failure in those with a severe, rapidly progressive illness
- Hospital admission to monitor respiratory status and begin prompt mechanical ventilation when needed[25]

The antitoxin is stockpiled regionally by the US Centers for Disease Control and Prevention (CDC) and can be accessed by notification on one's local health department. Antibiotics and wound debridement are additional measures for wound botulism.

Infant botulism is a distinct illness associated with the ingestion of *C botulinum* spores (vs direct ingestion of the toxin as seen in adult foodborne botulism) and is actually the most common form of botulism. As the name implies, it is seen in infants, and it is most commonly attributed to the ingestion of honey, which is why the American Academy of Pediatrics recommends no honey for children under the age of 12 months.[26] Clinical manifestations of infant botulism mirror those of adult foodborne botulism with signs such as inability to suck and swallow, weakened voice, ptosis, and floppy neck and that may progress to generalized flaccidity and respiratory compromise.[27] Infant botulism is treated with intravenous botulism immunoglobulin.[26]

FAMILIAL PERIODIC PARALYSES

The familial periodic paralyses are a group of hereditary diseases associated with abnormal ion channels.[28] This condition can be particularly difficult to diagnose, because examination between attacks may be completely normal until late the condition. The hallmark is a description of weakness that comes on randomly (not associated with any particular time of day or activity). Symptoms typically start before 20 years of age and can be triggered by certain foods (carbohydrates or potassium-rich foods) or rest after exercise.

Patients often show abnormal serum potassium (either hyperkalemia or hypokalemia) during the episode of weakness. Hypokalemic periodic paralysis is the most common type, and is a calcium channelopathy. Symptoms often follow exercise or a heavy carbohydrate meal. Acute treatment is supportive. Total body potassium is normal. Hyperkalemic periodic paralysis, which is much less common, is a sodium channelopathy, and the acute treatment consists of a carbohydrate meal/glucose. Electrodiagnostic testing shows a characteristic drop in compound muscle action potentials with exercise.[29]

POLIOMYELITIS

Poliovirus is an enterovirus that is transmitted by fecal-hand-oral transmission and can result in acute flaccid paralysis. Although poliovirus has been eradicated in much of the world, it remains endemic in sub-Saharan Africa and parts of Asia. It infects the anterior horn cells and can ultimately cause the death of these motor neurons, paralyzing the muscle fibers supplied by them. Only a few infections (<5%) experience paralytic poliomyelitis.[30] The infection commences with an influenza-like illness that leads to meningismus characterized by high fever, headache, and myalgia. Thereafter, asymmetric muscle spasms and muscle weakness set in, which gradually worsen over 2 to 3 days. Proximal muscle weakness is more common than distal muscle weakness with predominant involvement of the legs. Bulbar involvement can also be noted in a subgroup of these patients, more commonly in adults, with symptoms such as dysarthria and dysphagia.

Polymerase chain reaction (PCR) amplification of poliovirus is the most sensitive method for diagnosis. Poliovirus is most likely to be isolated from stool specimens. It may also be isolated from pharyngeal swabs. Isolation is less likely from blood or CSF.[31] Treatment recommendations for an acute attack are supportive, with a focus on pain relief and physiotherapy. Strict bed rest is required to prevent paralysis extension. Physical therapy assists in prevention of the development of contractures and joint ankylosis. In some patients, respiratory failure can also ensue, necessitating intubation and mechanical ventilation. Approximately 25% of polio survivors develop postpolio syndrome, characterized by progressive muscle weakness,[32] typically in previously affected muscles.

ORGANOPHOSPHATE AND CARBAMATE POISONING

Organophosphates (OPs) and carbamates are found in many pesticides and household products. These compounds cause weakness by binding to acetylcholinesterase and rendering it inactive, which leads to an excess of acetylcholine at the NMJ. OPs bind the receptor irreversibly, whereas carbamates bind it transiently. Symptoms of OP poisoning include muscarinic effects and nicotinic effects. The muscarinic effects are what one classically thinks of as the cholinergic toxidrome: salivation, lacrimation, urination, defecation, emesis, bronchorrhea, and miosis. The nicotinic manifestations are muscle weakness, fasciculations, and paralysis. In up to 20% of patients with OP poisoning, a new neuromuscular weakness sets in approximately 24 to 96 hours after initial exposure, and this phenomenon has been termed the intermediate syndrome.[33] It consists of proximal limb weakness and weakness of the respiratory muscles. The resulting respiratory distress needs to be aggressively managed, and when this is done most patients recover fully without sequelae.

Treatment of OP poisoning includes atropine (which only reverses the muscarinic effects) plus an oxime such as pyridoxime (which reverses both nicotinic and muscarinic effects).[34] They should be given together. The endpoint to atropine treatment is resolution of respiratory secretions and cessation of bronchoconstriction. Very large quantities of atropine, in the order of hundreds of milligrams are required. Pralidoxime is administered slowly at a dose of 30 mg/kg. If intubation is required, succinylcholine should be avoided, as OPs inhibit acetyl cholinesterase, the enzyme that metabolizes succinylcholine. Nondepolarizing neuromuscular blocking agents will work, but larger doses are required. Central nervous system (CNS) effects include seizures, and these should be treated with benzodiazepines, rather than phenytoin, which has not been shown to be effective.[35]

TRANSVERSE MYELITIS

Transverse myelitis is a monophasic immune-mediated condition restricted to the spinal cord. In children, up to 60% cases occur as an autoimmune phenomenon following an infection or vaccination. This association is less common in adults. Up to one-third of cases are idiopathic.[36] Multiple sclerosis is another relatively common cause; Lyme disease and schistosomiasis are 2 infectious causes. Symptoms depend on the spinal cord level involved, and can include motor symptoms such as paraparesis or quadraparesis, autonomic dysfunction such as bowel and bladder dysfunction, and a sensory level below the lesion. The symptoms are bilateral, and typically symmetric, but can occasionally be asymmetric. Leg flexors and arm extensors are more commonly affected. Symptoms evolve over hours to days, with an average of 4 to 21 days, with the nadir at 2 weeks. Progression to nadir within 4 hours excludes the diagnosis of transverse myelitis. In the acute phase, muscle flaccidity is observed; this converts into spasticity later in the disease course.[37] Pain is a common symptom both during and after an attack of traverse myelitis, and can be neuropathic or musculoskeletal in nature.

Diagnostics adjuncts include MRI, which demonstrates spinal cord inflammation, and lumbar puncture, which again demonstrates inflammation with pleocytosis and IgG. Treatment consists of high dose corticosteroids (eg, methylprednisolone 1000 mg intravenously daily for 3–5 days). Plasma exchange can be used for refractory cases. Deep venous thrombosis prophylaxis should be administered for patients who are immobile. In the occasional case caused by Lyme disease, antiborrelial antibiotics would be prescribed. Prognosis depends on the underlying etiology, timely diagnosis, and appropriate treatment; overall, the prognosis is fair. Spinal shock, back pain, and rapid symptom progression can result in dismal prognosis. Approximately 50% to 70% of patients have partial or full recovery.[38]

TICK PARALYSIS

Tick paralysis is an uncommon disorder that is caused by the neurotoxins present in the saliva of gravid female ticks. There are 40 species known to produce these toxins; of them, *Dermacentor andersonii* (the Rocky Mountain wood tick) and *D variabilis* (the American dog tick) are the most common causative agents in North America. The symptoms begin with paresthesias and gradually progress to unsteady gait and ultimately asymmetric ascending flaccid paralysis. The toxins are transmitted when ticks feed on human blood, and symptoms progress as long as the ticks feed. Treatment consists of tick removal, which requires a meticulous search for the tick on physical examination. Tick removal results in rapid improvement and is associated with an excellent prognosis.[39–41]

AMYOTROPHIC LATERAL SCLEROSIS

ALS, also known as Lou Gehrig's disease, is the most common form of degenerative motor neuron disease. It has an incidence of 2 to 3 cases per 100,000 individuals in the general population and is idiopathic in most instances. It affects both upper and lower motor neurons. There is progressive decrease in bulbar and limb function, with symptom onset more commonly seen in the limbs, and later progressing to the bulbar segment. Sensory symptoms including pain may be seen in only 20% of the patients. Cognitive dysfunction is frequently seen in ALS patients; frontotemporal dementia develops with disease progression. Muscle weakness, spasticity, and fasciculations are noted on the physical examination, as well as muscle atrophy.

Differential diagnosis for ALS includes MG, neurodegenerative disorders such as Parkinson disease, Huntington disease, and progressive muscular atrophy. There is no definitive diagnostic test for ALS; negative laboratory tests and imaging studies help in ruling out the differentials. Elaborate history and physical examination are key to the diagnosis. Electrodiagnostic tests such as electromyography can help in identification of the loss in lower motor neurons. There is no effective treatment for ALS. Riluzole is the only FDA approved disease-modifying drug that can provide symptomatic relief in ALS patients.[42] Respiratory failure is seen in approximately 60% of patients within 3 years of symptom onset and is the most common cause of death in ALS patients. Mechanical ventilation is necessary in patients who develop respiratory failure. Physical therapy and rehabilitation, along with gastrostomy, improve the quality of life of patients. Although the overall prognosis is poor, site of initial symptom onset (eg, the limbs) tends to have a better prognosis.

REFERENCES

1. Bingisser R. Weakness as presenting symptom in the emergency department. Swiss Med Wkly 2009;139(17–18):271–2.
2. Saguil A. Evaluation of the patient with muscle weakness. Am Fam Physician 2005;171(7):1327–36.
3. Valiyil R, Christopher-Stine L. Drug-related Myopathies of Which the Clinician Should Be Aware. Curr Rheumatol Rep 2010;12(3):213–20.
4. Bannwarth B. Drug-induced myopathies. Expert Opin Drug Saf 2002;1(1):65–70.
5. Mancall EL. Overview of the organization of the nervous system. In: Mancall EL, Brock DG, Gray H, editors. Gray's clinical neuroanatomy the anatomic basis for clinical neuroscience. 7th edition. Philadelphia: Elsevier Health Sciences; 2011. p. 3–10.
6. Greenberg DA, Aminoff MJ, Simon RP. Neurologic history & examination. In: Greenberg DA, Aminoff MJ, Simon RP, editors. Clinical neurology. 8th edition. New York: McGraw-Hill; 2012.
7. Medical Research Council. Aids to the investigation of peripheral nerves. London: Crown Publishing; 1976.
8. McGillicuddy DC, Walker O, Shapiro NI, et al. Guillain-Barré Syndrome in the Emergency Department. Ann Emerg Med 2006;47(4):390–3.
9. Sharshar T, Chevret S, Bourdain F, et al. Early predictors of mechanical ventilation in Guillain-Barré syndrome. Crit Care Med 2003;31:278.
10. Walgaard C, Lingsma HF, Ruts L, et al. Prediction of respiratory insufficiency in Guillain-Barré syndrome. Ann Neurol 2010;67:781.

11. Gronert GA. Cardiac arrest after succinylcholine: mortality greater with rhabdo-myolysis than receptor upregulation. Anesthesiology 2001;94(3):523–9.
12. So YT. Immune-mediated neuropathies. Continuum (Minneap Minn) 2012;18(1):85–105.
13. Raphael JC, Chvret S, Hughes RAC, et al. Plasma exchange for Guillain Barre Syndrome. Cochrane Database Syst Rev 2012;(7):CD001798.
14. Hughes RAC, Swan AV, van Doorn PA. Intravenous immunoglobulin for Guillain Barre Syndrome. Cochrane Database Syst Rev 2014;(9):CD002063.
15. Hughes RAC, van Doorn PA. Corticosteroids for Guillain Barre Syndrome. Cochrane Database Syst Rev 2012;(8):CD001446.
16. van Doorn PA. Diagnosis, treatment and prognosis of Guillain-Barré syndrome (GBS). Presse Med 2013;42(6 Pt 2):e193–201.
17. Phillips LH 2nd. The epidemiology of myasthenia gravis. Ann N Y Acad Sci 2003;998:407–12.
18. Sanders DB, Guptill JT. Myasthenia gravis and Lambert-Eaton myasthenic syndrome. Continuum (Minneap Minn) Oct 2014;20(5 Peripheral Nervous System Disorders):1413–25.
19. Sieb JP. Myasthenia gravis: an update for the clinician. Clin Exp Immunol 2014;175(3):408–18.
20. Rabinstein AA. Acute Neuromuscular Respiratory Failure. Continuum (Minneap Minn) 2015;21(5 Neurocritical Care):1324–45.
21. Flower O, Wainwright MS, Finley Caulfield AF. Emergency neurological life support: acute non-traumatic weakness. Neurocrit Care 2015;23:S23–47.
22. Ghasemi M, Norouzi R, Salari M, et al. Iatrogenic Botulism after the therapeutic use of botulinum toxin-A: a case report and review of the literature. Clin Neuropharmcol 2012;35(5):254–7.
23. Koussoulakos S. Botulinum Neurotoxin: The Ugly Duckling. Eur Neurol 2009;61:331–42.
24. Centers for Disease Control and Prevention (CDC). Investigational heptavalent botulinum antitoxin (HBAT) to replace licensed botulinum antitoxin AB and investigational botulinum antitoxin E. MMWR Morb Mortal Wkly Rep 2010;59(10):299.
25. Centers for Disease Control and Prevention. Botulism in the United States, 1899–1996. Handbook for epidemiologists, clinicians, and laboratory workers. Atlanta (GA): Centers for Disease Control and Prevention; 1998.
26. American Academy of Pediatrics. Botulism and infant botulism (Clostridium botulinum). In: Kimberlin DW, Brady MT, Jackson MA, et al, editors. Red book: 2015 report of the committee on infectious diseases. 30th edition. Elk Grove Village (IL): American Academy of Pediatrics; 2015. p. 294.
27. Sobel J. Botulism. Clin Infect Dis 2005;41(8):1167–73.
28. Venance SL, Cannon SC, Fialho D, et al. The primary periodic paralyses: diagnosis, pathogenesis, and treatment. Brain 2006;129:8.
29. Statland JM, Barohn RJ. Muscle channelopathies: the nondystrophic myotonias and periodic paralyses. Continuum (Minneap Minn) 2013;19(6):1598–614.
30. Flower O, Wainwright MS, Caulfield AF. Emergency Neurological Life Support: Acute Non-Traumatic Weakness. Neurocrit Care 2015;23:S23–47.
31. Available at: http://www.cdc.gov/polio/us/lab-testing/diagnostic.html. Accessed Ddecmber 29, 2015.
32. Howard RS. Poliomyelitis and the postpolio syndrome. BMJ Jun 2005;330(7503):1314–8.
33. Karalliedde L, Baker D, Marrs TC. Organophosphate-induced intermediate syndrome: etiology and relationships with myopathy. Toxicol Rev 2006;25(1):1–14.

34. Available at: http://www.uptodate.com/contents/organophosphate-and-carbamate-poisoning. Accessed December 29, 2015.
35. World Health Organization. Environmental health criteria No 63. Organophosphorus pesticides: a general introduction. Geneva (Switzerland): World Health Organization; 1986. Available at: http://www.inchem.org/documents/ehc/ehc/ehc63.htm#SubSectionNumber:7.4.3. Accessed December 29, 2015.
36. de Seze J, Lanctin C, Lebrun C, et al. Idiopathic acute transverse myelitis: application of the recent diagnostic criteria. Neurology 2005;65:1950–3.
37. West TW. Transverse myelitis–a review of the presentation, diagnosis, and initial management. Discov Med 2013;16(88):167–77.
38. Frohman EM, Wingerchuk DM. Transverse myelitis. N Engl J Med 2010;363:564–72.
39. Pecina CA. Tick Paralysis. Semin Neurol 2012;32(5):531–2.
40. Edlow JA. Tick Paralysis. Curr Treat Options Neurol 2010;12(3):167–77.
41. Salameh JS, Brown RH Jr, Berry JD. Amyotrophic lateral sclerosis: review. Semin Neurol 2015;35(4):469–76.
42. Hardiman O, van den Berg LH, Kiernan MC. Clinical diagnosis and management of amyotrophic lateral sclerosis. Nat Rev Neurol Nov 2011;7(11):639–49.

Transient Ischemic Attacks

Advances in Diagnosis and Management in the Emergency Department

Andrea Duca, MD[a], Andy Jagoda, MD[b],*

KEYWORDS

- Transient ischemic attack • Stroke • TIA

KEY POINTS

- Up to 50% of TIAs using the classic time-based definition show areas of infarction on brain MRI, hence the new definition of TIA is image-based.
- TIA shares the same pathophysiology as stroke, which occurs in up to 5% of patients within 48 hours of the TIA and 10% within 90 days.
- The use of clinical scores, such as the ABCD2 score, integrated with the clinical and radiological findings, help in stratifying the risk of stroke.
- Antiplatelet and anticoagulant therapies, as well as carotid endarterectomy/stenting, when indicated, reduce the risk of stroke after a TIA.
- The use of expedited assessment/management protocols for patients with TIA reduces stroke risk by up to 80%.

INTRODUCTION

Over the past decade, the diagnosis of a transient ischemic attack (TIA) has evolved from a clinical diagnosis to a tissue-based one based on neuroimaging results. Clinical scoring systems with or without neuroimaging has impacted decision making regarding timing and place of the diagnostic workup. Advances in pharmacotherapeutics have improved outcomes. Because up to 5% of TIAs will be followed by a stroke within 48 hours, facilitated evaluations should be tailored to the individual patient; these evaluations are often best accomplished through proactively designed protocols that provide patients with coordinated, multidisciplinary care. Many patients with TIA initially present to the emergency department (ED); consequently, knowledge of clinical presentations and diagnostic and management strategies is fundamental to

[a] Department of Emergency Medicine, Ospedale San Raffaele, via Olgettina 60, 20132 Milan, Italy; [b] Department of Emergency Medicine, Icahn School of Medicine at Mount Sinai, One Gustave Levy Place, Box 1620, New York, NY 10029, USA
* Corresponding author.
E-mail address: andy.jagoda@mssm.edu

Emerg Med Clin N Am 34 (2016) 811–835
http://dx.doi.org/10.1016/j.emc.2016.06.007
0733-8627/16/© 2016 Elsevier Inc. All rights reserved.

emed.theclinics.com

improve the outcome of stroke.[1,2] The class of evidence/graded recommendations, which are presented in this review, are based on the well-described methodology used by the American Stroke Association (ASA).[3]

DEFINITION

TIAs were defined in 1975 as "episodes of temporary and focal dysfunction of vascular origin, which are variable in duration, commonly lasting from 2 to 15 minutes, but occasionally lasting as long as a 24 hours; they leave no persistent neurologic deficit."[4] Advanced neuroimaging has shown that a subset of patients with TIA actually have evidence of clinically silent infarction. It is estimated that 30% of the events that were previously diagnosed as TIA actually have infarcted brain.[5] Thus, the definition of TIA has evolved into a tissue-based definition: "transient episode of neurologic dysfunction caused by focal brain, spinal cord, or retinal ischemia, without acute infarction."[5]

The new definition of TIA is dependent on the availability of either head computed tomography (CT) or MRI. CT is not nearly as sensitive as MRI and may require 12 hours after the event to demonstrate injury; diffusion-weighted imaging MRI (DWI MRI) is far more sensitive and more specific for acute injury and turns positive much sooner.[5] In the absence of imaging technology, it is accepted to use the old time-based definition of TIA, accepting that the probability of having a necrotic area is particularly high in patients with symptoms lasting more than 24 hours.[5] This approach is recommended because, although most TIAs last less than 1 hour, up to 50% of patients with TIA lasting 1 to 24 hours have negative DWI MRI, confirming the absence of stroke.[5]

The tissue-based definition of TIA has led to the creation of 2 stroke categories: the "nondisabling stroke," which is the transitory presence of neurologic symptoms with mild (National Institutes of Health Stroke Scale ≤3) to absence of persistent clinical deficits in the presence of imaging evidence of necrosis, and the "silent stroke," which is the radiologic finding of cerebral necrosis without neurologic findings. The importance of silent stroke is underscored by its high association with future strokes, cognitive sequelae, and mortality. There is ongoing discussion surrounding silent stroke and whether our current assessments are sensitive enough to identify subtle cognitive and behavioral deficits; there is a need to focus on this disease to better understand its pathophysiology and prognostic implications.[6]

EPIDEMIOLOGY

In 2013, stroke caused 130,000 deaths in the United States, making it the fifth leading cause of mortality after heart disease, cancer, chronic lower respiratory disease, and accidents.[7] The prevalence of stroke in the United States is 3% in patients older than 18 years, whereas the prevalence of silent stroke is estimated at 6% to 28% of the population, depending on age, sex, risk factors, and definition used.[8]

TIA prevalence in the United States is estimated at 2.3%, with an incidence of 0.7 to 0.8 per 1000 people evaluated.[8] The incidence of TIA increases with age and varies by sex and race/ethnicity. Men and African American and Mexican American individuals have higher rates of TIA than women and non-Hispanic white individuals. Approximately 15% of all strokes are preceded by a TIA; this rate has decreased over the past decade, possibly due to improved preventive strategies in patients at risk.[1]

Early outcome studies on the risk of stroke after TIA estimated an incidence of 3% to 10% at 2 days and 9% to 17% at 90 days[8]; however, recent studies have reported lower rates in the range of 1.5% at 2 days, 1.4% to 3.4% at 90 days, 4.8% at 1 year, and 9.0% at 5 years.[2,9] This lower incidence is most likely due to improvements in early diagnosis and management.[1] The combined 10-year stroke, myocardial infarction, or vascular death risk in patients who have had a stroke is 43%.[5] Most of the studies done so far, however, have used the old time-based definition of TIA; we expect that there will be a change in the epidemiologic estimates in the next years, when the tissue-based definition will become the standard.

ETIOLOGY AND PATHOPHYSIOLOGY

Both TIA and ischemic stroke share the same etiologies and pathophysiology. The final pathway is focal hypoperfusion, oligemia, and impairment of cerebral oxygenation and glucose metabolism. An individual's ability to tolerate short periods of cerebral hypoperfusion is variable and dependent on multiple factors, including collateral flow and oxygen delivery capacity.

Several systems have been developed to classify stroke etiology (**Table 1**; often referred to as the TOAST classification).[10–12] The importance of a standardized classification system is to achieve a framework for study design and outcome analyses that are appropriate for the type of disease process, for example, cardioembolic disease may respond differently to interventions than small vessel occlusion disease.

Cardioembolic etiologies account for approximately 34% of TIAs, followed by small artery occlusion/disease (10%–18%), large artery atherothrombosis (9%–13%), and other causes (3%–6%).[13] These causes must be put in the context of the patient, in which case the percentile may change; for example, in young patients without underlying disease, cervical artery dissection emerges as one of the most common causes of TIA. Nonetheless, in all classification schemes, the proportion of undetermined or cryptogenic causes remains as high as 25% to 50%.[13,14]

Atheromatous disease of large-sized to medium-sized arteries is often related to hypertension. It usually forms at branch points or in tortuous vessels where endothelial damage can progress to smooth muscle proliferation and fibrolipid plaque formation. Common sites of plaque formation are the aortic arch, proximal subclavian arteries, carotid bifurcation, and vertebral artery origins.[15] An ulcerated plaque can result in emboli or it can directly propagate and obstruct flow to a branching vessel; it can

Table 1
Stroke/TIA classification of etiology

Etiology	Example
Large artery atherosclerosis	Cervical artery (carotid or vertebral) stenosis; aortic atherosclerosis
Cardioembolic	Cardiac dysrhythmia (atrial fibrillation); cardiac thrombosis; valve disease, patent foramen ovale; impaired left ventricular function (such as recent myocardial infarction), dilated cardiomyopathies, infective endocarditis, mechanical valvular prostheses, septal aneurysm, myxomas
Small artery occlusion	Intracranial atherosclerosis (hypertension and diabetes)
Other defined mechanisms	Hypercoagulable states (eg, protein C disease, inherited thrombophilias, protein S deficiency, antithrombin III deficiency, plasminogen deficiency, activated protein C resistance/factor V Leiden mutation, anticardiolipin antibodies, lupus anticoagulant, ptothrombin mutation, thrombocytosis), arterial dissection, vasculitis, and so forth
Undetermined causes	

also result in local stenosis to the point of reducing flow to susceptible tissue or to the point of complete occlusion. Individuals with large artery atherosclerosis have a high all-cause mortality at 2 years.[16]

Small vessel disease refers to hyaline arteriosclerosis (lipohyalinosis, which is pathologically distinct from extracranial atherothromboembolic disease) that forms in small penetrating arteries (<0.5 mm in thickness) within the brain. It results in small-volume and lacunar strokes, often at the lenticulo-striate branches of the middle cerebral artery and perforating vessels of the anterior and posterior cerebral arteries. Intracranial vessels are less elastic than their extracranial parent vessels, and they are more prone to narrowing from collagen deposition that occurs with aging. Cortical lacunar strokes and TIAs may present with minor deficits or may be clinically silent.

Cardioembolism has been associated with severely debilitating strokes, and is an independent predictor of mortality.[16–18] Atrial fibrillation is the most common cause. It has a highly variable average annual risk of first-time stroke in patients who are not anticoagulated, ranging from 0.2% to 23.6%, depending on the clinical characteristic, as defined by CHA_2DS_2-VASc criteria (**Table 2**).[19,20] This high risk of stroke underscores the importance of expedited management of new-onset atrial fibrillation, although, as discussed in the therapy section, there are limited data on the 1-week and 1-month stroke risk in newly diagnosed atrial fibrillation.

DIAGNOSIS

Differentiating TIAs from alternative diagnoses that cause focal neurologic symptoms is a challenge in emergency medicine. Considerations of high priority include hypoglycemia, stroke, central nervous system (CNS) mass lesions, CNS vasculitis, and CNS infections (**Table 3**).[21–23] Although rare, hypokalemia has been reported in case reports to present with focal deficits.[24]

Table 2 By CHA$_2$DS$_2$-VASc score	
Comorbidity	**Value**
Congestive heart failure	1
Hypertension	1
Age >75	2
Diabetes	1
Prior TIA, stroke, or VTE	2
Vascular disease (PAD, MI, aortic plaque)	1
Age 65–74	1
Female sex	1

Low risk = 0: Thromboembolic risk at 1 year 0.2%.
  Moderate risk = 1: Thromboembolic risk at 1 year 0.6%.
  High risk greater than 1: Thromboembolic risk at 1 year 2.2% to 23.6%.
  Abbreviations: MI, myocardial infarction; PAD, peripheral artery disease; TIA, transient ischemic attack; VTE, venous thromboembolism.
  Data from Lip GY, Nieuwlaat R, Pisters R, et al. Refining clinical risk stratification for predicting stroke and thromboembolism in atrial fibrillation using a novel risk factor-based approach: the Euro Heart Survey on Atrial Fibrillation. Chest 2010;137(2):263–72; and Friberg L, Rosenqvist M, Lip GY, et al. Evaluation of risk stratification schemes for ischaemic stroke and bleeding in 182 678 patients with atrial fibrillation: the Swedish Atrial Fibrillation cohort study. Eur Heart J 2012;33(12):1500–10.

Table 3
Differential diagnosis of new acute onset of focal neurologic symptoms

Diagnosis	Common Characteristics
Emergent diagnosis	
Transient ischemic attack	Vascular/cardioembolic risk factors. More frequent negative symptoms (numbness, weakness, visual loss), diplopia, does not spread into other sensory modalities. Alteration/loss of consciousness (LOC) rare. Abrupt onset, lasting often <1 h. Headaches may occur, usually during attacks.
Ischemic or hemorrhagic stroke	Evidence of cerebral necrosis or bleeding on imaging. In hemorrhagic stroke, sudden onset of severe headache, can have sentinel events in the previous days.
Hypoglycemia	History of diabetes mellitus, hypoglycemic medications. Negative symptoms, decreased level of consciousness. Low serum glucose.
Hypertensive encephalopathy	History of uncontrolled hypertension, recent suspension of medications. Headache, delirium, cortical blindness, seizure, cerebral edema. Significant hypertension.
Central nervous system infections	Immunocompromised patient, intravenous drug use, persistent/worsening symptoms, can have fever, headache, meningismus, increased inflammatory markers, electroencephalographic/radiologic findings.
Cerebral venous thrombosis	Procoagulant risk factors; for example, pregnancy; headache, nausea/vomiting, can develop seizures and altered level of consciousness.
Chronic or subacute subdural hematoma	Common history of previous head trauma, elderly patients, antiplatelet/anticoagulant medications, subacute onset, and persistent/worsening symptoms.
Urgent diagnosis	
Central nervous system mass lesions	History of neoplasia (eg, breast or lung neoplasia, melanoma), persistent/worsening symptoms over days, can be associated with seizure/have positive symptoms, alteration on cerebral imaging.
Central nervous system vasculitis	Usually young, persistent/worsening negative symptoms, can be associated with headache, can be multifocal, alteration on MRI.
Central nervous system inflammatory disease	History of multiple sclerosis, previous episodes, usually young, multiple alterations on MRI.
System infections	Elderly, frail patients, variable and fluctuant neurologic findings often associated with confusion/delirium, fever, increased inflammatory markers. This may represent "unmasking" of a prior stroke that is asymptomatic under normal circumstances.
Seizure	History of seizure, witnessed seizure activity. Positive symptoms (pain, limb jerking, lip smacking), frequent loss of awareness and amnesia, symptoms usually brief but Todd paresis may persist for hours). Incontinence, tongue bite, muscle pain, postictal period.
Less urgent diagnosis	
Migraine	History of similar events, visual symptoms most common, symptoms may spread into other sensory modalities, headache follows symptoms, frequent nausea/vomiting, alteration/LOC rare, confusion possible.

(continued on next page)

Table 3
(continued)

Diagnosis	Common Characteristics
Transient global amnesia	Paroxysmal, transient loss of memory. Remote and immediate memory spared, attention and visual-spatial skills intact. No neurologic signs on physical examination.
Psychogenic (conversion disorder, somatization, hyperventilation)	Usually young, emotional stress. Most frequent isolated sensory symptoms in nonvascular distribution, recurrent. Can have dyspnea, anxiety. In hyperventilation, peripheral bilateral tingling and cramps. Lack of neurologic signs. Diagnosis is rarely made in the emergency department.
Syncope	Previous episodes, cardiologic risk factors, emotional stress. Faint, dizziness, light head (presyncope), loss of awareness, blurred vision/may darken, muffled hearing. Lasting seconds to <1 min. Rapid recovery to full alertness, pallor, sweating, palpitation, chest pain, nausea, dyspnea.
Acute vestibular syndrome due to peripheral cause	Variable onset of vertigo with fluctuating symptoms, associated with nausea/vomiting, gait impairment, horizontal/torsional nystagmus, absence of dysmetria/neurologic findings, Head Impulse Test positive, test of Skew negative.
Peripheral nervous system lesion/ compression	Subacute onset, weakness and numbness often preceded by pain/ paresthesia, previous episodes with same characteristic, radicular/single nerve distribution, can be persistent. Alteration on medullar MRI, electromyography/electroneurography.
Drug toxicity (Lithium, phenytoin, carbamazepine)	History of medication use, tingling/numbness with nonvascular distribution.

History

TIA almost always produces focal symptoms that can be attributed to a specific vessel. The history should characterize the event, as in most cases the symptoms have resolved by the time the patient is seen. Indeed, if the symptoms have not resolved, TIA cannot be diagnosed and the patient should be assumed to have a stroke, or a stroke mimic. The history focuses on the positive or negative features of the symptoms (see the following paragraph), the outset and time course, comorbidities, risk factors, and medications. Nonfocal symptoms, such as loss of consciousness, confusion, lightheadedness, generalized weakness, or incontinence, are much less often caused by TIAs and tend not to be predictive of future stroke.[25]

The symptoms experienced in a that TIA are predominantly "negative", are associated with a loss of a function, such as motor (weakness), speech (decreased or altered speech), visual (diminished vision), or sensation (anesthesia). "Positive" symptoms are associated with the presence of something that is not normal, such as motor (involuntary motions), speech (increased volume of incomprehensible speech), visual (flashes of light or scintillating scotoma), or sensation (dysesthesias), and sometimes pain. As a general rule, negative symptoms suggest ischemia or infarction, whereas positive symptoms suggest migraine or seizure-related diagnoses. An important exception is "dizziness," which, at least in the case of vertigo, is a positive symptom and can be due to posterior circulation ischemia; in particular, even without any other neurologic sign, it has been associated with TIA or stroke in 0.7% of dizzy patients.[26] Taken from the other perspective, in a series of 1141 cases of stroke, a preceding episode of isolated transient vertigo was found in 2% of patients (and 8% in the 275 patients with posterior circulation strokes).[27]

TIA generally occurs suddenly and without prodrome. Stuttering symptoms, over hours to days, are of particular concern and warn of a highly unstable plaque. Although the component of time has been removed from the definition of TIA, the duration of symptoms remains an important aspect of the diagnosis. Most TIAs are brief, most lasting less than 1 hour[28,29]; in up to 50% of patients with symptoms lasting more than 1 hour, radiologic evidence of infarction can be found.[5]

Physical Examination

By definition, the physical examination is expected to be normal in a patient with a TIA; the presence of neurologic deficits should be treated as a stroke until proven otherwise. The physical examination must be systematic and comprehensive, addressing strength, sensation, coordination, balance, vision, and cognition. The examination assesses both the neurologic function and also assesses findings that might be associated with TIA risk, including irregular heart rate and carotid bruit, or alternative diagnoses, such as hyperventilation or presence of a heart murmur.

The use of scales, such as the National Institute of Health Stroke Scale (NIHSS) are useful only if the patient has an ongoing deficit; in a patient with TIA, the score will be zero. The NIHSS is of less value in assessing small posterior lesions and lesions on the nondominant side of the brain. Truncal ataxia, decreased visual acuity, Horner syndrome, and memory impairment are just a few focal neurologic deficits that would be missed by the NIHSS.[30,31] For all these reasons, a full neurologic examination is required before diagnosing a TIA.

Laboratory Tests

There are no laboratory tests that are diagnostic for TIA but there are several tests needed to assess risk for TIA, and to eliminate other processes that may mimic TIA. Serum blood sugar and electrolytes are indicated in all patients. A complete blood count with platelet count evaluates for inflammation, thrombocytosis, and myelodysplastic disease.[3] Evaluation of prothrombin time and international normalized ratio (INR) is useful in the evaluation of patients that are taking warfarin or who have liver dysfunction.[3] Although the 2013 ASA guidelines recommend a troponin level in patients with stroke, its value in the assessment of TIA is not identified.[3,32]

Other laboratory tests are performed on a case-by-case basis related to pretest risk assessment and suspected etiology of the TIA (eg, pregnancy test, toxicology screening). Diagnostic and prognostic TIA markers have been suggested; for example, C-reactive protein, S100B; however, at this time, none have been identified as useful during clinical practice.[33–41]

Electrocardiogram and Cardiac Monitoring

An electrocardiogram (ECG) is recommended to assess for a cardioembolic mechanism, including atrial fibrillation, ventricular hypertrophy, or signs of cardiac ischemia (Class of evidence IB). The 2013 stroke American Heart Association (AHA) guidelines recommend 24-hour telemetry to investigate for paroxysmal atrial fibrillation; this time limit can be extended to up to 30 days in case of suspected embolic or cryptogenic cause. Trials have reported paroxysmal atrial fibrillation during 21-day telemetry monitoring in up to 23% of patients thought to have a cryptogenic etiology.[42–45]

Cardiac Echocardiography

Transthoracic echocardiography (TTE) is used to assess for evidence of cardiac hypertrophy, ventricular hypokinesis or thrombus, mitral stenosis, endocarditis, and valve disease (Class of evidence IIaA).[3] In one retrospective study of 186 individuals with stroke or TIA without obvious cause of cardioembolism, TTE detected a source of embolism in 19% of patients.[46] The transesophageal echocardiography is particularly useful as a secondary examination in the cohort of patients thought to have an embolic cause that is hard to see on the transthoracic examination, such as left atrial appendage thrombosis or patent foramen ovale.[3,46]

Brain Imaging

The 2013 ASA guidelines state that patients with transient ischemic neurologic symptoms should undergo neuroimaging evaluation within 24 hours of symptom onset or as soon as possible in patients with delayed presentations using MRI (including diffusion-weighted imaging) as the preferred brain diagnostic imaging modality. If MRI is not available, head CT should be performed. (Class of evidence IB).[42] The sensitivity of CT scan in identifying stroke within 12 hours of symptom onset is only 0.39, while the sensitivity of DWI MRI is 0.99.[47] The availability of an MRI is therefore of great importance during the first hours to evaluate for cerebral infarction and hence defining the event as stroke versus TIA (**Fig. 1**).

The perfusion (for CT and MRI) and fluid-attenuated inversion recovery (for MRI) techniques are helpful to further increase the specificity and sensitivity of MRI and CT and, in the case of a stroke, can identify the area of the brain eventually salvageable by reperfusion therapies (ie, the "ischemic penumbra").[5,42]

Magnetic resonance angiography (MRA) or CT angiography (CTA) is recommended to assess the intracranial vessels for intracranial stenosis and guides the need for

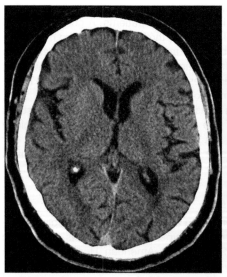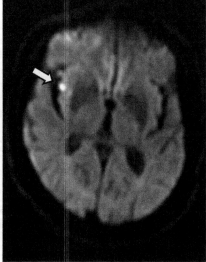

Fig. 1. A 78-year-old man with episode of dysarthria lasting 20 minutes. Head CT scan (*on the left*) done after 3 hours from episode showing no acute alteration. DWI MRI (*on the right*) done right after the CT revealing punctate area of restricted diffusion in the right insula (*arrow*) compatible with infarction.

endovascular interventions (Class of evidence IA). Angiography is indicated when intracranial stenosis is identified.[42]

Cervical Vessel Imaging

The evaluation of patient with suspected TIA includes the noninvasive imaging of cervical vessels (Class of evidence IA) using Doppler-ultrasound, MRA, or CTA (**Fig. 2, Table 4**).[42]

RISK STRATIFICATION

Many instruments have been developed for risk stratification, including the Stroke Prognosis Instrument,[48,49] the California score[50] and the ABCD score,[51] and more recently the ABCD2 score,[52] the ABCD2-I score,[53] and the ABCD3-I score.[54] The most used score at this time is the ABCD2 score (**Table 5**), which stratifies patients as low, moderate, or high risk for stroke at 2, 7, and 90 days following TIA, in an effort to guide appropriate triage and disposition. Despite widespread acceptance of these scores and their incorporation into guidelines, a meta-analysis of the literature failed to find sufficient evidence to validate this instrument. Limitations of the ABCD2 score include the finding that up to 41% of the patients with a high score (>4) have been found to have TIA mimics, and at the same time up to 21% of patients with low score have a high-risk etiology, such as atrial fibrillation or carotid stenosis.[55] Another

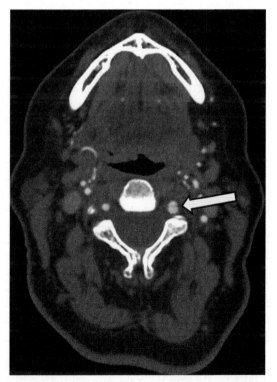

Fig. 2. A 37-year-old woman with neck pain and episode of vertigo and dysmetria lasting 30 minutes. CTA demonstrates a transverse flap across the left vertebral artery (*arrow*) compatible with dissection.

Table 4
Carotid imaging

Imaging Technique	Sens and Spec for Detecting Stenosis >70%	Limitations	Cost
Duplex Doppler	Sens 83%–86%, Spec 87%–99%	Limited ability to image vasculature proximal and distal to bifurcation; operator-dependent	Low
CTA	Sens 83%, Spec 93%	Radiation exposure Contrast administration	Medium
MRA	Sens 93%, Spec 88% Sens 86%–97%, Spec 62%–91% if contrast enhanced	Limited availability, contraindicated in patients with some forms of indwelling hardware, time-consuming	High

Abbreviations: CTA, computed tomography angiography; MRA, magnetic resonance angiography; Sens, sensitivity; Spec, specificity.

Data from Jauch EC, Saver JL, Adams HP Jr, et al. American Heart Association Stroke Council; Council on Cardiovascular Nursing; Council on Peripheral Vascular Disease; Council on Clinical Cardiology. Guidelines for the early management of patients with acute ischemic stroke: a guideline for healthcare professionals from the American Heart Association/American Stroke Association. Stroke 2013;44:870–947.

limitation is that the clinical measurements favor identifying anterior circulation strokes and miss posterior circulation findings, such as dizziness or sensory loss. Regardless, the ABCD2 score does provide a framework for approaching clinical decision making in these patients.

In an attempt to improve on the ABCD2 score, the ABCD2-I score has been proposed in which neuroimaging is added to the formula.[53,56] This score adds the finding of radiologic features (CT or DWI MRI) of cerebral infarction to the ABCD2 clinical findings with better results in prediction of risk for stroke (area under the curve 0.78 vs 0.66 at 7 days; 0.80 vs 0.68 at 90 days).[53] Other scores have been developed, including the ABCD3-I score that adds the presence of a previous TIA

Table 5
ABCD2 score

Predictor	Points
Age >60 y	1
Blood pressure >140/90	1
Unilateral weakness	2
Speech difficulty without weakness	1
Duration <10 min	0
Duration 10–59 min	1
Duration >60 min	2
Diabetes	1

Low risk: <4 (stroke risk 1.0% at 2 days, 1.2% at 7 days, and 3.1% at 90 days).
    Moderate risk: 4–5 (stroke risk 4.1% at 2 days, 5.9% at 7 days, and 9.8% at 90 days).
    High risk: >5 (stroke risk 8.1% at 2 days, 11.7% at 7 days, and 17.8% at 90 days).
    Data from Johnston SC, Rothwell PM, Nguyen-Huynh MN, et al. Validation and refinement of scores to predict very early stroke risk after transient ischaemic attack. Lancet 2007;369(9558): 283–92.

within 7 days to the ABCD2 and the presence of carotid stenosis or abnormal DWI MRI,[54] or the ABCDE+ score that adds DWI MRI finding and etiology to the ABCD2 score.[57]

The premise underlying the various risk stratification scores is that the more components incorporated, the more accurate it will be for prognosis. Unfortunately, the perfect scoring system has yet to be developed, and clinical acumen based on a careful history and physical must be incorporated into the clinical decision making.[58] Some have suggested that the addition of various imaging components to risk stratification renders the very concept of risk stratification meaningless, as the newer comprehensive tools are simply doing the entire workup.[59] This is analogous to "risk stratifying" patients with potential pulmonary embolism by doing a CTA in all of them.

TREATMENT

The goal in TIA treatment is to prevent subsequent stroke. Therefore, treatment aims to optimize the cerebral blood flow and cerebral oxygenation; at the same time, special attention is given to identify and treat underlying predisposing pathologies and conditions. Once stabilized, specific interventions are directed toward the suspected underlying etiology. There are 3 main therapeutic actions that reduce stroke occurrence: antiplatelet therapy, anticoagulant therapy, and surgical or endovascular treatment of significant arterial stenosis.

Immediate Treatment

There are no specific guidelines for immediate treatment of TIA; indeed, findings have generally resolved by the time the patient is seen. In those cases in which findings are present, treat the patients as if they have a stroke, trying to promote CNS oxygenation and perfusion.[42] In one trial it has been shown that the supine position ensures an increased cerebral flow compared with the seating or standing position; therefore, in patients at high risk of stroke without signs of hypoxia, we recommend that the patient be supine.[42] Oxygen administration is recommended only in case of hypoxia (ie, oxygen saturation <94% on room air) and should be avoided in nonhypoxic patients (Class of evidence IIIB).[42]

Anticoagulant Therapy

In cases of nonvalvular atrial fibrillation, the 2013 ASA stroke guidelines recommend starting an anticoagulant within 14 days of the event (**Table 6**). The newest factor Xa inhibitor edoxaban has not yet been included in the ASA guidelines. For patients who have contraindications to anticoagulant therapy, acetylsalicylic acid plus clopidogrel is recommended.[42] TIA has a lower risk for intracranial hemorrhage and therefore, unlike stroke benefit, favors early treatment after diagnosis.[60]

At the present time, a vitamin K antagonist (VKA) is the only indicated treatment for valvular atrial fibrillation or situation at high risk for thrombus, such as apical ventricular akinesia. The same indication is valid for patients with ventricular assisted devices, mechanical aortic valve (INR target 2,5) or mechanical mitral valve (INR target 3).[42]

An antiplatelet agent can be added to the anticoagulant therapy in particular cases, such as atrial fibrillation in the context of coronary artery disease, new TIA in the presence of rheumatic valve disease already on anticoagulant therapy, or aortic or mitral mechanical valve.[42]

Table 6
Oral anticoagulant in nonvalvular atrial fibrillation

Drug	Mechanism of Action	Dose	Major Contraindications	Stroke or Systemic Embolism Risk Reduction	Major Bleeding Rate	Major Bleeding Treatment
Warfarin	Interferes with synthesis of vitamin K–dependent clotting factors	Depending on INR	Hypersensitivity, hemorrhagic tendencies/active bleeding, recent surgery of CNS or eye, thrombocytopenia, pregnancy	RR reduction of 68% (95% CI 50%–79%)	1.3% per year	• PCC or fresh frozen plasma if PCC not available • IV vitamin K
Dabigatran	Direct thrombin inhibitor	75-150 mg q 12h	Severe hypersensitivity, active pathologic bleeding; mechanical prosthetic valve	RR 0.65 (95% CI 0.52–0.81 $P<.001$) vs warfarin	RR 0.93 (95% CI 0.81–1.07 $P = .31$) vs warfarin	• Idarucizumab • Tranexamic acid (grade of evidence 2C) • FEIBA (grade of evidence 2C)
Rivaroxaban	Factor Xa inhibitor	20 mg q 24 h	Severe hypersensitivity, active pathologic bleeding	HR 0.79 (95% CI 0.66–0.96 $P<.001$ for noninferiority) vs warfarin	HR 1.03 (95% CI 0.96–1.11 $P = .44$) vs warfarin	• Tranexamic acid (grade of evidence 2C) • 4-factor PCC • Oral activated charcoal if recent assumption • Under development: adexanet alfa

| Apixaban | Factor Xa inhibitor | 2.5–5 mg q 12 h | Severe hypersensitivity, active pathologic bleeding | HR 0.45 (95% CI 0.32–0.62 $P<.001$) vs aspirin
HR 0.89 (95% CI 0.66–0.95 $P<.001$ for noninferiority; $P = .01$ for superiority) vs warfarin | HR 1.13 (95% CI, 0.74–1.75 $P = .57$) vs aspirin
HR 0.69 (95% CI 0.60–0.80 $P<.001$) vs warfarin | • Tranexamic acid (grade of evidence 2C)
• 4 factor PCC (grade of evidence 2C)
• Oral activated charcoal if recent assumption (grade of evidence 2C)
• Under development: adexanet alfa |
| Edoxaban | Factor Xa inhibitor | 30–60 mg q 24 h (only if creatinine clearance <95 mL/min) | Hypersensitivity, active pathologic bleeding | HR 0.79 (97.5% CI 0.63–0.99; $P<.001$ for noninferiority; $P = .02$ for superiority) vs warfarin | HR 0.80 (95% CI 0.71–0.91; $P<.001$) vs warfarin | • Tranexamic acid (grade of evidence 2C)
• 4 factor PCC (grade of evidence 2C)
• Oral activated charcoal if recent assumption (grade of evidence 2C)
• Under development: adexanet alfa, PER977 |

Abbreviations: CI, confidence interval; CNS, central nervous system; FEIBA, Factor eight inhibitor bypassing agent; HR, hazard ratio; INR, international normalized ratio; IV, intravenous; PCC, prothrombin complex concentrate; q, every; RR, relative risk.
Data from Refs.[41,61–65]

Antiplatelet Therapy

Antiplatelet therapy is recommended in all cases of noncardioembolic TIA (Level of evidence IA).[66]

Aspirin, aspirin plus dipyridamole, clopidogrel, and ticlopidine are currently the 4 antiplatelet therapies approved by the Food and Drug Administration for secondary prevention in acute ischemic stroke and TIA. Acetylsalicylic acid is the best studied and most widely prescribed of the approved antiplatelet medications, and it is first line for initial therapy. Overall, it confers a 2-year stroke risk reduction of approximately 15% compared with placebo, at a variety of doses ranging from 50 mg to 1500 mg.[67] Lower doses (61 mg to 325 mg per day) appear to be as effective, with a lower incidence of gastrointestinal bleeding. However, even low-dose ($\leq$325 mg/d) aspirin users are 2.5 times more likely to have a serious gastrointestinal hemorrhage than nonusers (annual risk 0.4%) and have a small absolute increase in the risk of hemorrhagic stroke (12 events per 10,000 persons).[68,69]

Aspirin plus dipyridamole has been evaluated in 4 large randomized controlled trials showing that this combination is more effective than aspirin alone, but less well tolerated[70–73]; for this reason, it is recommended for initial treatment after TIA as an alternative to aspirin by the ASA guidelines (Level of evidence IB).[66]

There are 5 conditions when double antiplatelet therapy with aspirin and clopidogrel should be considered: high-risk TIA (large artery atherosclerosis and cardioembolic disease) within the first 24 hours, TIA associated with severe (70%–99%) intracranial arterial stenosis within the first 3 days, TIA with intracranial or carotid symptomatic stenosis with microembolic signs within 7 days, extracranial vertebral stenting with bare metal stents, or TIA with aortic arch atherosclerotic plaque or mobile thrombosis or patches.[66,74–86] See **Table 7** for a summary of trials.

Carotid Endarterectomy and Carotid Stenting

Carotid endarterectomy is indicated in cases of 50% to 90% carotid stenosis when the estimated intervention morbidity and mortality is lower than 6%. Ideally the procedure should be done within 2 weeks of diagnosis (Class of evidence IA for severe stenosis, IB for moderate stenosis).[66] For the same pathology, therapy with statins and antihypertensive therapy is recommended.

Endovascular carotid artery stenting versus endarterectomy has been the focus of several studies and the findings synthesized in a 2012 Cochrane review and by the ASA. The reviews concluded that overall endovascular treatment is associated with an increased risk of periprocedural stroke or death compared with endarterectomy, although this excess risk appears to be limited to older patients. In fact, in patients younger than 70 years, the odds ratio of death or stroke at 30 days for endovascular treatment compared with endarterectomy was 1.16 (95% confidence interval [CI] 0.8–1.67), whereas it was 2.20 (95% CI 1.47–3.29 $P = .02$) for patients older than 70 years.[87]

Treatment of Risk Factors

Adjunctive to stroke-prevention treatments is assessing risk factors for stroke and implementing a strategy to manage them. The first risk factor to assess is arterial blood pressure. Antihypertensive treatment is recommended in all patients having an arterial blood pressure greater than 140/90 mm Hg, with the goal to lower the pressure under that value (Level of evidence IB); the guidelines do not specify the speed with which one should treat the hypertension, and our opinion is that this should be done with oral agents slowly.[66]

Table 7
Double antiplatelet therapy with acetylsalicylic acid and clopidogrel

Study	Population	Therapy	Results	Major Bleeding Risk
CHANCE 2013[75] + 1-y follow-up[76]	Nondisabling stroke/high risk of TIA within 24 h of onset	Aspirin 75–300 mg on day 1, then 75 mg day 2–21 + clopidogrel 300 mg on day 1, then 75 mg day 2–90 vs aspirin 300 mg on day 1, then 75 mg on days 2–90	Stroke recurrence/occurrence Dual antiplatelet vs aspirin: HR 0.67 (95% CI 0.56–0.81 P<.001) at 90 d, HR 0.78 (95% CI 0.65–0.93 P = .005) at 1 y	HR 1.41 (95% CI 0.95–2.10 P = .09) at 90 d, HR 0.67 (95% CI 0.24–1.87 P = .44) at 1 y
FASTER,[77] 2004	Minor stroke/high risk TIA within 24 h of onset	Clopidogrel 300 mg on day 1, then 75 mg day 2–90 + aspirin vs aspirin	Stroke (ischemic + hemorrhagic) reduction –3.8% (–9.4–1.9, P = .19)	Risk increase 1.0% (–0.4–2.4, P = .5)
SPS3,[79] 2012	Nondisabling lacunar stroke after at least 14 d of onset (mean 62 d)	Aspirin 325 mg + clopidogrel 75 mg vs aspirin 325 mg	Ischemic stroke recurrence HR 0.82 (95% CI, 0.63–1.09, P = .13) at 1 y	HR 1.97 (95% CI 1.14–2.04, P = .004) at 1 y
MATCH,[78] 2004	Ischemic stroke/TIA within 3 mo with risk factors (53% lacunar strokes)	Aspirin 75 mg + clopidogrel 75 mg vs clopidogrel 75 mg	Occurrence of ischemic stroke, 8% vs 9%; relative risk reduction 7.1% (95% CI –8.5–20.4, P = .353) mean follow-up 18 mo	2% vs 1%, difference +1.36% (95% CI 0.86%–1.86%, P<.0001)
WASID,[82] 2005	TIA or stroke with intracranial arterial stenosis 70%–99%	WASID: aspirin 1300 mg/d	WASID: Stroke or death 10.7% at 30 d; 25% at 1 y	WASID: major bleeding 3.2% at 1 y
SAMMPRIS,[81] 2011	TIA or stroke with intracranial arterial stenosis 70%–99%	SAMMPRIS: aspirin 375 mg/d + clopidogrel 75 mg/d per 90 d + aggressive medical management	SAMMPRIS probability of stroke or death 5.8% (3.4%–9.7%) at 30 d; 17.5% (12.8%–23.6%) at 1 y	SAMMPRIS: probability of major bleeding 0.9% (0.2%–3.5%) at 30 d; 1.8% at 1 y (0.7%–4.8%)

(continued on next page)

Table 7
(continued)

Study	Population	Therapy	Results	Major Bleeding Risk
CARESS,[83] 2005	Symptomatic carotid stenosis with asymptomatic MES detected by transcranial Doppler	Aspirin 75 mg vs aspirin 75 mg + clopidogrel 300 mg day 1, 75 mg days 2–7	Relative reduction of MES of 39.8% (95% CI 13.8–58.0; $P = .005$) at 7 d	
CLAIR,[84] 2010	Symptomatic carotid or cerebral artery stenosis with MES detected by transcranial Doppler	Aspirin 75–160 mg vs aspirin 75–160 mg + clopidogrel 300 mg day 1, 75 mg days 2–7	Relative reduction of MES of 42.4% (95% CI 4.6–65.2; $P = .025$) at day 2; 54.4% (95% CI 16.4%–75.1%; $P = .006$) at day 7	
ARCH,[86] 2014	TIA or nondisabling stroke or peripheral embolism and atherosclerotic plaque in thoracic aorta	Aspirin 75–150 mg + clopidogrel 75 mg vs warfarin (INR 2–3)	Recurrent stroke, myocardial infarction, peripheral embolism, vascular death HR 0.76 (95% CI 0.36–1.61; $P = .5$) at 3.4 y. Reduction of vascular death from 3.4% to 0% ($P = .013$) at 3.4 y	2.3% (aspirin + clopidogrel) vs 3.45% (warfarin) $P = .17$

Abbreviations: CI, confidence interval; HR, hazard ratio; INR, international normalized ratio; MES, microembolic signals; TIA, transient ischemic attack.

Statin therapy is recommended for patients with presumed arteriosclerotic-related TIA who have a low density lipoprotein (LDL) level greater than 100 mg/dL (Class of evidence IB), and even in cases of LDL less than 100 mg/dL in the absence of evidence of other atherosclerotic cardiovascular disease (Class of evidence IC).[66] Other risk factors that should be assessed are diabetes, obesity, nutrition, cigarette smoke, alcohol consumption, and physical inactivity.[66]

Table 8
Transient ischemic attack clinic and outpatient evaluation studies

Study	Design	Main Results
OTTAWA,[89] 2010	• ECG, blood tests and head CT in the emergency department • Carotid Doppler, echocardiogram, 24-h ECG, lipid profile as outpatients • Neurology visit at 7, 14, or >14 d based on ABCD2 score	• 90-d stroke rate of 3.2% compared with the ABCD2 predicted score of 9.2% • 48-h stroke rate of 1%
SOS-TIA,[90] 2007	24-h access hospital clinic (SOS-TIA) with neurologic, arterial, cardiac assessment and blood tests within 4 h from admission	• 26% of patients admitted to stroke unit after clinic evaluation • 90-d stroke rate of 1.24% compared with the ABCD2 predicted score of 5.96%
Marti'nez-Marti'nez et al,[95] 2013	TIA clinic (8 AM–3 PM) for patients with low to moderate risk compared with previous model involving hospitalization for all patients	• 9.6% of patients admitted after evaluation in the clinic • 90-d stroke recurrence rate 2.4% vs 1.2% ($P = .65$)
TWO ACES,[96] 2011	• Head CT, blood tests, ECG, and neurology evaluation in the emergency department • Discharge to be seen in TIA clinic within 1–2 business day if ABCD2 score 0–3; vascular imaging if ABCD2 score 4–5; admit if ABCD2 score >5	• 30% of patients admitted to hospital • 90-d stroke rate of 0.9% compared with the ABCD2 predicted score of 7.1%
M3T,[97] 2012	• Head CT, ECG, carotid Doppler, blood tests in the emergency department, phone referral to stroke team and discharge with therapy and follow-up • If outpatients: faxed referral to TIA clinic, priority of evaluation based on presence of atrial fibrillation or carotid stenosis	• 17.4% of patients admitted after evaluation • 90-d stroke rate of 1.50%
EXPRESS,[101] 2007	Stroke/TIA clinic vs standard outpatient care of previous study (OXVASC[94]). Patients with stroke or TIA referred by primary physician	90-d risk of recurrent stroke of 2.1% vs 10.3% HR 0.20 (95% CI 0.08–0.49, $P = .0001$)

Abbreviations: CI, confidence interval; CT, computed tomography; ECG, electrocardiogram; HR, hazard ratio; TIA, transient ischemic attack.

DISPOSITION

Outpatient versus observation unit versus inpatient admission decision is usually based on the ABCD2-I score or some variation of it, the patient's resources, and the access to follow-up. Guidelines have tried to address the issue of which patients are at higher risk of stroke, thus deserving of an inpatient admission. In particular, the 2009 AHA guidelines used the ABCD2 score recommending that hospitalization be considered for patients with an ABCD2 score greater than 2, evidence of focal ischemia, or for any patient in whom rapid follow-up as an outpatient cannot realistically be obtained within 2 days.[4]

However, as previously explained, the ABCD2 score is imperfect in identifying both high-risk and low-risk individual patients, and cannot be used alone to determine the disposition of a patient.

Another criterion to take into account is the time elapsed from the symptoms to the medical evaluation, because after 2 days the risk of stroke recurrence is lower than in

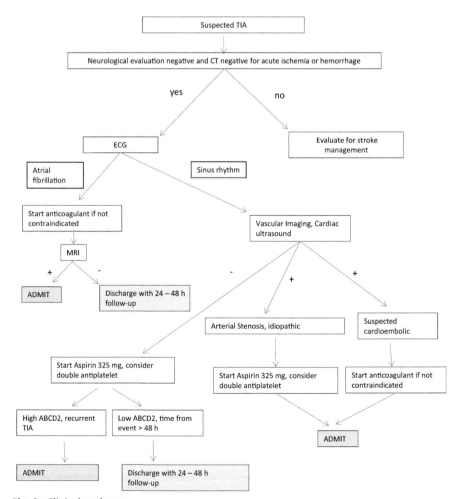

Fig. 3. Clinical pathway.

the immediate days following the TIA and the urgency of the clinical assessment is then lower.

Some investigators have evaluated electronic decision tools more detailed than the ABCD2 score that can help general practitioners to identify high-risk patients who need to be referred urgently to specialist and/or in-hospital evaluations.[88]

On the other hand, other organizational models than hospital admission have been tried, such as TIA clinics and observation units. TIA clinics ensure that a comprehensive evaluation is provided within 24 hours. Observation units provide the advance of a facilitated evaluation plus cardiac monitoring, plus access to emergent therapy in the event of a stroke. Both these options have shown good results and to be noninferior to hospital admission in reducing the occurrence of stroke following TIA in patients with medium and low risk of stroke recurrence (**Table 8**).[89–102]

In conclusion, whatever the local pathway, we recommend that the patient with a TIA receive a comprehensive evaluation within the first 24 hours from the event to identify the treatable causes and to educate the patients regarding the modifiable risk factors: it is the timing of the workup rather than its location that is most important.[59] Based on the identification of the pathogenetic factors of the event, for patients at particularly high risk, such as patients with severe arterial stenosis, we recommend admission for inpatient monitoring and treatment. For patients referred for an outpatient follow-up, we recommend a clear hand-off to the physician taking responsibility for the patient's evaluation, with well-defined instructions to the patient on where to go for the outpatient care and when to return to the ED. Regardless of where patients with TIA receive their evaluation, health care providers should take the opportunity to educate the patient and family on risk modulation and engage in a discussion introducing thrombolytic therapy in the event that the emergency arises (**Fig. 3**).

REFERENCES

1. Hong KS, Yegiaian S, Lee M, et al. Declining stroke and vascular event recurrence rates in secondary prevention trials over the past 50 years and consequences for current trial design. Circulation 2011;123:2111–9.

2. Wasserman JK, Perry JJ, Sivilotti ML, et al. Computed tomography identifies patients at high risk for stroke after transient ischemic attack/nondisabling stroke: prospective, multicenter cohort study. Stroke 2015;46:114–9.

3. Easton JD, Saver JL, Albers GW, et al. Definition and evaluation of transient ischemic attack: a scientific statement for healthcare professionals from the American Heart Association/American Stroke Association Stroke Council; Council on Cardiovascular Surgery and Anesthesia; Council on Cardiovascular Radiology and Intervention; Council on Cardiovascular Nursing; and the Interdisciplinary Council on Peripheral Vascular Disease. The American Academy of Neurology affirms the value of this statement as an educational tool for neurologists. Stroke 2009;40:2276–93.

4. Advisory Council for the National Institute of Neurological and Communicative Disorders and Stroke. A classification and outline of cerebrovascular diseases, II. Stroke 1975;6:564–616.

5. Sacco RL, Kasner SE, Broderick JP, et al, American Heart Association Stroke Council, Council on Cardiovascular Surgery and Anesthesia. An updated definition of stroke for the 21st century: a statement for healthcare professionals from the American Heart Association/American Stroke Association. Stroke 2013;44:2064–89.

6. Fanning JP, Wesley AJ, Wong AA, et al. Emerging spectra of silent brain infarction. Stroke 2014;45:3461–71.

7. Center for Disease Control. Mortality multiple cause micro-data files. 2013. Available at: www.cdc.gov/nchs/data/nvsr/nvsr64/nvsr64_02.pdf.

8. Mozaffarian D, Benjamin EJ, Go AS, et al, American Heart Association Statistics Committee and Stroke Statistics Subcommittee. Heart disease and stroke statistics–2015 update: a report from the American Heart Association. Circulation 2015;131(4):e29–322.

9. Anticoli S, Pezzella FR, Pozzessere C, et al. Transient ischemic attack fast-track and long-term stroke risk: role of diffusion-weighted magnetic resonance imaging. J Stroke Cerebrovasc Dis 2015;24(9):2110–6.

10. Adams HP Jr, Bendixen BH, Kappelle LJ, et al. Classification of subtype of acute ischemic stroke. Definitions for use in a multicenter clinical trial. TOAST. Trial of Org 10172 in Acute Stroke Treatment. Stroke 1993;24:35–41.

11. Ay H, Benner T, Arsava EM, et al. A computerized algorithm for etiologic classification of ischemic stroke: the Causative Classification of Stroke System. Stroke 2007;38:2979–84.

12. Amarenco P, Bogousslavsky J, Caplan LR, et al. New approach to stroke subtyping: the A-S-C-O (phenotypic) classification of stroke. Cerebrovasc Dis 2009;27:502–8.

13. Marnane M, Duggan CA, Sheehan OC, et al. Stroke subtype classification to mechanism-specific and undetermined categories by TOAST, A-S-C-O, and causative classification system: direct comparison in the North Dublin population stroke study. Stroke 2010;41:1579–86.

14. Desai JA, Abuzinadah AR, Imoukhuede O, et al. Etiologic classification of TIA and minor stroke by A-S-C-O and causative classification system as compared to TOAST reduces the proportion of patients categorized as cause undetermined. Cerebrovasc Dis 2014;38(2):121–6.

15. Pendlebury ST, Giles MF, Rothwell PM. Transient ischemic attack and stroke: diagnosis, investigation, and management. 1st edition. New York: Cambridge University Press; 2009. p. 55–90.

16. Redfors P, Jood K, Holmegaard L, et al. Stroke subtype predicts outcome in young and middle-aged stroke sufferers. Acta Neurol Scand 2012;126(5): 329–35.

17. Stead LG, Gilmore RM, Bellolio MF, et al. Cardioembolic but not other stroke subtypes predict mortality independent of stroke severity at presentation. Stroke Res Treat 2011;2011:281496.

18. Arboix A, Alio J. Cardioembolic stroke: clinical features, specific cardiac disorders and prognosis. Curr Cardiol Rev 2010;6(3):150–61.

19. Lip GY, Nieuwlaat R, Pisters R, et al. Refining clinical risk stratification for predicting stroke and thromboembolism in atrial fibrillation using a novel risk factor-based approach: the Euro Heart Survey on Atrial Fibrillation. Chest 2010;137(2):263–72.

20. Friberg L, Rosenqvist M, Lip GY, et al. Evaluation of risk stratification schemes for ischaemic stroke and bleeding in 182 678 patients with atrial fibrillation: the Swedish Atrial Fibrillation cohort study. Eur Heart J 2012;33(12):1500–10.

21. Nadarajan V, Perry RJ, Johnson J, et al. Transient ischaemic attacks: mimics and chameleons. Pract Neurol 2014;14:23–31.

22. Hand PJ, Kwan J, Lindley RI, et al. Distinguishing between stroke and mimic at the bedside: the Brain Attack Study. Stroke 2006;37(3):769–75.

23. Amort M, Fluri F, Schäfer J, et al. Transient ischemic attack versus transient ischemic attack mimics: frequency, clinical characteristics and outcome. Cerebrovasc Dis 2011;32(1):57–64.

24. Negrotto L, Barroso FA. Focal hypokalemic paralysis: report of 2 cases and review of the literature. J Clin Neuromuscul Dis 2012;14(1):21–7.

25. Landi G. Clinical diagnosis of transient ischaemic attacks. Lancet 1992; 339(8790):402–5.

26. Kerber KA, Brown DL, Lisabeth LD, et al. Stroke among patients with dizziness, vertigo, and imbalance in the emergency department: a population-based study. Stroke 2006;37(10):2484–7.

27. Paul NL, Simoni M, Rothwell PM. Transient isolated brainstem symptoms preceding posterior circulation stroke: a population-based study. Lancet Neurol 2013;12(1):65–71.

28. Levy DE. How transient are transient ischemic attacks? Neurology 1988;38(5): 674–7.

29. Kimura K, Minematsu K, Yasaka M, et al. The duration of symptoms in transient ischemic attack. Neurology 1999;52(5):976–80.

30. Pendlebury ST, Wadling S, Silver LE, et al. Transient cognitive impairment in TIA and minor stroke. Stroke 2011;42(11):3116–21.

31. Moreau F, Jeerakathil T, Coutts SB, FRCPC for the ASPIRE Investigators. Patients referred for TIA may still have persisting neurological deficits. Can J Neurol Sci 2012;39(2):170–3.

32. Casaubon LK, Boulanger JM, Blacquiere D, et al, Heart and Stroke Foundation of Canada Canadian Stroke Best Practices Advisory Committee. Canadian Stroke Best Practice Recommendations: hyperacute stroke care guidelines, update 2015. Int J Stroke 2015;10(6):924–40.

33. George PM, Mlynash M, Adams CM, et al. Novel TIA biomarkers identified by mass spectrometry-based proteomics. Int J Stroke 2015;10(8):1204–11.

34. Jickling GC, Zhan X, Stamova B, et al. Ischemic transient neurological events identified by immune response to cerebral ischemia. Stroke 2012;43(4): 1006–12.

35. Cucchiara BL, Messe SR, Sansing L, et al. Lipoprotein-associated phospholipase A2 and C-reactive protein for risk-stratification of patients with TIA. Stroke 2009;40(7):2332–6.

36. Rosell A, Alvarez-Sabín J, Arenillas JF, et al. A matrix metalloproteinase protein array reveals a strong relation between MMP-9 and MMP-13 with diffusion-weighted image lesion increase in human stroke. Stroke 2005;36(7):1415–20.

37. Nash DL, Bellolio MF, Stead LG, et al. Neuron-specific enolase as a marker for acute ischemic stroke: a systematic review. Cerebrovasc Dis 2005;20(4):213–9.

38. Dambinova SA, Khounteev GA, Izykenova GA, et al. Blood test detecting autoantibodies to N-methyl-D-aspartate neuroreceptors for evaluation of patients with transient ischemic attack and stroke. Clin Chem 2003;49(10):1752–62.

39. Whiteley W, Wardlaw J, Dennis M, et al. Blood biomarkers for the diagnosis of acute cerebrovascular diseases: a prospective cohort study. Cerebrovasc Dis 2011;32(2):141–7.

40. Laskowitz DT, Blessing R, Floyd J, et al. Panel of biomarkers predicts stroke. Ann N Y Acad Sci 2005;1053:30.

41. Welsh P, Barber M, Langhorne P, et al. Associations of inflammatory and haemostatic biomarkers with poor outcome in acute ischaemic stroke. Cerebrovasc Dis 2009;27(3):247–53.

42. Jauch EC, Saver JL, Adams HP Jr, et al, American Heart Association Stroke Council, Council on Cardiovascular Nursing, Council on Peripheral Vascular Disease, Council on Clinical Cardiology. Guidelines for the early management of patients with acute ischemic stroke: a guideline for healthcare professionals from the American Heart Association/American Stroke Association. Stroke 2013;44:870–947.

43. Tayal AH, Tian M, Kelly KM, et al. Atrial fibrillation detected by mobile cardiac outpatient telemetry in cryptogenic TIA or stroke. Neurology 2008;71(21): 1696–701.

44. Gaillard N, Deltour S, Vilotijevic B, et al. Detection of paroxysmal atrial fibrillation with transtelephonic EKG in TIA or stroke patients. Neurology 2010;74(21): 1666–70.

45. Culebras A, Messé SR, Chaturvedi S, et al. Summary of evidence-based guideline update: prevention of stroke in nonvalvular atrial fibrillation: report of the Guideline Development Subcommittee of the American Academy of Neurology. Neurology 2014;82(8):716–24.

46. Zhang L, Harrison JK, Goldstein LB. Echocardiography for the detection of cardiac sources of embolism in patients with stroke or transient ischemic attack. J Stroke Cerebrovasc Dis 2012;21(7):577–82.

47. Brazzelli M, Sandercock PA, Chappell FM, et al. Magnetic resonance imaging versus computed tomography for detection of acute vascular lesions in patients presenting with stroke symptoms. Cochrane Database Syst Rev 2009;(4):CD007424.

48. Kernan WN, Horwitz RI, Brass LM, et al. A prognostic system for transient ischemia or minor stroke. Ann Intern Med 1991;114(7):552–7.

49. Kernan WN, Viscoli CM, Brass LM, et al. The Stroke Prognosis Instrument II (SPI-II): a clinical prediction instrument for patients with transient ischemia and non-disabling ischemic stroke. Stroke 2000;31(2):456–62.

50. Johnston SC, Gress DR, Browner WS, et al. Short-term prognosis after emergency department diagnosis of TIA. JAMA 2000;284(22):2901–6.

51. Rothwell PM, Giles MF, Flossmann E, et al. A simple score (ABCD) to identify individuals at high early risk of stroke after transient ischaemic attack. Lancet 2005;366(9479):29–36.

52. Johnston SC, Rothwell PM, Nguyen-Huynh MN, et al. Validation and refinement of scores to predict very early stroke risk after transient ischaemic attack. Lancet 2007;369(9558):283–92.

53. Giles MF, Albers GW, Amarenco P, et al. Addition of brain infarction to the ABCD2 Score (ABCD2I): a collaborative analysis of unpublished data on 4574 patients. Stroke 2010;41(9):1907–13.

54. Merwick A, Albers GW, Amarenco P, et al. Addition of brain and carotid imaging to the ABCD[2] score to identify patients at early risk of stroke after transient ischaemic attack: a multicentre observational study. Lancet Neurol 2010;9(11): 1060–9.

55. Wardlaw JM, Brazzelli M, Chappell FM, et al. ABCD2 score and secondary stroke prevention: meta-analysis and effect per 1,000 patients triaged. Neurology 2015;85(4):373–80.

56. Coutts SB, Eliasziw M, Hill MD, et al. An improved scoring system for identifying patients at high early risk of stroke and functional impairment after an acute transient ischemic attack or minor stroke. Int J Stroke 2008;3(1):3–10.

57. Engelter ST, Amort M, Jax F, et al. Optimizing the risk estimation after a transient ischaemic attack—the ABCDE⊕ score. Eur J Neurol 2012;19(1):55–61.

58. Kiyohara T, Kamouchi M, Kumai Y, et al. ABCD3 and ABCD3-I scores are superior to ABCD2 score in the prediction of short- and long-term risks of stroke after transient ischemic attack. Stroke 2014;45(2):418–25.

59. Edlow JA. Risk stratification in TIA patients: 'It's the vascular lesion, stupid!'. Neurology 2012;79:958.

60. Hahn C, Hill MD. Early anti-coagulation after ischemic stroke due to atrial fibrillation is safe and prevents recurrent stroke. Can J Neurol Sci 2015;42(2):92–5.

61. Connolly SJ, Ezekowitz MD, Yusuf S, et al. Dabigatran versus warfarin in patients with atrial fibrillation. N Engl J Med 2009;361:1139–51.

62. Patel MR, Mahaffey KW, Garg J, et al. Rivaroxaban versus warfarin in nonvalvular atrial fibrillation. N Engl J Med 2011;365:883–91.

63. Connolly SJ, Eikelboom J, Joyner C, et al. Apixaban in patients with atrial fibrillation. N Engl J Med 2011;364:806–17.

64. Granger CB, Alexander JH, McMurray JJV, et al. Apixaban versus warfarin in patients with atrial fibrillation. N Engl J Med 2011;365:981–92.

65. Giugliano RP, Ruff CT, Braunwald E, et al. Edoxaban versus warfarin in patients with atrial fibrillation. N Engl J Med 2013;369:2093–104.

66. Kernan WN, Ovbiagele B, Black HR, et al, American Heart Association Stroke Council, Council on Cardiovascular and Stroke Nursing, Council on Clinical Cardiology, Council on Peripheral Vascular Disease. Guidelines for the prevention of stroke in patients with stroke and transient ischemic attack: a guideline for healthcare professionals from the American Heart Association/American Stroke Association. Stroke 2014;45:2160–236.

67. Johnson ES, Lanes SF, Wentworth CE 3rd, et al. A metaregression analysis of the dose-response effect of aspirin on stroke. Arch Intern Med 1999;159(11): 1248–53.

68. Weisman SM, Graham DY. Evaluation of the benefits and risks of low-dose aspirin in the secondary prevention of cardiovascular and cerebrovascular events. Arch Intern Med 2002;162(19):2197–202.

69. He J, Whelton PK, Vu B, et al. Aspirin and risk of hemorrhagic stroke: a meta-analysis of randomized controlled trials. JAMA 1998;280(22):1930–5.

70. The European Stroke Prevention Study: principal end-points. The ESPS Group. Lancet 1987;2:1351–4.

71. Diener H, Cunha L, Forbes C, et al. European Stroke Prevention Study 2: dipyridamole and acetyl-salicylic acid in the secondary prevention of stroke. J Neurol Sci 1996;143:1–13.

72. The ESPRIT Study Group, Halkes PH, van Gijn J, et al. Aspirin plus dipyridamole versus aspirin alone after cerebral ischaemia of arterial origin (ESPRIT): randomised controlled trial. Lancet 2006;367:1665–73 [Erratum appears in Lancet 2007;369:274].

73. Dengler R, Diener HC, Schwartz A, et al. Early treatment with aspirin plus extended-release dipyridamole for transient ischaemic attack or ischaemic stroke within 24 h of symptom onset (EARLY trial): a randomised, open-label, blinded-endpoint trial. Lancet Neurol 2010;9:159–66.

74. Wang Y, Chen W, Wang Y. Dual antiplatelet therapy with clopidogrel and aspirin for secondary stroke prevention. Curr Cardiol Rep 2015;17(10):642.

75. Wang Y, Wang Y, Zhao X, et al. Clopidogrel with aspirin in acute minor stroke or transient ischemic attack. N Engl J Med 2013;369(1):11–9.

76. Wang Y, Pan Y, Zhao X, et al. Clopidogrel with aspirin in acute minor stroke or transient ischemic attack (CHANCE) trial: one-year outcomes. Circulation 2015;132(1):40–6.

77. Kennedy J, Hill MD, Ryckborst KJ, et al. Fast assessment of stroke and transient ischaemic attack to prevent early recurrence (FASTER): a randomised controlled pilot trial. Lancet Neurol 2007;6(11):961–9.

78. Diener HC, Bogousslavsky J, Brass LM, et al. Aspirin and clopidogrel compared with clopidogrel alone after recent ischaemic stroke or transient ischaemic attack in high-risk patients (MATCH): randomised, double-blind, placebo-controlled trial. Lancet 2004;364(9431):331–7.

79. SPS3 Investigators, Benavente OR, Hart RG, et al. Effects of clopidogrel added to aspirin in patients with recent lacunar stroke. N Engl J Med 2012;367(9): 817–25.

80. Bhatt DL, Fox KA, Hacke W, et al. Clopidogrel and aspirin versus aspirin alone for the prevention of atherothrombotic events. N Engl J Med 2006;354(16): 1706–17.

81. Chimowitz MI, Lynn MJ, Derdeyn CP, et al. Stenting versus aggressive medical therapy for intracranial arterial stenosis. N Engl J Med 2011;365:993–1003.

82. Chimowitz MI, Lynn MJ, Howlett-Smith H, et al. Comparison of warfarin and aspirin for symptomatic intracranial arterial stenosis. N Engl J Med 2005;352: 1305–16.

83. Markus HS, Droste DW, Kaps M, et al. Dual antiplatelet therapy with clopidogrel and aspirin in symptomatic carotid stenosis evaluated using Doppler embolic signal detection: the clopidogrel and aspirin for reduction of emboli in symptomatic carotid stenosis (CARESS) trial. Circulation 2005;111:2233–40.

84. Wong KS, Chen C, Fu J, et al. Clopidogrel plus aspirin versus aspirin alone for reducing embolisation in patients with acute symptomatic cerebral or carotid artery stenosis (CLAIR study): a randomised, open-label, blinded-endpoint trial. Lancet Neurol 2010;9:489–97.

85. Brott TG, Halperin JL, Abbara S, et al. 2011 ASA/ACCF/AHA/AANN/AANS/ACR/ ASNR/CNS/SAIP/SCAI/SIR/SNIS/SVM/SVS guideline on the management of patients with extracranial carotid and vertebral artery disease: a report of the American College of Cardiology Foundation/American Heart Association Task Force on Practice Guidelines, and the American Stroke Association, American Association of Neuroscience Nurses, American Association of Neurological Surgeons, American College of Radiology, American Society of Neuroradiology, Congress of Neurological Surgeons, Society of Atherosclerosis Imaging and Prevention, Society for Cardiovascular Angiography and Interventions, Society of Interventional Radiology, Society of NeuroInterventional Surgery, Society for Vascular Medicine, and Society for Vascular Surgery. J Am Coll Cardiol 2011; 57(8):e16–94.

86. Amarenco P, Davis S, Jones EF, et al. Clopidogrel plus aspirin versus warfarin in patients with stroke and aortic arch plaques. Stroke 2014;45:1248–57.

87. Bonati LH, Lyrer P, Ederle J, et al. Percutaneous transluminal balloon angioplasty and stenting for carotid artery stenosis. Cochrane Database Syst Rev 2012;(9):CD000515.

88. Ranta A, Dovey S, Weatherall M, et al. Cluster randomized controlled trial of TIA electronic decision support in primary care. Neurology 2015;84:1545–51.

89. Mijalski C, Silver B. TIA management: should TIA patients be admitted? Should TIA patients get combination antiplatelet therapy? Neurohospitalist 2015;5(3): 151–60.

90. Wasserman J, Perry J, Dowlatshahi D, et al. Stratified, urgent care for transient ischemic attack results in low stroke rates. Stroke 2010;41(11):2601–5.

91. Lavallée P, Meseguer E, Abboud H, et al. A transient ischaemic attack clinic with round-the-clock access (SOS-TIA): feasibility and effects. Lancet Neurol 2007; 6(11):953–60.
92. Ranta A, Barber PA. Transient ischemic attack service provision: a review of available service models. Neurology 2016;86(10):947–53.
93. Amarenco P. Not all patients should be admitted to the hospital for observation after a transient ischemic attack. Stroke 2012;43(5):1448–9.
94. Lavallée P, Amarenco P. TIA clinic: a major advance in management of transient ischemic attacks. Front Neurol Neurosci 2014;33:30–40.
95. Martınez-Martınez MM, Martınez-Sanchez P, Fuentes B, et al. Transient ischaemic attacks clinics provide equivalent and more efficient care than early in-hospital assessment. Eur J Neurol 2013;20(2):338–43.
96. Olivot JM, Wolford C, Castle J, et al. Two aces: transient ischemic attack work-up as outpatient assessment of clinical evaluation and safety. Stroke 2011;42(7): 1839–43.
97. Sanders LM, Srikanth VK, Jolley DJ, et al. Monash transient ischemic attack tri-aging treatment: safety of a transient ischemic attack mechanism-based outpatient model of care. Stroke 2012;43(11):2936–41.
98. Molina CA, Selim MM. Hospital admission after transient ischemic attack: unmasking wolves in sheep's clothing. Stroke 2012;43(5):1450–1.
99. Joshi JK, Ouyang B, Prabhakaran S. Should TIA patients be hospitalized or referred to a same-day clinic? A decision analysis. Neurology 2011;77(24): 2082–8.
100. Nguyen-Huynh MN, Johnston SC. Is hospitalization after TIA cost-effective on the basis of treatment with tPA? Neurology 2005;65(11):1799–801.
101. Rothwell PM, Giles MF, Chandratheva A, et al. Effect of urgent treatment of transient ischaemic attack and minor stroke on early recurrent stroke (EXPRESS study): a prospective population-based sequential comparison. Lancet 2007; 370:1432–42.
102. Rothwell PM, Coull AJ, Silver LE, et al. Population-based study of event-rate, incidence, case fatality and mortality for all acute vascular events in all arterial territories (Oxford Vascular Study). Lancet 2005;366:1773–83.

Diagnosis of Acute Ischemic Stoke

Lauren M. Nentwich, MD[a,b]

KEYWORDS

- Community detection • Prehospital diagnosis • ED evaluation • Stroke scales
- Brain imaging

KEY POINTS

- Public education and awareness of the signs and symptoms of acute ischemic stroke (AIS), via education campaigns such as the FAST mnemonic or the "suddens" message, is an essential first step in making a timely diagnosis in patients suffering an AIS.
- In their determination of whether a patient is suffering an AIS, emergency medical service providers should use focused tools, such as the Cincinnati Prehospital Stroke Scale or the Los Angeles Prehospital Stroke Screen. Prehospital scales to further evaluate for stroke severity are currently being developed and studied.
- The diagnosis of AIS is made using a combination of patient history, clinical examination, and brain imaging.
- Time of symptom onset, or time that the patient was last symptom-free, is the most important piece of historical data obtained in the evaluation of a patient with suspected AIS.
- The primary goal of brain imaging in the evaluation of a patient with suspected AIS is to exclude intracranial hemorrhage. The benefit of treatment with endovascular therapy in selected patients has expanded the role of imaging to also evaluate for the presence of an intravascular thrombus, the size of irreversible infarcted tissue, and potentially the amount of hypoperfused tissue at risk for infarction.

INTRODUCTION

Acute ischemic stroke (AIS) is defined as an episode of neurologic dysfunction caused by focal cerebral, spinal, or retinal cell death attributable to ischemia, based on (1) pathologic, imaging or other objective evidence of cerebral, spinal cord, or retinal focal ischemic injury in a defined vascular distribution; or (2) clinical evidence of cerebral, spinal cord, or retinal focal ischemic injury based on symptoms persisting 24 or more hours or until death, and other causes excluded.[1] (**Fig. 1**).

Approximately 795,000 people per year suffer from a new or recurrent stroke, and 87% of all strokes are due to acute brain ischemia. Stroke is the leading cause of

Disclosure: The author has nothing to disclose.
[a] Department of Emergency Medicine, Boston University School of Medicine, Boston, MA, USA;
[b] Department of Emergency Medicine, Boston Medical Center, Dowling 1 South, 1 Boston Medical Center Place, Boston, MA 02118, USA
E-mail address: lauren.nentwich@bmc.org

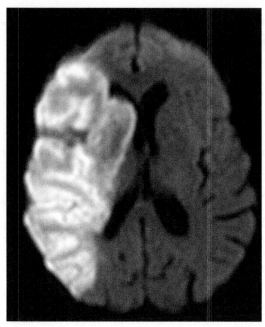

Fig. 1. Large right middle cerebral artery territory AIS on diffusion-weighted imaging.

long-term disability and the fourth leading cause of death in the United States.[2] Treatment of patients suffering an AIS is time-dependent and early treatment is associated with reduced morbidity and mortality.[3] Rapid detection and diagnosis of patients suffering an AIS is paramount to improving outcomes in these patients. (See Matthew S. Siket's article, "Treatment of Acute Ischemic Stroke," in this issue.) This article focuses on the rapid and accurate diagnosis of patients suffering an AIS, starting with initial detection in the community, leading to the prehospital evaluation, and finally resulting in a rapid work-up by the acute stroke team in the emergency department (ED).

Community Awareness and Education

The first link in the stroke chain of recovery is detection, or the rapid recognition and identification of stroke symptoms by the patient or bystanders.[4] Unfortunately, public knowledge of symptoms of AIS is poor.[5–7] In a meta-analysis evaluating the delay in care in patients suffering an AIS, 21 of the 54 studies identified lack of recognition of symptoms of AIS or delay in seeking care if symptoms were recognized by patients and their families as the primary limitation in obtaining timely and urgent care. **Box 1** lists the most common factors associated with this early delay in care by patients and their family members.[8]

To improve access to treatment and, thereby, have better outcomes in patients suffering an AIS, community education on the symptoms of AIS and community-wide coordination of stroke care is paramount. Ideally, patients, family members, bystanders, and the general public should recognize the signs and symptoms of a potential AIS and understand the urgent need to seek treatment. In particular, patients at high risk for AIS and groups of patients that are more likely to delay seeking medical attention, as well as family members, coworkers, and caregivers of these patients, should be the target of community education interventions.[9]

> **Box 1**
> **Common factors associated with early delay in care by patients suffering an acute ischemic stroke**
>
> - Patient living alone or retired
> - Symptoms of AIS not recognized
> - No bystander witness on symptom onset
> - Patient or family did not seek help or did not think it urgent to seek help at symptom onset
> - Stroke at home
> - Patient refused to go to the hospital
> - Patient or family thought symptoms would improve spontaneously
>
> *Adapted from* Sandercock P, Berge E, Dennis M, et al. A systematic review of the effectiveness, cost effectiveness and barriers to implementation of thrombolytic and neuroprotective therapy for acute ischaemic stroke in the NHS. Health Technol Assess 2002;6(26):1–112.

A recent review evaluating the question of whether or not public educational interventions were successful in reducing patient delays to hospital presentation in patients with suspected AIS found that 10 of the 13 studies showed statistically significant reduction in prehospital delay after public education. Successful educational interventions used included mass media campaigns, role-modeling with public advertising of stroke survivors, targeted community intervention, and professional education.[10]

Currently, 2 of the most accepted public stroke education messages are the FAST (**Box 2**) mnemonic and the "suddens" (**Box 3**) message. The simple mnemonic FAST is based on the Cincinnati Prehospital Stroke Scale (CPSS).[11] The "suddens" message is a list of 5 stroke warning signs created by the Brain Attack Coalition and used in the National Institutes of Health (NIH) educational campaign, *Know Stroke. Know the Signs. Act in Time.*[12] A retrospective review of patients who suffered an AIS showed that a much larger percentage of strokes are missed when using the FAST message versus the "suddens" message (16.8% vs 0.1%).[13] Though the "suddens" message misses fewer strokes, it is longer and may be more difficult for the general public to remember when compared with the simplified FAST mnemonic. Though the message that provides the most benefit remains highly debated, public education on the signs and symptoms of an acute stroke remain an important key in the early diagnosis and treatment of patients suffering an AIS.

PREHOSPITAL IDENTIFICATION AND DIAGNOSIS

When a patient or bystander recognizes that a patient may be suffering from an AIS, it is important that patient be transported rapidly to the closest available hospital with

> **Box 2**
> **FAST message for stroke warning signs**
>
> F, face: does the *face* look uneven?
>
> A, arm, does 1 *arm* drift down?
>
> S, speech, does their *speech* sound strange?
>
> T, *time*, if any of these signs observed, it is *time* to call 911.

Box 3
The 5 "suddens" stroke warning signs

- Sudden numbness or weakness of face, arm, or leg, especially on 1 side of the body
- Sudden confusion, trouble speaking or understanding speech
- Sudden trouble seeing in 1 or both eyes
- Sudden trouble walking, dizziness, loss of balance or coordination
- Sudden severe headache with no known cause

From NINDS Know Stroke Campaign - Know Stroke Home [Internet]. Available at: http://stroke.nih.gov/index.htm. Accessed November 29, 2015.

---

the necessary resources and capabilities to provide exceptional stroke care. This rapid transport should be initiated by calling an emergency medical service (EMS), such as 9-1-1 in the United States, because patients with suspected AIS who arrived at the hospital by EMS received faster physician evaluation and were more likely to receive brain imaging than those patients who arrive via private transport.[14] As soon as an EMS call for suspected AIS is received, the call center should prioritize the EMS response at the highest level of triage available, equivalent to trauma or acute myocardial infarction. The target time between the receipt of the call and the dispatch of the EMS response team is less than 90 seconds. Target time for EMS response to the suspected AIS call is less than 9 minutes, and on-scene time should be less than 15 minutes.[15]

Prehospital Identification of Stroke

On arrival, EMS providers have the difficult job of rapidly determining whether the patient is likely suffering an AIS or a stroke mimic so they can facilitate transport to the highest necessary level of care in the shortest possible time. Stroke mimics are conditions that present with stroke-like symptoms not caused by focal ischemia of the central nervous system and are important in the differential diagnosis of patients presenting with focal neurologic deficits (**Box 4**).[16–21]

EMS personnel should begin with obtaining a brief and focused history from the patient or bystanders, including the last time the patient was seen well and whether the patient suffered a recent seizure, illness, or trauma. EMS providers should attempt to obtain relevant past medical history, including diabetes mellitus, atrial fibrillation, hypertension, or prior stroke, as well as the medications that the patient is currently taking, specifically anticoagulants. The attempts to gather information should not delay transport the proper facility. After their initial evaluation, EMS providers should perform a focused tool to aid in the diagnosis and differentiation of an AIS. The 2 most accepted and used prehospital stroke tools are the CPSS and the Los Angeles Prehospital Stroke Screen (LAPSS).

CPSS is a 3-item scale that is a simplification of the NIH Stroke Scale (NIHSS) score assessing facial weakness, arm weakness, and speech (**Box 5**). Developed in 1997, it has been prospectively studied in physicians and prehospital providers and has been shown to have high sensitivity and specificity in identifying patients with stroke, with the presence of a single abnormality having a sensitivity of 66% and specificity of 87% for patients suffering from acute stroke. It is easily taught and can be performed in less than 1 minute.[11,22] The CPSS and its variations are used by many prehospital providers to identify potential acute strokes in the field.

Box 4
Stroke mimics

- Toxic-metabolic
  - Hypoglycemia or hyperglycemia
  - Hyponatremia or hypernatremia
  - Ingestion or overdose
  - Drug toxicity
  - Intoxication (alcohol, illicit drugs)
  - Hepatic encephalopathy

- Intracranial hemorrhage
  - Intracerebral hemorrhage
  - Subarachnoid hemorrhage
  - Subdural hematoma

- Infectious
  - Sepsis
  - Encephalitis
  - Meningitis

- Structural lesions
  - Brain mass or tumor
  - Spinal cord lesion

- Demyelinating disease (ie, multiple sclerosis)

- Seizure or Todd paralysis

- Migraine

- Idiopathic intracranial hypertension

- Reversible cerebral vasoconstrictive syndrome

- Central nervous system vasculitis

- Vestibular dysfunction

- Hypertensive encephalopathy

- Peripheral neuropathy

- Dementia

- Conversion disorder

Data from Refs.[16–21]

The LAPSS is a single-page instrument consisting of 4 history items with assessment for unilateral motor weakness and was developed to best identify patients suffering an AIS while excluding common stroke mimics (**Box 6**). It has been prospectively validated with a high sensitivity and specificity, 91% and 97%, respectively. It takes less than 3 minutes to complete but is slightly more complicated and difficult to remember than the CPSS.[23,24]

Prehospital Assessment of Stroke Severity

In 2015, 5 new randomized controlled studies were published that provide high-quality evidence on the clinical benefit of endovascular therapy using a second-generation stent retriever within 6 hours of symptom onset for patients with large vessel occlusive stroke.[25–30] Because this new treatment must be performed at hospitals with endovascular capabilities, systems of care now need to be organized to facilitate the delivery of patients with suspected large vessel occlusive AIS to comprehensive stroke

---

Box 5
The Cincinnati Prehospital Stroke Scale

Facial droop: the patient shows teeth or smiles
  Normal: both sides of face move equally
  Abnormal: 1 side of face does not move as well as the other

Arm drift: the patient closes his or her eyes and extends both arms straight out for 10 seconds
  Normal: both arms move the same, or both arms do not move at all
  Abnormal: 1 arm either does not move, or 1 arm drifts down compared with the other

Speech: the patient repeats "The sky is blue in Cincinnati."
  Normal: the patient says correct words with no slurring of words
  Abnormal: the patient slurs words, says the wrong words, or is unable to speak

Data from Kothari RU, Pancioli A, Liu T, et al. Cincinnati Prehospital Stroke Scale: reproducibility and validity. Ann Emerg Med 1999;33(4):373–8; and Kothari R, Hall K, Brott T, et al. Early stroke recognition: developing an out-of-hospital NIH Stroke Scale. Acad Emerg Med 1997;4(10):986–90.

---

centers with this endovascular capability. As such, prehospital providers must begin to use stroke severity scales to try to properly triage these patients in the field. Various stroke severity scales have been created, including the shortened NIHSS (sNIHSS), the 3-Item Stroke Scale (3I-SS), the Los Angeles Motor Scale (LAMS), the Rapid Arterial oCclusion Evaluation (RACE) scale, and the Cincinnati Prehospital Stroke Severity Scale (CPSSS); however, most are awaiting prospective validation.

The sNIHSS versions were derived and validated from data sets from acute stroke clinical trials in which the full version of the NIHSS (15 neurologic examination testing items) was shortened. The shortened versions used 8 items (sNIHSS-8) or 5 items (sNIHSS-5) **(Table 1)** for measuring stroke severity and predicting outcome for use

---

Box 6
The Los Angeles Prehospital Stroke Scale

Screening criteria:

• Age greater than 45

• History of seizures or epilepsy absent

• Symptoms duration less than 24 hours

• At baseline, patient is not wheelchair bound or bedridden

• Blood glucose between 60 and 400 mg/dL

Examination: look for obvious asymmetry in:

• Facial smile or grimace

• Grip

• Arm strength

Confirm that patient has only unilateral (and not bilateral) weakness.

If the answer to all screening criteria is yes or unknown, and the patient has obvious asymmetric weakness on examination, then the patient should be presumed to be having a stroke.

From Kidwell CS, Starkman S, Eckstein M, et al. Identifying Stroke in the Field: Prospective Validation of the Los Angeles Prehospital Stroke Screen (LAPSS). Stroke 2000;31(1):71–6; and Kidwell CS, Saver JL, Schubert GB, et al. Design and retrospective analysis of the Los Angeles Prehospital Stroke Screen (LAPSS). Prehospital Emerg Care 1998;2(4):267–73.

Table 1
Shortened National Institutes of Health Stroke Scale

NIHSS Questions Included	sNIHSS-8	sNIHSS-5
1a. Level of consciousness	X	—
2. Gaze	X	X
3. Visual fields	X	X
4. Facial paresis	X	—
6a. Motor leg, right	X	X
6b. Motor leg, left	X	X
9. Language	X	X
10. Dysarthria	X	—

From Tirschwell DL, Longstreth WT, Becker KJ, et al. Shortening the NIH Stroke scale for use in the prehospital setting. Stroke 2002;33(12):2801–6.

in the prehospital setting. In the derivation and validation paper, much of the predictive performance of the full NIHSS was retained with the shortened scale with no significant difference between the sNIHSS-8 or the sNIHSS-5.[31]

The 3I-SS (**Table 2**) was designed to establish a simple scale with that predicts initial stroke severity and middle cerebral artery occlusion. In a prospective hospital-based study in which a neurologist assessed the 3I-SS and NIHSS, the 3I-SS was strongly associated with the NIHSS and a score higher than or equal to 4 had a sensitivity and specificity of 0.67 and 0.92, respectively, for detecting proximal hyperdense middle cerebral artery (MCA) occlusion.[32]

The LAMS (**Table 3**) is a 3-item, 0-point to 5-point motor stroke deficit scale derived from the motor examination portion of the LAPSS developed for prehospital and ED use. The LAMS takes approximately 30 seconds to perform.[33] A retrospective study showed that LAMS had high sensitivity and specificity for predicting large artery

Table 2
The 3-item stroke scale

Disturbance of Consciousness	
No	0
Mild	1
Severe	2
Gaze and head deviation	
Absent	0
Incomplete gaze or head deviation	1
Forced gaze or head deviation	2
Hemiparesis	
Absent	0
Moderate	1
Severe	2

*** 3I-SS greater than or equal to 4 has a high predictive value of proximal vessel occlusion.
From Singer OC, Dvorak F, du Mesnil de Rochemont R, et al. A Simple 3-Item Stroke Scale: Comparison with the National Institutes of Health Stroke Scale and Prediction of Middle Cerebral Artery Occlusion. Stroke 2005;36(4):773–6.

Table 3	
Los Angeles Motor Scale	
Facial Droop	
Absent	0
Present	1
Arm drift	
Absent	0
Drifts down	1
Falls repeatedly	2
Grip strength	
Normal	0
Weak grip	1
No grip	2

***LAMS greater than or equal to 4 concerning for a large vessel occlusion.**
From Nazliel B, Starkman S, Liebeskind DS, et al. A brief prehospital stroke severity scale identifies ischemic stroke patients harboring persisting large arterial occlusions. Stroke 2008;39(8):2264–7.

anterior circulation occlusion, a LAMS score higher than or equal to 4 increases the likelihood that an AIS patient has a large vessel occlusion by 7-fold.[34]

The RACE scale (**Table 4**) was derived using data to identify the items on the NIHSS with the highest predictive value of large vessel occlusion with the exclusion of items that had high correlation with large vessel occlusion but were difficult or inconsistent for paramedic personnel to perform (eg, visual field, sensory). The RACE scale was evaluated prospectively by prehospital providers with a strong correlation between the RACE scale and the NIHSS assessed by the hospital on admission. The best predictive value of the RACE score for large vessel occlusion was established as higher than or equal to 5, with a sensitivity of 0.85 and a specificity of 0.68.[35]

The CPSSS was retrospectively derived and validated to identify a severe stroke (defined as NIHSS higher than or equal to 15) with anticipation of ease of administration by prehospital providers (**Box 7**). CPSSS evaluates 3 individual items with scores ranging from 0 to 4 and a score higher than or equal to 2 was found to be 83% sensitive and 40% specific in identifying patients with large vessel occlusion.[36]

EMERGENCY DEPARTMENT EVALUATION

On arrival to the ED, the diagnosis of AIS is made using a combination of patient history, clinical examination, and brain imaging. It is important to make the diagnosis of AIS quickly on ED arrival because patients suffering an AIS who receive early treatment to restore cerebral perfusion have better clinical outcomes.[37] Before January 2015, the only recommended treatment of patients suffering an AIS was intravenous (IV) recombinant tissue plasminogen activator (rt-PA) given within 0 to 4.5 hours from symptoms onset.[38] IV rt-PA improves outcomes in 1 in 3 patients treated within 3 hours of symptoms onset and 1 in 6 patients treated within 3 to 4.5 hours of symptoms onset.[4,39–42] Due to the recent positive trials for endovascular therapy in certain populations with AIS, the current guidelines recommend endovascular therapy with a stent retriever for large vessel occlusive AIS if therapy can be initiated within 6 hours of symptom onset.[30] Given the narrow therapeutic treatment windows for patients

Table 4
Rapid Arterial oCclusion Evaluation Scale

Facial Palsy	
Absent	0
Mild	1
Moderate to severe	2
Arm motor function	
Normal to mild	0
Moderate	1
Severe	2
Leg motor function	
Normal to mild	0
Moderate	1
Severe	2
Head and gaze deviation	
Absent	0
Present	1
Aphasia (if right hemiparesis), ask the patient to: (1) close eyes and (2) make a fist	
Performs both tasks correctly	0
Performs 1 task correctly	1
Performs neither task	2
Agnosia (if left hemiparesis), ask the patient: (1) while showing his or her paretic arm, "Whose are is this?" and (2) "Can you lift both arms and clap?"	
Patient recognizes his/her arm and the impairment	0
Does not recognize his or her arm or the impairment	1
Does not recognize his or her arm nor the impairment	2

***RACE scale greater than or equal to 5 has high prediction for a large vessel occlusion.

From Pérez de la Ossa N, Carrera D, Gorchs M, et al. Design and validation of a prehospital stroke scale to predict large arterial occlusion: the rapid arterial occlusion evaluation scale. Stroke 2014;45(1):87–91.

suffering an AIS and that "time is brain" in the treatment of patients suffering an AIS,[43] rapid ED evaluation and diagnosis is of the utmost importance.

Hospitals caring for patients with AIS should have a rapid and efficient response system and streamlined pathway for patients suffering a suspected AIS who present

Box 7
Cincinnati Prehospital Stroke Severity Scale

2 points: conjugate gaze deviation

1 point: incorrectly answers at least 1 of 2 level of consciousness questions on NIHSS and does not follow at least 1 of 2 commands

1 point: cannot hold arm (either right, left, or both) up for 10 seconds before arm falls to the bed

*** CPSSS greater than or equal to 2 has a high likelihood of prediction large vessel occlusion.

From Katz BS, McMullan JT, Sucharew H, et al. Design and validation of a prehospital scale to predict stroke severity: Cincinnati Prehospital Stroke Severity Scale. Stroke 2015;46(6):1508–12.

to the ED. During the stabilization and initial evaluation of a patient presenting with suspected AIS, stroke team notification and implementation of the hospital's stroke pathway should occur.[4] Hospitals that are designated stroke centers should have an acute stroke expert at the bedside of a patient with suspected AIS within 15 minutes, via either in-person patient-bedside stroke expertise or telephone or telemedicine consultation.[39] A consensus panel convened by the National Institute of Neurological Disorders and Stroke (NINDS) established time goals in the ED evaluation of patients presenting with AIS (**Table 5**).[40] Adherence to these goals in the care of patients suffering an AIS remind providers of the time-sensitive nature of the diagnosis and management of AIS and assist in the optimization of acute stroke care.[4,33,40]

Target: Stroke[SM] is a national quality improvement initiative organized by the American Heart Association/American Stroke Association (AHA/ASA) that was started in 2010 to introduce key best practice strategies associated with achieving faster treatment times in AIS.[41] After its introduction, there was substantial improvement in IV rt-PA treatment times with resulting improved clinical outcomes. These outcomes include lower in-hospital mortality, more frequent discharge to more independent functioning environment, and lower complications, including symptomatic intracranial hemorrhage (ICH).[3] Due to the success of the initial phase, the AHA/ASA has recently begun Target: Stroke[SM] Phase II to continue to continue to eliminate delays in the treatment of patients suffering AIS. Use of key best practice strategies from Target: Stroke[SM] Phase II will aid in more rapid diagnosis and timely treatment of patients presenting with suspected AIS (**Box 8**).[42]

Patient History

A precise history should be obtained from any possible source, including the patient, family, or bystander witnesses. The most important piece of historical data is the time of symptom onset, also known as the "last known well" time (LKW). This LKW time is defined as when the patient was at his or her previous baseline or symptom-free state. For patients who awaken with symptoms or are unable to provide an accurate history, the LKW is defined as the time when the patient was last awake and symptom-free or without acute focal neurologic symptoms.

Additional history should include circumstances surrounding the development of the acute focal neurologic symptoms and features that may point to other potential causes of these symptoms. It is important to review the patient's prior medical history. Special consideration should be focused on risk factors for AIS, including

Table 5	
National Institute of Neurologic Disorders and Stroke time goals of care BOCH—39	
ED Action	**Time (minutes)**
Door to physician evaluation	<10
Door to stroke team notification	<15
Door to CT scan initiation	<25
Door to CT scan interpretation	<45
Door to thrombolytic drug	<60
Door to monitored bed	<360

From Bock BF. Response system for patients presenting with acute stroke. Paper presented at: Proceedings of a National Symposium on Rapid Identification and Treatment of Acute Stroke; December 12-13, 1996; Bethesda, MD. Available at: http://www.ninds.nih.gov/news_and_events/proceedings/stroke_proceedings/bock.htm. Accessed September 23, 2014.

Box 8
11 Key best practice strategies in the American Heart Association/American Stroke Association target: Stroke^{SM} Phase II

1. EMS notification to the receiving hospital when stroke is recognized in the field
2. Stroke toolkit containing rapid triage protocol, clinical decision support, stroke-specific order sets, guidelines, hospital-specific algorithms, critical pathways, NIHSS
3. Rapid triage protocol and stroke team notification
4. Single call activation of the entire stroke team by the ED
5. Triage of eligible stroke patients directly from ED triage to the CT scanner, bypassing the ED bed
6. Rapid acquisition (within 25 minutes) and interpretation (within 45 minutes) of brain imaging
7. Rapid laboratory testing (within 30 minutes), including glucose as well as international normalized ratio (INR), prothrombin time (PT), or partial prothrombin time (PTT) in patients with suspected coagulopathy or warfarin treatment
8. Mix rt-PA as soon as the patient is recognized as a potential rt-PA candidate, even before brain imaging is completed.
9. Rapid access and administration of IV rt-PA, with consideration of initial bolus being given on the CT table.
10. Team-based approach with an interdisciplinary collaborative stroke team.
11. Accurate tracking of stroke performance or quality measures with a process for timely feedback and recommendations for improvement.

From Target: Stroke [Internet]. Available at: http://www.strokeassociation.org/STROKEORG/Professionals/Target-Stroke_UCM_314495_SubHomePage.jsp. Accessed September 23, 2014.

Box 9
Risk factors for acute ischemic stroke

- Hypertension
- Diabetes mellitus
- Atrial fibrillation
- High total cholesterol
- Smoking
- Physical inactivity
- Unhealthy diet
- Family history of AIS (parent before age 65)
- Chronic kidney disease
- Early natural menopause (before age 42)
- Obstructive sleep apnea

From Mozaffarian D, Benjamin EJ, Go AS, et al. Heart disease and stroke statistics–2015 Update: a report from the American Heart Association. Circulation 2015;131(4):e29–322.

arteriosclerosis or cardiac disease, as well as any history of drug abuse, migraine, seizure disorder, infections, trauma, or pregnancy (**Box 9**).[33] Medications should be reviewed, and it should be determined if the patient is currently taking warfarin or any other oral anticoagulants, specifically the direct thrombin inhibitors or direct factor Xa inhibitors because they are contraindications to IV rt-PA. Other major contraindications to IV rt-PA should be screened for during the patient history, including neurologic surgery, serious head trauma, previous stroke in the past 3 months, history of ICH, known arteriovenous malformation, neoplasm or aneurysm, suspected or confirmed endocarditis, and known coagulopathy.

Physical Examination

Primary assessment
On initial assessment of the patient with suspected AIS, the physician should immediately evaluate and stabilize the patient's airway, breathing, and circulation (ABCs). After an AIS, the ventilatory drive usually remains intact, with the exception of patients suffering from medullary injury or massive hemispheric infarction, and most patients suffering an AIS do not have airway compromise. The ability to protect the airway may be impaired in patients with decreased consciousness or brain stem dysfunction due to impaired oropharyngeal mobility and loss of protective reflexes.[33] Intubation with mechanical ventilation may be necessary in these patients.[44] Patients with an intact airway may suffer from hypoxemia after a stroke, and AHA guidelines recommend using supplemental oxygen via the least invasive method possible to maintain the patients' oxygen saturation greater than 94%.[4] Patients with oxygen saturation greater than 94% should not be empirically given supplemental oxygen.

Secondary assessment
Once the patient's primary assessment has been completed and stabilized, vital signs (eg, blood pressure, heart rate, oxygen saturation, and temperature) should be obtained. A rapid and thorough physical examination should be performed to assess for trauma as well as other potential causes of the patient's symptoms (ie, stroke mimics; see **Box 4**). The evaluation should include examination for prior seizure activity, coexisting comorbidities, or issues that may impact the management of an AIS. A fingerstick blood glucose should be checked to rule out hypoglycemia, a common and treatable stroke mimic that can cause focal neurologic deficits.

Concurrently, a focused neurologic examination should be performed on the patient to assess for presence and severity of focal neurologic deficits. Patients suffering an AIS may present with any number of focal neurologic deficits, including motor weakness or hemiparesis, sensory loss, aphasia or dysarthria neglect, vertigo, ataxia, altered mental status, gaze deficits, or visual field deficits.[45]

The neurologic examination is enhanced by the use of a formal stroke scale, such as the NIHSS (https://www.ninds.nih.gov/doctors/NIH_Stroke_Scale.pdf).[46] The NIHSS is an 11-item scale scored from 0 to 42 that assesses for level of consciousness, language, neglect, visual-field loss, extraocular movements, motor strength, ataxia, dysarthria, and sensory loss. It can be easily learned, quickly administered, and has been shown to have good interrater reliability by both neurologists and nonneurologists.[47,48] The standardization of the NIHSS ensures that the major components of the neurologic examination are performed in a timely fashion, and the entire scale can be completed in about 5 to 7 minutes. It allows for rapid assessment of the patient's level of impairment and quantifies the degree of neurologic deficit, with a NIHSS score lower than 5 representing a minor stroke and a NIHSS score higher than 20 representing severe stroke. The NIHSS score facilitates communication between health care providers, and the baseline NIHSS score on admission has prognostic value and has been shown to strongly predict the likelihood of recovery after an AIS in untreated patients.[49–51]

Diagnostic Tests

Basic laboratory tests should be emergently performed in all patients presenting with suspected AIS (**Box 10**). As previously discussed, a fingerstick blood glucose should be obtained on arrival because hypoglycemia is a common stroke mimic and hyperglycemia is associated with poor outcomes. Coagulation studies and platelets, especially in patients with concern for bleeding abnormality, thrombocytopenia, or anticoagulant use, are important because abnormal results will affect treatment. However, due the time-sensitive nature, treatment with IV rt-PA should not be delayed while awaiting coagulation studies or platelets unless the patient has been taking anticoagulants or a coagulopathy or thrombocytopenia is suspected based on patient history or examination.[33] Retrospective studies of patients receiving IV thrombolysis for AIS showed very low rates of unsuspected coagulopathies or thrombocytopenia in patients that would have precluded treatment.[52,53]

Specific laboratory tests may be useful in the emergency evaluation of select patients with suspected AIS. Particularly in young patients suffering AIS, toxicology screens for sympathomimetic use (ie, amphetamine, cocaine) may identify the underlying cause of the stroke.[54] A pregnancy test should be checked in all women of childbearing age because the results may impact overall management.

Due to a close association between AIS and cardiac abnormalities, all patients with suspected AIS should undergo cardiovascular evaluation, including a 12-lead electrocardiogram, ongoing cardiac monitoring, and cardiac biomarkers. Atrial fibrillation is a common cause of AIS and should be assessed for on initial electrocardiogram and ongoing telemetry. AIS and acute myocardial infarction can present together, each precipitating the other.[33] Elevated troponin is common in patients suffering an AIS and is associated with increased risk of death.[55] Though recommended in the initial assessment, baseline electrocardiogram should not delay rapid imaging or treatment with IV rt-PA.

Box 10
Emergency department laboratory tests for patient presenting with acute ischemic stroke

Necessary:

- Blood glucose
- Coagulation studies
- Complete blood count (including platelets)
- Renal function tests
- Liver function tests
- Serum electrolytes
- Cardiac biomarkers

Consider, based on presentation:

- Toxicology screen
- Pregnancy test

Neuroimaging

The primary goal of brain imaging in the management of patients suffering a potential AIS is to exclude the presence of hemorrhage. Brain imaging, using either computed tomography (CT) or MRI, in patients presenting with a history and clinical examination consistent with AIS is essential in differentiating AIS from hemorrhagic stroke and often helps to guide therapy. Additionally, with the new evidence supporting the treatment of patients with large vessel occlusive strokes with endovascular therapy,[25–30] the goals of brain imaging have expanded to include the evaluation for an intravascular thrombus, the identification of the size of the core of irreversibly infarcted tissue, and the determination of the amount of hypoperfused tissue at risk for subsequent infarction unless adequate perfusion is restored.[56] As previously discussed, AHA guidelines recommend that neuroimaging on all patients with suspected AIS should be completed within 25 minutes and interpreted within 45 minutes of ED arrival.[4]

Computed tomography

Noncontrast brain CT (NCCT) is typically the first imaging choice for patients with suspected AIS because of its accuracy in excluding hemorrhage, speed in acquisition, general safety for both stable and unstable patients, and widespread availability in most US EDs.[56–58] NCCT may be used as the primary and only brain imaging for the evaluation of patients presenting with suspected AIS because it accurately diagnoses most cases of ICH and may identify nonvascular causes of focal neurologic deficits.[33] Multimodal CT imaging adds CT angiography (CTA) and CT perfusion (CTP) to NCCT and may be able to identify intravascular thrombus or vascular narrowing, as well as differentiate between the penumbra and irreversibly infarcted brain tissue (**Table 6**).[58,59]

NCCT can accurately identify hemorrhage because blood from an acute ICH is hyperdense (bright), whereas ischemic brain should appear normal on an NCCT scan during the first few hours after stroke (**Fig. 2**). Evidence of arterial occlusion on NCCT, known as the hyperdense artery sign, is due to the increased density within the occluded vessel representing visualization of the thrombus.[58,60] The most commonly identified hyperdense artery sign is the hyperdense MCA[61] (**Fig. 3**), which is highly specific for MCA occlusion but with variable sensitivity.[62,63] NCCT may demonstrate visible ischemic damage within 3 hours.[33] Early ischemic changes that may be seen on NCCT include loss of grey-white differentiation, hypodensity, or

Table 6 Multimodal computed tomography	
Imaging Modality	**Clinical Use**
Noncontrast Head CT	Excludes or diagnoses ICH May identify certain stroke mimics (eg, tumor, infection), arterial occlusion, or early signs of infarction Diagnoses SAH
CTA	Evaluates the intracranial and extracranial arterial circulation for occlusion or stenosis Evaluates for some secondary causes of ICH and vascular abnormalities in SAH (eg, aneurysms, arteriovenous malformations)
CTP	Quantifies cerebral blood volume, cerebral blood flow, and mean transit time for blood flow through brain tissue

Abbreviation: SAH, subarachnoid hemorrhage.
Adapted from Nentwich LM, Veloz W. Neuroimaging in acute stroke. Emerg Med Clin North Am 2012;30(3):660; with permission.

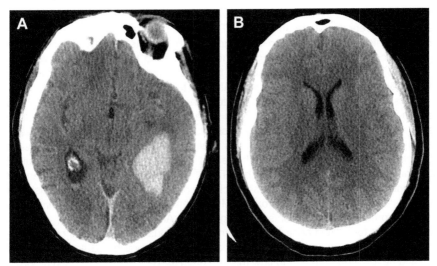

Fig. 2. Noncontrast brain CT with left temporal hemorrhage (*A*) and normal brain (*B*).

hypoattenuation of the brain parenchyma, and sulcal effacement due to swelling of the gyri.[64–69] Early ischemic changes may be subtle but are highly specific for AIS and are more likely to be seen in more severe stroke and in longer times from symptom onset.[65] Detection and quantification of early ischemic changes in patients with AIS of the anterior circulation can be performed through a structured scoring system such as the Alberta Stroke Program Early CT Score (ASPECTS). The ASPECTS is

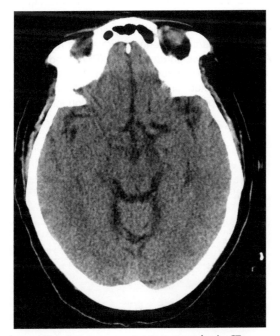

Fig. 3. Left hyperdense MCA sign as seen on noncontrast brain CT.

simple and reliable and identifies patients with severe stroke unlikely to make an independent recovery despite treatment.[70,71] The recent endovascular trials used an ASPECTS of higher than 5 to 6 to determine which patients may best benefit from thrombectomy.[25–30] Current AHA guidelines recommend that patients should have an ASPECTS of greater than or equal to 6 to be considered for endovascular therapy with a stent retriever if suffering from an AIS due to a large vessel occlusion.[30]

CTA is a rapid, minimally invasive tool for imaging of the vessels of the head and neck in patients with suspected AIS, and advances in multidetector CT technology have made CTA the preferred noninvasive alternative to conventional catheter-based cerebral arteriography.[59] CTA can evaluate the intracranial vessels for sites of occlusion or stenosis (**Fig. 4**).[72] The recent positive endovascular trials required documentation of a vessel occlusion by CTA.[25–29] As such, CTA should be performed in patients with suspected large vessel occlusion because a documented occlusion of the distal internal carotid or the proximal MCA is a main prerequisite for offering intra-arterial thrombectomy to patients suffering from an AIS.[30,73]

CTP allows for a rapid noninvasive, quantitative evaluation of dynamic brain perfusion and is able to quantify cerebral blood volume, cerebral blood flow, and mean transit time required for blood to flow through brain tissue.[74] It has also been reported to identify alteration in cerebral perfusion in patients with suspected AIS and can delineate ischemic core from penumbra.[59] Despite these data, CTP remains investigational and the clinical value of the information that CTP provides has yet to be established.[75]

MRI

Both CT and MRI are highly sensitive in the detection of acute ICH,[76,77] but MRI is much more sensitive than CT in detecting acute ischemic changes and, as such, is more accurate in diagnosing patients with AIS.[77] MRI also has a higher sensitivity and specificity than CT for detection of other neurologic diseases that mimic stroke, such as cerebral edema, vascular malformations, neoplasms, infection, inflammatory diseases, and toxic-metabolic disorders.[78]

Multimodal MRI includes the following sequences: diffusion-weighted imaging (DWI), T2-weighted sequences/fluid-attenuated inversion recovery (T2W/FLAIR), MR angiography (MRA), perfusion-weighted imaging (PWI), and gradient-recalled echo (GRE) (**Table 7**). It is able to provide excellent anatomic detail of the brain, differentiate between ischemic and infarcted brain tissue, exclude intracerebral hemorrhage, and provide angiographic, spectroscopic, and perfusion information of the cerebral

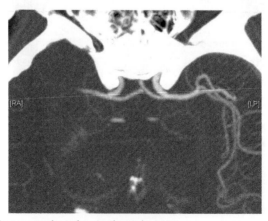

Fig. 4. CTA showing acute thrombus in the right MCA.

Table 7
Multimodal MRI

Sequence	Clinical Use
DWI	Diagnoses AIS within minutes of onset of ischemic injury
FLAIR	Diagnoses subAIS within 3–8 h after symptom onset Identifies older ischemic strokes and small vessel disease May diagnose SAH (decreased accuracy compared with NCCT)
MRA	Identifies intracranial occlusions and stenosis Allows for the evaluation of the cranial circulation without IV contrast Evaluates for some secondary causes of ICH and vascular abnormalities in SAH (eg, aneurysms, arteriovenous malformations)
PWI	Depicts areas of brain tissue with reduced cerebral blood flow DWI-PWI mismatch may estimate an area of brain tissue at risk of infarction if blood flow is not restored
GRE	Diagnoses acute ICH Detects chronic ICH

Adapted from Nentwich LM, Veloz W. Neuroimaging in acute stroke. Emerg Med Clin North Am 2012;30(3):659–80.

vasculature and tissue bed.[33,59] Multimodal MRI can be performed in 10 to 20 minutes in the acute setting, thus making it feasible within the 3-hour thrombolysis time window and competitive with multimodal CT study acquisition time in the accurate diagnosis of patients presenting with suspected AIS.[78]

DWI is the imaging modality of choice for diagnosing acute ischemia and has been shown to detect physiologic changes within 15 minutes of ischemic injury.[79] Hyperacute ischemic brain lesions have increased signal intensity of DWI (**Fig. 5**).[79] T2W/FLAIR imaging diagnoses sub-AISs with an ischemic infarction appearing as a

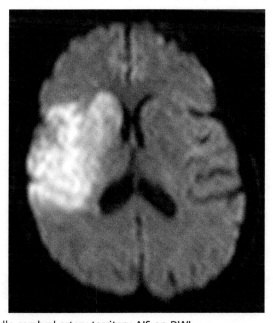

Fig. 5. Right middle cerebral artery territory AIS on DWI.

hyperintense lesion usually within 3 to 8 hours after stroke onset.[58] GRE is the preferred MRI sequence for detecting acute or chronic ICH, and hemorrhage appears hypointense (dark) on GRE (**Fig. 6**).[80] GRE is as accurate as CT for the diagnosis of acute ICH and more accurate than CT in the detection of chronic hemorrhage.[76,77] Noncontrast 3-dimensional time-of-flight (TOF) MRA produces flow-dependent luminal imaging and is the mainstay of intracranial arterial evaluation by MRI.[81] It has the benefit of not requiring a timed contrast agent but, compared with CTA, TOF MRA has limitations due to its sensitivity to patient motion artifact and flow artifact that can result in overestimation of vessel stenosis.[82] Like CTA, TOF MRI may also be used evaluate for a distal internal carotid or proximal MCA occlusion to identify patients suffering an AIS who may benefit form intra-arterial thrombectomy. PWI allows for visualization of capillary blood flow. Unlike, the other MRI sequences performed in the evaluation of suspected AIS, PWI requires administration of a gadolinium-based contrast agent. PWI depicts areas of brain tissue with reduced cerebral blood flow, whereas DWI is thought to represent severely injured tissue. The DWI-PWI mismatch may estimate the extent of an ischemic penumbra, defined as brain tissue that is dysfunctional because of low blood flow but potentially salvageable if blood flow is restored.[78] However, like CTP, the clinical utility of the information obtained from PWI and the DWI-PWI mismatch remains investigational.

DIAGNOSIS AND DISPOSITION

The patient, the community, the EMS providers, and the ED and hospital personnel are all important members of the acute stroke team working in collaboration to make a rapid and accurate diagnosis in a patient suffering an AIS. Once the diagnosis is made, a decision should also be made regarding the patients' eligibility for treatment with IV thrombolysis or intra-arterial thrombectomy. After the acute treatment, the patient suffering an AIS should be rapidly admitted to the hospital, preferentially to a stroke unit or neurocritical care unit for further treatment and care.[33]

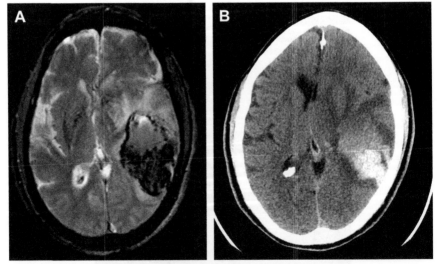

Fig. 6. Left temporoparietal intraparenchymal hemorrhage as depicted on GRE (*A*) and CT (*B*).

The diagnosis of AIS can be difficult and highly time-sensitive. It requires the teamwork of everyone who interacts with the patient suffering an AIS, from the bystanders at the onset of symptoms, to the EMS providers, to ED providers who quickly get involved in the patients' care. Continued education and improved diagnostic tools can make the difference between an excellent outcome and death in these critical patients.

REFERENCES

1. Sacco RL, Kasner SE, Broderick JP, et al. An updated definition of stroke for the 21st century: a statement for healthcare professionals from the American Heart Association/American Stroke Association. Stroke 2013;44(7):2064–89.
2. Mozaffarian D, Benjamin EJ, Go AS, et al. Heart disease and stroke statistics–2015 update: a report from the American Heart Association. Circulation 2015; 131(4):e29–322.
3. Fonarow GC, Zhao X, Smith EE, et al. Door-to-needle times for tissue plasminogen activator administration and clinical outcomes in acute ischemic stroke before and after a quality improvement initiative. JAMA 2014;311(16):1632.
4. Jauch EC, Cucchiara B, Adeoye O, et al. Part 11: adult stroke 2010 American Heart Association Guidelines for Cardiopulmonary Resuscitation and Emergency Cardiovascular Care. Circulation 2010;122(18 Suppl 3):S818–28.
5. Pancioli AM, Broderick J, Kothari R, et al. Public perception of stroke warning signs and knowledge of potential risk factors. JAMA 1998;279(16):1288–92.
6. Schneider AT, Pancioli AM, Khoury JC, et al. Trends in community knowledge of the warning signs and risk factors for stroke. JAMA 2003;289(3):343–6.
7. Kleindorfer D, Khoury J, Broderick JP, et al. Temporal trends in public awareness of stroke: warning signs, risk factors, and treatment. Stroke 2009;40(7):2502–6.
8. Sandercock P, Berge E, Dennis M, et al. A systematic review of the effectiveness, cost-effectiveness and barriers to implementation of thrombolytic and neuroprotective therapy for acute ischaemic stroke in the NHS. Health Technol Assess 2002;6(26):1–112.
9. Crocco TJ. Streamlining stroke care: from symptom onset to emergency department. j Emerg Med 2007;33(3):255–60.
10. Mellon L, Doyle F, Rohde D, et al. Stroke warning campaigns: delivering better patient outcomes? A systematic review. Patient Relat Outcome Meas 2015;6:61.
11. Kothari RU, Pancioli A, Liu T, et al. Cincinnati Prehospital Stroke Scale: reproducibility and validity. Ann Emerg Med 1999;33(4):373–8.
12. NINDS Know Stroke Campaign - Know Stroke Home [Internet]. Available at: http://stroke.nih.gov/index.htm. Accessed November 29, 2015.
13. Kleindorfer DO, Miller R, Moomaw CJ, et al. Designing a Message for Public Education Regarding Stroke Does FAST Capture Enough Stroke? Stroke 2007; 38(10):2864–8.
14. Mohammad YM. Mode of arrival to the emergency department of stroke patients in the United States. J Vasc Interv Neurol 2008;1(3):83–6.
15. Acker JE, Pancioli AM, Crocco TJ, et al. Implementation strategies for emergency medical services within stroke systems of care: a policy statement from the American Heart Association/American Stroke Association Expert Panel on Emergency Medical Services Systems and the Stroke Council. Stroke 2007;38(11):3097–115.
16. Hand PJ, Kwan J, Lindley RI, et al. Distinguishing between stroke and mimic at the bedside the brain attack study. Stroke 2006;37(3):769–75.

17. Libman RB, Wirkowski E, Alvir J, et al. Conditions that mimic stroke in the emergency department. Implications for acute stroke trials. Arch Neurol 1995;52(11): 1119–22.

18. Hemmen TM, Meyer BC, McClean TL, et al. Identification of nonischemic stroke mimics among 411 code strokes at the University of California, San Diego, Stroke Center. J Stroke Cerebrovasc Dis 2008;17(1):23–5.

19. Artto V, Putaala J, Strbian D, et al. Stroke mimics and intravenous thrombolysis. Ann Emerg Med 2012;59(1):27–32.

20. Förster A, Griebe M, Wolf ME, et al. How to identify stroke mimics in patients eligible for intravenous thrombolysis? J Neurol 2012;259(7):1347–53.

21. Magauran BG, Nitka M. Stroke mimics. Emerg Med Clin North Am 2012;30(3): 795–804.

22. Kothari R, Hall K, Brott T, et al. Early stroke recognition: developing an out-of-hospital NIH Stroke Scale. Acad Emerg Med 1997;4(10):986–90.

23. Kidwell CS, Starkman S, Eckstein M, et al. Identifying Stroke in the Field: Prospective Validation of the Los Angeles Prehospital Stroke Screen (LAPSS). Stroke 2000;31(1):71–6.

24. Kidwell CS, Saver JL, Schubert GB, et al. Design and retrospective analysis of the Los Angeles Prehospital Stroke Screen (LAPSS). Prehosp Emerg Care 1998;2(4):267–73.

25. Berkhemer OA, Fransen PSS, Beumer D, et al. A randomized trial of intraarterial treatment for acute ischemic stroke. N Engl J Med 2015;372(1):11–20.

26. Goyal M, Demchuk AM, Menon BK, et al. Randomized assessment of rapid endovascular treatment of ischemic stroke. N Engl J Med 2015;372(11):1019–30.

27. Saver JL, Goyal M, Bonafe A, et al. Stent-retriever thrombectomy after intravenous t-PA vs. t-PA alone in stroke. N Engl J Med 2015;372(24):2285–95.

28. Campbell BCV, Mitchell PJ, Kleinig TJ, et al. Endovascular therapy for ischemic stroke with perfusion-imaging selection. N Engl J Med 2015;372(11):1009–18.

29. Jovin TG, Chamorro A, Cobo E, et al. Thrombectomy within 8 hours after symptom onset in ischemic stroke. N Engl J Med 2015;372(24):2296–306.

30. Powers WJ, Derdeyn CP, Biller J, et al. 2015 American Heart Association/American Stroke Association Focused Update of the 2013 Guidelines for the Early Management of Patients With Acute Ischemic Stroke Regarding Endovascular Treatment: A Guideline for Healthcare Professionals From the American Heart Association/American Stroke Association. Stroke 2015;46(10):3020–35.

31. Tirschwell DL, Longstreth WT, Becker KJ, et al. Shortening the NIH Stroke scale for use in the prehospital setting. Stroke 2002;33(12):2801–6.

32. Singer OC, Dvorak F, du Mesnil de Rochemont R, et al. A simple 3-item stroke scale: comparison with the National Institutes of Health Stroke Scale and prediction of middle cerebral artery occlusion. Stroke 2005;36(4):773–6.

33. Jauch EC, Saver JL, Adams HP, et al. Guidelines for the early management of patients with acute ischemic stroke: a guideline for healthcare professionals from the American Heart Association/American Stroke Association. Stroke 2013; 44(3):870–947.

34. Nazliel B, Starkman S, Liebeskind DS, et al. A brief prehospital stroke severity scale identifies ischemic stroke patients harboring persisting large arterial occlusions. Stroke 2008;39(8):2264–7.

35. Pérez de la Ossa N, Carrera D, Gorchs M, et al. Design and validation of a prehospital stroke scale to predict large arterial occlusion: the rapid arterial occlusion evaluation scale. Stroke 2014;45(1):87–91.

36. Katz BS, McMullan JT, Sucharew H, et al. Design and validation of a prehospital scale to predict stroke severity: Cincinnati Prehospital Stroke Severity Scale. Stroke 2015;46(6):1508–12.

37. Emberson J, Lees KR, Lyden P, et al. Effect of treatment delay, age, and stroke severity on the effects of intravenous thrombolysis with alteplase for acute ischaemic stroke: a meta-analysis of individual patient data from randomised trials. Lancet 2014;384(9958):1929–35.

38. Tissue Plasminogen Activator for Acute Ischemic Stroke. The National Institute of Neurological Disorders and Stroke rt-PA Stroke Study Group. N Engl J Med 1995; 333(24):1581–8.

39. Higashida R, Alberts MJ, Alexander DN, et al. Interactions within stroke systems of care a policy statement from the American Heart Association/American Stroke Association. Stroke 2013;44(10):2961–84.

40. NINDS: Stroke Proceedings: Bock : National Institute of Neurological Disorders and Stroke (NINDS) [Internet]. Available at: http://www.ninds.nih.gov/news_and_events/proceedings/stroke_proceedings/bock.htm. Accessed September 23, 2014.

41. Fonarow GC, Smith EE, Saver JL, et al. Improving door-to-needle times in acute ischemic stroke: the design and rationale for the American Heart Association/American Stroke Association's Target: Stroke initiative. Stroke 2011;42(10): 2983–9.

42. Target: Stroke [Internet]. Available at: http://www.strokeassociation.org/STROKEORG/Professionals/Target-Stroke_UCM_314495_SubHomePage.jsp.   Accessed September 23, 2014.

43. Saver JL. Time is brain–quantified. Stroke 2006;37(1):263–6.

44. Grotta J, Pasteur W, Khwaja G, et al. Elective intubation for neurologic deterioration after stroke. Neurology 1995;45(4):640–4.

45. Pare JR, Kahn JH. Basic neuroanatomy and stroke syndromes. Emerg Med Clin North Am 2012;30(3):601–15.

46. NINDS Know Stroke Campaign - NIH Stroke Scale [Internet]. Available at: http://stroke.nih.gov/resources/scale.htm. Accessed December 10, 2015.

47. Goldstein LB, Bertels C, Davis JN. Interrater reliability of the NIH stroke scale. Arch Neurol 1989;46(6):660–2.

48. Goldstein LB, Samsa GP. Reliability of the National Institutes of Health Stroke Scale. Extension to non-neurologists in the context of a clinical trial. Stroke 1997;28(2):307–10.

49. Adams HP, Davis PH, Leira EC, et al. Baseline NIH Stroke Scale score strongly predicts outcome after stroke A report of the Trial of Org 10172 in Acute Stroke Treatment (TOAST). Neurology 1999;53(1):126.

50. Sato S, Toyoda K, Uehara T, et al. Baseline NIH Stroke Scale Score predicting outcome in anterior and posterior circulation strokes. Neurology 2008;70(24 Pt 2): 2371–7.

51. Frankel MR, Morgenstern LB, Kwiatkowski T, et al. Predicting prognosis after stroke: a placebo group analysis from the National Institute of Neurological Disorders and Stroke rt-PA Stroke Trial. Neurology 2000;55(7):952–9.

52. Rost NS, Masrur S, Pervez MA, et al. Unsuspected coagulopathy rarely prevents IV thrombolysis in acute ischemic stroke. Neurology 2009;73(23):1957–62.

53. Cucchiara BL, Jackson B, Weiner M, et al. Usefulness of checking platelet count before thrombolysis in acute ischemic. Stroke 2007;38(5):1639–40.

54. Westover AN, McBride S, Haley RW. Stroke in young adults who abuse amphetamines or cocaine: a population-based study of hospitalized patients. Arch Gen Psychiatry 2007;64(4):495–502.
55. Kerr G, Ray G, Wu O, et al. Elevated troponin after stroke: a systematic review. Cerebrovasc Dis 2009;28(3):220–6.
56. Latchaw RE, Alberts MJ, Lev MH, et al. Recommendations for imaging of acute ischemic stroke: a scientific statement from the American Heart Association. Stroke 2009;40(11):3646–78.
57. Ginde AA, Foianini A, Renner DM, et al. Availability and quality of computed tomography and magnetic resonance imaging equipment in U.S. emergency departments. Acad Emerg Med 2008;15(8):780–3.
58. Leiva-Salinas C, Wintermark M. Imaging of acute ischemic stroke. Neuroimaging Clin N Am 2010;20(4):455–68.
59. Nentwich LM, Veloz W. Neuroimaging in acute stroke. Emerg Med Clin North Am 2012;30(3):659–80.
60. Lövblad K-O, Baird AE. Computed tomography in acute ischemic stroke. Neuroradiology 2010;52(3):175–87.
61. Schuknecht B, Ratzka M, Hofmann E. The "dense artery sign"–major cerebral artery thromboembolism demonstrated by computed tomography. Neuroradiology 1990;32(2):98–103.
62. Leys D, Pruvo JP, Godefroy O, et al. Prevalence and significance of hyperdense middle cerebral artery in acute stroke. Stroke 1992;23(3):317–24.
63. Tomsick TA, Brott TG, Chambers AA, et al. Hyperdense middle cerebral artery sign on CT: efficacy in detecting middle cerebral artery thrombosis. AJNR Am J Neuroradiol 1990;11(3):473–7.
64. von Kummer R, Meyding-Lamadé U, Forsting M, et al. Sensitivity and prognostic value of early CT in occlusion of the middle cerebral artery trunk. AJNR Am J Neuroradiol 1994;15(1):9–15 [discussion: 16–8].
65. Patel SC, Levine SR, Tilley BC, et al. Lack of clinical significance of early ischemic changes on computed tomography in acute stroke. JAMA 2001;286(22):2830–8.
66. von Kummer R, Holle R, Gizyska U, et al. Interobserver agreement in assessing early CT signs of middle cerebral artery infarction. AJNR Am J Neuroradiol 1996; 17(9):1743–8.
67. Truwit CL, Barkovich AJ, Gean-Marton A, et al. Loss of the insular ribbon: another early CT sign of acute middle cerebral artery infarction. Radiology 1990;176(3): 801–6.
68. Sarikaya B, Provenzale J. Frequency of various brain parenchymal findings of early cerebral ischemia on unenhanced CT scans. Emerg Radiol 2010;17(5): 381–90.
69. Tomura N, Uemura K, Inugami A, et al. Early CT finding in cerebral infarction: obscuration of the lentiform nucleus. Radiology 1988;168(2):463–7.
70. Barber PA, Demchuk AM, Zhang J, et al. Validity and reliability of a quantitative computed tomography score in predicting outcome of hyperacute stroke before thrombolytic therapy. Lancet 2000;355(9216):1670–4.
71. Pexman JHW, Barber PA, Hill MD, et al. Use of the Alberta Stroke Program Early CT Score (ASPECTS) for assessing CT scans in patients with acute stroke. AJNR Am J Neuroradiol 2001;22(8):1534–42.
72. Prokop M. Multislice CT angiography. Eur J Radiol 2000;36(2):86–96.
73. Grotta JC, Hacke W. Stroke neurologist's perspective on the new endovascular trials. Stroke 2015;46(6):1447–52.

74. Eastwood JD, Lev MH, Provenzale JM. Pertusion CT with iodinated contrast material. AJR Am J Roentgenol 2003;180(1):3–12.
75. Merino JG, Warach S. Imaging of acute stroke. Nat Rev Neurol 2010;6(10): 560–71.
76. Kidwell CS, Chalela JA, Saver JL, et al. Comparison of MRI and CT for detection of acute intracerebral hemorrhage. JAMA 2004;292(15):1823–30.
77. Chalela JA, Kidwell CS, Nentwich LM, et al. Magnetic resonance imaging and computed tomography in emergency assessment of patients with suspected acute stroke: a prospective comparison. Lancet 2007;369(9558):293–8.
78. Xavier AR, Qureshi AI, Kirmani JF, et al. Neuroimaging of stroke: a review. South Med J 2003;96(4):367–79.
79. Wu O, Nentwich L, Chutinet A. Diffusion in acute stroke. In: Diffusion MRI: theory, methods, and applications. New York: Oxford University Press; 2011. p. 518–28.
80. Linfante I, Llinas RH, Caplan LR, et al. MRI features of intracerebral hemorrhage within 2 hours from symptom onset. Stroke 1999;30(11):2263–7.
81. Miyazaki M, Lee VS. Nonenhanced MR angiography. Radiology 2008;248(1): 20–43.
82. Yoo AJ, Pulli B, Gonzalez RG. Imaging-based treatment selection for intravenous and intra-arterial stroke therapies: a comprehensive review. Expert Rev Cardiovasc Ther 2011;9(7):857–76.

Treatment of Acute Ischemic Stroke

Matthew S. Siket, MD, MS

KEYWORDS

- Acute ischemic stroke • Reperfusion • Intravenous thrombolysis
- Endovascular therapy • Tissue plasminogen activator

KEY POINTS

- The treatment of acute ischemic stroke is aimed at reperfusing ischemic tissue, halting progression of infarction, and preventing recurrence.
- Brain parenchyma is sensitive to brief periods of oligemia and hypoperfusion, and the success of reperfusion therapies are highly time dependent.
- Intravenous thrombolysis may benefit patients experiencing an acute ischemic stroke up to 4.5 hours from symptom onset.
- Emergency medicine systems of care should focus on the availability and speed of access to reperfusion therapies to maximize the benefit for as many patients as possible.
- Extended time window reperfusion, neuroprotection, and adjunctive therapies remain exciting areas of acute ischemic stroke research.

INTRODUCTION

The treatment of acute ischemic stroke (AIS) shares similarities with other vascular emergencies, in that reperfusion of ischemic tissue, halt in propagation of infarction, and prevention of recurrence are the 3 primary early goals of care. Even more than myocardial and other tissue, however, brain parenchyma is exquisitely sensitive to short periods of oligemia and hypoperfusion. In fact, radiographically proven acute cerebral infarction has been reported in patients with as little as 10 seconds of symptoms.[1] The term "time is brain" has been popularized to emphasize the rapidity by which neurons are irretrievably lost during an ischemic stroke.[2] Although dependent on several factors, including degree of ischemic preconditioning, site of occlusion, perfusion of collateral vessels, blood pressure, and glucose and oxygen delivery, on average 1.9 million neurons are destroyed with each passing minute that a stroke evolves.[2] When translated into patient lifetime benefits from expeditious thrombolysis, each minute saved in stroke onset to treatment led to an average of 1.8 days of additional healthy life (95% prediction interval, 0.9–2.7).[3]

Department of Emergency Medicine, The Warren Alpert Medical School of Brown University, 55 Claverick Street, 2nd Floor, Providence, RI 02903, USA
E-mail address: Matthew_Siket@brown.edu

Emerg Med Clin N Am 34 (2016) 861–882
http://dx.doi.org/10.1016/j.emc.2016.06.009   emed.theclinics.com

Although stroke recently declined from the third to the fifth most common cause of death in the United States, the annual incidence and overall prevalence continue to increase and it remains a leading cause of long-term disability.[4] Since the available US Food and Drug Administration (FDA)–approved treatment options are time dependent, improving stroke care in the early moments may have more of a public health impact than any other phase of care. Timely and efficient stroke treatment should be a priority for emergency department (ED) and prehospital providers. This article discusses the currently available and emerging treatment options in AIS focusing on the preservation of salvageable brain tissue, minimizing complications, and secondary prevention.

PATIENT EVALUATION OVERVIEW

The initial evaluation of AIS should be focused on the efficient detection of functionally disabling neurologic deficits to optimize eligibility for time-dependent treatment options. A detailed discussion of AIS diagnosis is discussed elsewhere in this issue (See Lauren M. Nentwich's article, "Diagnosis of Acute Ischemic Stroke," in this issue). In short, an expedited neurologic examination should be performed including, but not limited to the National Institutes of Health Stroke Scale (NIHSS). Documentation of a NIHSS before stroke treatment and at the time of initial evaluation is a quality metric per The Joint Commission for Primary and Comprehensive Stroke Centers, which becomes the responsibility of the emergency medicine provider, unless neurologic expertise is available in house or via remote video telestroke services. Although formal NIHSS training and certification is not currently required per The Joint Commission, it is encouraged and freely available (https://secure.trainingcampus.net/uas/modules/trees/windex.aspx?rx=nihss-english.trainingcampus.net). Perhaps more important than a full NIHSS, at least initially, is to perform a brief stroke detection and severity screen, which can be performed in the ambulance or while being triaged in the ED. Prehospital stroke detection screens such as FAST (Facial drooping, Arm weakness, Speech difficulties and Time), CPSS (Cincinnati Prehospital Stroke Scale), LAPSS (Los Angeles Prehospital Stroke Screen), MASS (Massachusetts Stroke Scale), Med-PACS (Medic Prehospital Assessment for Code Stroke), OPSS (Ontario Prehospital Stroke Screening Tool), and ROSIER (Recognition of Stroke in the Emergency Room) have been linked with improved thrombolytic treatment rates and door-to-needle times.[5] Severity scales such as the LAMS (Los Angeles Motor Scale), KPSS (Kurashiki Prehospital Stroke Scale), sNIHSS (Short NIHSS), CPSSS (Cincinnati Prehospital Stroke Severity Scale), VAN (vision, aphasia, neglect), and RACE (Rapid Arterial oCclusion Evaluation) have proven reasonably sensitive and specific tools to detect patients with emergent large vessel occlusion (ELVO) and may be used to trigger neurointerventional team activation, prehospital diversion, or interfacility transfer to a comprehensive stroke center.[6–10]

Emphasis should be given to establishing the time the patient was "last known well," that is, without symptoms, which is distinct from the time symptoms were first noted. The time last known well should be used in all cases as the equivalent of symptom onset unless the patient or witness is clearly able to recall the time symptoms began. This is important to ensure that symptom duration is not underestimated, resulting in treatment of the patient with thrombolytics beyond the approved treatment window.

It is also important to gain a sense of the patient's premorbid functional status immediately before the stroke onset. This becomes important when weighing and discussing the risks and benefits of treatment options for reperfusion. This can usually be done by simply asking if the patient was functionally independent before stroke onset. A number of easy-to-use disability scales have been developed for this purpose,[11] but the clinician often assesses a 'gestalt' version at the bedside. The modified Rankin Scale (mRS) is the most commonly used measure in stroke trials and measures global disability on a 6-point ordinal scale as shown in **Table 1**.

EMERGENT AND SUPPORTIVE CARE

Once the diagnosis of AIS has been made, it should go without saying that the basics of patient resuscitation, including the ABCs (airway, breathing, and circulation) take precedence, just as with any other ED patient. Especially important are temperature and glucose regulation, prevention of hypoxia, and optimization of blood pressure, and should remain priorities in all stroke patients. Cerebral perfusion pressure is the difference between the mean arterial pressure and intracranial pressure and is influenced by patient positioning and the progression of vasogenic edema in large territory infarcts. Unless the patient will, is, or has just received thrombolytic therapy, permissive hypertension ($\leq$220 mm Hg systolic) should be allowed to promote cerebral autoregulation and perfusion of collateral vessels. Patients receiving thrombolytics should have their blood pressure maintained at or below 185/110 mm Hg in accordance with the American Heart Association/American Stroke Association (AHA/ASA) recommendations.[12] Patients should be positioned with their heads in the midline position to promote optimal venous return and supine as tolerated, except in cases where impaired swallowing is noted, or there is concern for increased intracranial pressure or impaired cardiopulmonary function wherein the supine position may induce hypoxia. In these cases, elevating the head of the bed 15° to 30° is recommended.[12] Hyperthermia (>38°C) is associated with poor neurologic outcomes and should be quickly corrected. The QASC (Quality in Acute Stroke Care) trial showed that hospital-wide supportive protocols focusing on the management of fever, hyperglycemia, and swallowing dysfunction were associated with improved 90-day functional outcomes (absolute difference, 15.7%; 95% confidence interval [CI], 5.8–25.4; P = .002) with a number needed to treat of 6.[13] Empiric supplementary oxygen need not be administered unless it is required to maintain oxygen saturation of greater

Table 1
The modified Rankin scale

Score	Description
0	No symptoms at all
1	No significant disability despite symptoms; able to carry out all usual duties and activities
2	Slight disability; unable to carry out all previous activities, but able to look after own affairs without assistance
3	Moderate disability; requiring some help, but able to walk without assistance
4	Moderately severe disability; unable to walk without assistance, unable to attend to needs without assistance
5	Severe disability; bedridden, incontinent, and requiring constant nursing care and attention
6	Dead

than 94%.[12] Normoglycemia should be maintained, but the degree to which tight adherence is required remains unresolved.

REPERFUSION WITH INTRAVENOUS THROMBOLYSIS

The concept of thrombolysis in AIS is neither new nor without sustained controversy. Initial studies in the 1950s used streptokinase and urokinase, isolated from *Streptococcus* strains and human urine, respectively.[14] Intracerebral hemorrhage (ICH) was a leading cause of death in these early investigations, which preceded computed tomography (CT) technology. In the 1960s, Meyer and colleagues[15,16] used diagnostic angiography to perform investigations, first comparing intravenous (IV) plasmin with placebo, then combination therapy with streptokinase and heparin versus heparin alone. Although the former showed no benefit of the plasmin treated group, the latter showed greater mortality and ICH in the streptokinase-treated group. The MAST-E (Multicenter Acute Stroke Trial-Europe) and MAST-I (Multicenter Acute Stroke Trial-Italy) trials of streptokinase in the 1990s further confirmed increased risk of ICH and mortality, leading to the eventual abandonment of it as a treatment for AIS.[17,18]

Concurrently, tissue plasminogen activator (t-PA) emerged as a clinically superior fibrinolytic to streptokinase in myocardial ischemia,[19] which quickly translated into new investigations in AIS. This culminated in the landmark NINDS-II (National Institute of Neurological Disorders and Stroke) trial of 624 stroke patients published in 1995, which showed improved clinical outcome at 3 months for AIS patients treated with t-PA within 3 hours, despite a risk of symptomatic ICH of 6.4%, compared with 0.6% of controls ($P<.001$).[20] Earlier the same year, the ECASS (European Cooperative Acute Stroke Study)-I trial failed to demonstrate the same benefit among 620 patients randomized to t-PA versus placebo treated within 6 hours of symptom onset, which the authors attributed to a large number of protocol violations, accounting for 17.4% of the study population.[21] Regardless, 1 year later the FDA approved t-PA for the treatment of AIS up to 3 hours after symptom onset.

The NINDS-II study has been criticized for having significant imbalances between treatment groups.[22] However, the benefits of t-PA when given between 0 and 3 hours have been reinforced in post hoc analyses.[23–25] Moreover, an independent commission concluded that there was no significant difference in treatment effect based on these imbalances.[24] Overall, the NINDS trial found that t-PA–treated patients were 30% more likely to have minimal or no disability at 3 months for a number needed to treat of 7 to 8 for a favorable outcome.

Multiple subsequent studies in the following years either failed to demonstrate the treatment effect of the NINDS trial or were terminated owing to harm, including ECASS II and ATLANTIS (Alteplase Thrombolysis for Acute Noninterventional Therapy in Ischemic Stroke) Part A (0–6 hours), and ATLANTIS Part B (3–5 hours).[26–28] The 0- to 3-hour treatment window remained the standard of care until publication of ECASS III in 2008, which showed clinical efficacy in treatment up to 4.5 hours (OR, 1.34; 95% CI, 1.02–1.76; $P = .04$).[29] There was no difference in mortality, despite an increased risk of symptomatic ICH (7.9% for t-PA vs 3.5% for placebo; $P<.001$). The number needed to treat for a favorable outcome was 14 to 15. Unfortunately, these results were not replicated in the EPITHET (Echoplanar Imaging Thrombolytic Evaluation Trial) trial, which was published the same year and randomly assigned patients to t-PA or placebo with symptoms between 3 to 6 hours' duration and a perfusion–diffusion mismatch on emergency MRI.[30] Although EPITHET failed to achieve its primary endpoint (radiographic infarct growth at day 90), the t-PA–treated group was significantly associated with reperfusion, which correlated with improved neurologic outcomes.

The benefits of t-PA were further reinforced in 2009 in a metaanalysis inclusive of patients from ECASS 1, 2, and 3, and ATLANTIS showing an increased odds of a favorable outcome without difference in mortality (OR, 1.31; 95% CI, 1.10–1.56; $P = .002$).[31] This led to the AHA/ASA revising its stroke guidelines accordingly the same year, recommending t-PA treatment up to 4.5 hours of symptom onset (class 1, level of evidence B).[32] An updated pooled analysis was published in 2010 adding NINDS and EPITHET subjects totaling 3670 patients further supporting the time-dependent treatment effect with favorable outcomes up to 4.5 hours.[23] In 2013, a joint recommendation by the AHA/ASA, American Academy of Neurology, American College of Emergency Physicians (ACEP), American Nurses Association, and Neurocritical Care Society supported the use of t-PA from 0 to 3 hours with a Level A recommendation and between 3 and 4.5 hours with a level B recommendation.[12,33] The use of t-PA beyond 3 hours remains off-label in the United States, however, because it is FDA-approved only up to 3 hours of symptoms.

The IST-3 (Third International Stroke Trial) is the most recent large clinical trial to investigate the efficacy of IV t-PA up to 6 hours of symptom duration.[34] The study had intended to enroll 6000 subjects in a 1:1 open, controlled design. However, owing to slow subject recruitment, the target was adjusted and in total, 3035 patients were enrolled. Because thrombolysis was already considered standard of care from 0 to 4.5 hours during the enrollment period, only patients for whom there remained clinical equipoise as to the efficacy of t-PA were recruited.[35] Even among this population who were enrolled despite classical exclusion criteria and up to 6 hours after symptom onset, a significant ordinal reduction in disability was noted at 6 months. Most important, the subgroup of patients treated within 3 hours of onset showed a significant benefit of t-PA (OR, 1.64; 95% CI, 1.03–2.62). In a separate publication of 18-month follow-up of IST-3 subjects, the favorable shift in functional status persisted (OR, 1.3; 95% CI, 1.10–1.55; $P = .002$) and t-PA–treated patients self-reported better overall health ($P = .019$).[36] This trial is sometimes dismissed because it did not achieve its primary aim, namely, demonstration of improvement in the primary outcome, at the P <.05 level.[37] It should be emphasized, however, that this is not the same as showing harm, simply that our confidence in the benefit of t-PA (outside of traditional NINDS criteria) is not as strong. When combined with the pool of all available trials of thrombolytics for stroke, IST-3 provided further evidence that t-PA treatment in stroke is not life saving, but rather autonomy preserving.

Although subject to methodologic heterogeneity, pooled analyses do provide valuable insight as to the overall efficacy and safety of IV t-PA. Systemic thrombolysis has, for some time, been considered the worldwide standard of care in AIS; thus, the replication of the landmark clinical trials that have been subject to heavy criticism would be unethical given a universal lack of clinical equipoise. The most robust of the pooled analyses performed to date is a Cochrane review published in 2014 inclusive of 10,187 patients from 27 different clinical trials.[38] Of the subjects in this pooled analysis, 7012 were randomized to IV t-PA versus placebo, whereas the others involved other thrombolytics. The key findings reinforced the individual studies' conclusions, namely that "time is brain" and faster treatment is better.[39] Not surprisingly, dichotomized treatment from 0 to 3 hours outperformed treatment between 3 and 6 hours (OR, 1.56 [95% CI, 1.28–1.90] vs OR 1.07 [95% CI 0.96–1.2]). The authors' conclusion that treatment with t-PA improves outcomes for patients if given up to 4.5 hours after stroke onset has been criticized and led to some debate.[40,41] Although heterogeneous in total, a homogeneous subgroup of 1779 patients across 6 trials showed clear benefit of t-PA when given early, within the first 3 hours (OR, 0.65; 95% CI, 0.54–0.80; P<.0001).[38] Moreover, an individual patient data metaanalysis from 6756 patients conducted in 2014 by the Stroke Thrombolysis Trialists' Collaboration in 2014 concluded that the benefit of t-PA extends to sometime beyond 4.5 hours.[42] Ninety-day mortality was 1.4% higher among those receiving t-PA (hazard ratio, 1.11; 95% CI, 0.99–1.25; P = .07), but was offset by an absolute increase in disability-free survival of 10% if treated within 0 to 3 hours or 5% if treated within 3 to 4.5 hours.

Nevertheless, the methodology and conclusions of recent pooled analyses have been called into question and has resulted in the recent revised grading of evidence supporting the use of t-PA by both the ACEP and the Canadian Association of Emergency Physicians.[33,40,43] Whereas ACEP supports the use of t-PA up to 4.5 hours (level B recommendation), the Canadian Association of Emergency Physicians has issued a conditional recommendation against the use of t-PA in the 3- to 4.5-hour window, largely owing to the increased risk of ICH and possible increase in 90-day mortality until further research is available.

Clearly, the lack of consensus regarding the use of t-PA continues to be the subject of debates, extending to the highest levels of health care policy. What should not be lost in these debates, however, is the patient's preference. Although the risk of ICH is relatively small, it is by no means insignificant (4.9%–7.7%)[34,44] and the decision to risk a potentially expedited death for a reduced likelihood of long-term disability is a highly personal one.[45] Hence, a brief discussion of risks and benefits, and, when feasible, the use of shared-decision making between the patient/surrogate and health care provider is recommended (ACEP level C recommendation).[33]

THE ISSUE OF INFORMED CONSENT AND INFORMED REFUSAL

Whether informed consent for IV t-PA is needed in acute stroke is medicolegally and ethically unclear, and has been the source of a fair amount of debate. Because it has been established that "time is brain," deferring treatment until risks and benefits have been discussed adequately could be viewed by some as withholding the established standard of care. Additionally, the acute stress of the event on the patient and family often impedes comprehension and may quickly lead to paternalistic decision making.[46] Although t-PA use in ischemic stroke is not accepted universally as an emergency exception to informed consent, a survey in JAMA suggests that overall rates favoring t-PA treatment in stroke is similar to rates for cardiopulmonary resuscitation for cardiac arrest.[47] Yet, the unique risk/benefit profile of t-PA draws no parallel or precedent in medicine and so general consensus among the stroke community favors obtaining informed consent. The use of a visual aid such as the one proposed by Gadhia and colleagues[48] may facilitate a balanced and efficient discussion. Implied consent may be invoked per an institutional standard of care when the patient lacks decision-making capacity and no surrogate can be located after a reasonable effort.[45]

Because t-PA is considered standard of care in certain circumstances, it has been proposed that the risks/benefits discussion be focused on informed refusal rather than informed consent.[49] This model preserves patient autonomy and the right of self-determination, while emphasizing the substantial, yet time-dependent benefit of t-PA. Patient-centered decision support tools aimed to streamline a brief summary of risks/benefits have been developed, and, among focus groups of stroke survivors, caregivers, emergency physicians, and advanced practice nurses are well-received when framed positively and displayed as simplified graphs.[50] The Rapid Evaluation for Stroke Outcomes using Lytics in a Vascular Event (RESOLVE) decision aid is currently being tested and consists of a 3-page patient tool and single page clinician tool summarizing individualized risk prediction models.

SAFETY OF TISSUE PLASMINOGEN ACTIVATOR IN STROKE MIMICS

The emphasis on shortening door-to-needle times to expedite stroke thrombolysis comes at some expense to the specificity of stroke diagnosis. Certainly, some of the stroke mimics like hemiplegic migraine and Todd's paralysis may be indistinguishable from stroke in the early moments of care. In a recent metaanalysis of reported case series inclusive of 8942 total patients treated with t-PA, 392 were found to be stroke mimics.[51] Symptomatic ICH rates (defined as imaging evidence of hemorrhage as well as a NIHSS increase of $\geq$4 points) were 0.5% (95% CI, 0%-2%) and the risk was significantly lower in stroke mimics (risk ratio 0.33; 95% CI, 0.14–0.77; P = .010). The rate of orolingual edema was also low (0.3%; 95% CI, 0%-2%) and favorable outcomes were 3-fold higher among stroke mimics. From a medicolegal perspective, a systematic review of malpractice litigation cases in AIS revealed that of 40 cases related to IV t-PA, only 2 (5%) were related to complications of administration, whereas 38 (95%) were related to failure to administer.[52]

ALTERNATIVE AND EMERGING THROMBOLYTIC AGENTS

Alteplase remains the thrombolytic of choice in clinical practice, but is not the ideal agent. Its short half-life (5 minutes) requires a continuous infusion after initial bolus and its fibrin selectivity is moderate on the spectrum of thrombolytic agents.[14] Its limited efficacy in causing reperfusion, particularly in large vessels, as well as its associated risk of ICH and postulated neurotoxicity has kept researchers searching for newer and better thrombolytics.[53,54] Tenecteplase (TNK) is a genetically engineered alternative to alteplase that has more than twice the half-life and is 15 times more fibrin specific.[55] It also is more resistant to plasminogen activator inhibition, which is an endogenous counteraction to thrombolytic effect, and is associated with less degradation of apolipoprotein A-1, the main protein component of high-density lipoprotein.[56] For these reasons, it is currently the preferred lytic in patients with ST-elevation myocardial infarction.[57] TNK may be even more appealing in AIS because it causes less hypofibrinogenemia, and early degradation of fibrinogen is associated with ICH.[58,59] Three multicenter RCTs comparing TNK to alteplase are currently underway (TEMPO-2 [A Randomized Controlled Trial of TNK-tPA Versus Standard of Care for Minor Ischemic Stroke With Proven Occlusion], NOR-TEST [Norwegian Tenecteplase Stroke Trial], and EXTEND-IA TNK [Tenecteplase Versus Alteplase Before Endovascular Therapy for Ischemic Stroke]), but multiple phase II trials have shown promise and no increase in risk for symptomatic ICH.[60–64] One study found that TNK at a dose of 0.25 mg/kg was superior to alteplase in reperfusion and clinical outcome at 90 days.[60]

Desmoteplase, a recombinant fibrinolytic isolated from the saliva of the vampire bat, has an even longer half-life and is more fibrin selective than either TNK or alteplase. In fact, desmoteplase activity was found to be 105,000 times higher in the presence of fibrin than without, compared with alteplase, which showed only a 550-fold increase.[14,65] Phase II clinical trials (DEDAS [Dose Escalation of Desmoteplase for Acute Ischemic Stroke]/DIAS [Desmoteplase in Acute Ischemic Stroke Trial]) suggested safety and efficacy of desmoteplase in stroke patients treated 3 to 9 hours from symptom onset, but these findings were not replicated in the subsequent DIAS 2 or 3 trials.[66–69] However, despite a median time to treatment of 7 hours in DIAS 3, there were no safety concerns and symptomatic ICH rates were low (3%) and similar to placebo.[69] Although these trials were unable to extend the therapeutic window of systemic thrombolysis, desmoteplase remains an appealing alternative thrombolytic agent. Several other agents, including retaplase and microplasmin, are showing promise in the preclinical phase.[70]

INTERVENTIONAL STROKE TREATMENT

The history of endovascular stroke treatment began with intraarterial (IA) administration of fibrinolytic agents. In 1999, the PROACT (Intra-arterial Prourokinase for Acute Ischemic Stroke) II trial showed improved functional outcomes at 90 days in patients treated with IA prourokinase within 6 hours of onset of large middle cerebral artery occlusion ($P = .04$).[71] Catheter-directed thrombolysis offers the theoretic advantage of targeted drug delivery directly at the site of the thrombus to achieve recanalization at a lesser total drug dose.[72] Although prohibited in the PROACT II trial, in clinical practice recanalization was further augmented through guidewire-mediated mechanical clot disruption during IA thrombolysis.[73]

Mechanical clot retrieval devices were first developed to recover displaced coils from endovascular procedures. The first device to gain FDA approval was the MERCI retriever in August 2004, after the device was shown to successfully recanalize 43% of large vessel occlusions when used alone, or 64% in combination with IA t-PA.[74,75] Suction thrombectomy using an aspiration device such as the Penumbra System gained FDA approval in 2007 after showing recanalization in 82% of patients in a prospective, single-arm study of 125 subjects.[76] It should be noted, however, that FDA approval was granted solely based on the ability of these devices to successfully recanalize thrombosed vessels in acute stroke patients, not from efficacy in improving functional outcomes.

The initial randomized, controlled trials investigating the efficacy of interventional stroke treatment on functional outcomes included 3 studies: IMS (Interventional Management of Stroke) III, MR RESCUE (Mechanical Retrieval and Recanalization of Stroke Clots Using Embolectomy) and SYNTHESIS (Local Versus Systemic Thrombolysis for Acute Ischemic Stroke), all published in the same issue of the *New England Journal of Medicine* on February 8, 2013.[77–79] None of the studies showed a statistically significant difference in clinical outcome of patients treated with endovascular therapy (EVT) versus systemic thrombolysis alone. SYNTHESIS remains the only trial to date that directly compared EVT without IV t-PA with t-PA alone. 362 AIS patients within 4.5 hours of onset were randomized to IV t-PA or EVT (IA or clot disruption/retrieval, or both) and the proportion alive without disability (mRS 0–1) at 3 months were similar between groups (30.4% vs 34.8%; adjusted OR 0.71; 95% CI, 0.44–1.14; $P = .16$). The rates of symptomatic ICH were similar between groups (~6%).

IMS III and MR RESCUE were similar in comparing IV t-PA alone with IV t-PA + EVT. MR RESCUE used perfusion-weighted imaging (CT or MRI) to differentiate patients thought to have a "favorable" imaging pattern, in whom a greater portion of potentially salvageable tissue was present.[78] A "favorable" imaging pattern was defined as the infarct core was 90 mL or less and the proportion of predicted infarct was 70% or less of the at-risk region. Patients were randomized to EVT + IV t-PA or IV t-PA alone, regardless of the imaging pattern and embolectomy was not found to be superior in reducing 90-day mRS scores among penumbral ($P = .23$) or nonpenumbral ($P = .32$) imagining patterned patients. IMS III, on the other hand, did not require perfusion imaging or even vessel imaging showing evidence of large vessel occlusion before randomization. In this study, stroke patients who had received IV t-PA within 3 hours of onset were randomized 2:1 to EVT (mechanical thrombectomy or IA) or no adjunctive therapy. The study was terminated prematurely owing to futility after 656 of an anticipated 900 patients were enrolled. The primary outcome measure was the proportion of patients with a mRS of 0 to 2 at 90 days, which did not differ between groups (40.8% for EVT vs 38.7% for t-PA alone; absolute adjusted difference, 1.5%; 95% CI, -6.1–9.1). Mortality and symptomatic ICH rates were similar as well. A trend toward a favorable outcome was noted in patients with a carotid T-type or L-type occlusion of the internal carotid artery, M1/A1 or tandem internal carotid artery and M1 occlusion in a subgroup analysis of 306 subjects (47%) with baseline CT or MR angiographic data.[80] This finding may have contributed to baseline vessel imaging becoming standard in all subsequent EVT trials.

Collectively, the negative results of IMS III, SYNTHESIS, and MR RESCUE helped to reestablish clinical equipoise to a stroke treatment strategy that had become pervasive without any compelling outcome data from a randomized, controlled trial.[81] This set the stage for a new round of EVT trials, which benefitted from the advent of third-generation devices, called stent retrievers or "stent-trievers," which were felt to more consistently, efficiently, and safely establish recanalization.[82,83] These devices include the SOLITAIRE and TREVO devices, which received FDA approval in 2012. Simultaneously, stroke systems of care continued to evolve, thereby allowing for more rapid identification of ELVO strokes. These advances helped to fuel the second round of clinical trials that would prove revolutionary to acute stroke treatment.

The second wave of EVT trials came in early 2015 with 5 prospective, randomized multicenter studies from around the world demonstrating benefit of EVT over IV t-PA alone. These include MR CLEAN (Multicenter Randomized Clinical trial of Endovascular treatment for Acute ischemic stroke in the Netherlands), EXTEND-IA, ESCAPE (Endovascular Treatment for Small Core and Proximal Occlusion Ischemic Stroke), SWIFT PRIME (Solitaire With the Intention For Thrombectomy as PRIMary Endovascular Treatment), and REVASCAT (Endovascular Revascularization With Solitaire Device Versus Best Medical Therapy in Anterior Circulation Stroke Within 8 Hours). Partial results of 2 additional studies, THRACE (Trial and Cost Effectiveness Evaluation of Intra-arterial Thrombectomy in Acute Ischemic Stroke) and THERAPY (Assess the PENUMBRA System in the Treatment of Acute Stroke) have also been reported, but remain in prepublication phase.[84–89] Despite variations in inclusion/exclusion criteria across studies, all 5 shared several similarities, most notably the confirmation of ELVO via vascular imaging acquisition (CTA or MRA) at baseline, as well as a common outcome measure, the mRS at 90 days. A favorable outcome was considered an mRS of 0 to 2. Of note, only the first trial to report its results, MR CLEAN, completed enrollment; all other trials were halted prematurely owing to meeting predetermined efficacy endpoint or owing to lack of equipoise in light of other positive trials.

The MR CLEAN study concluded in March 2014 after enrolling 500 subjects across 16 sites in the Netherlands.[8] The Dutch Ministry of Health was a motivating factor in trial completion by provisionally reimbursing for EVT only in the setting of this trial on the heels of the prior negative studies. Patients were enrolled within 6 hours of symptom onset if NIHSS was 2 or greater. Of the 233 patients in the interventional arm, 33% had a favorable outcome compared with 19% of the 267 in the control group. This was an absolute difference of 14% (adjusted OR, 1.67; 95% CI, 1.2–2.3).

The ESCAPE study was conducted primarily in Canada, including 22 sites that enrolled 316 of an intended 500 subjects.[84] Patients with an NIHSS of 6 or greater were included up to 12 hours after symptom onset. Of the 165 patients in the intervention arm, 53% had a favorable outcome compared with 29% in the control arm, for an absolute difference of 24% (P<.001).

The EXTEND-IA trial was conducted in Australia and New Zealand across 14 different sites. Only 70 of the planned 100 patients (35 intervention, 35 control) were enrolled. Patients with an NIHSS of 2 or greater were included up to 6 hours from symptom onset. Although the 90-day mRS was an outcome measure, this was a secondary endpoint in this study, and the coprimary endpoints were radiographic reperfusion at 24 hours and early neurologic recovery (improvement of NIHSS by ≥ 8 points).[89] The absolute difference in favorable outcomes at 90 days between treatment groups was 31% favoring EVT (71% vs 40%; $P = .009$).

The SWIFT PRIME trial enrolled only 196 of an intended 833 patients across 39 sites, primarily in the United States, before being halted owing to efficacy.[85] This trial used a cutoff of 8 on the NIHSS and enrolled up to 6 hours from symptom onset. All patients received baseline CT/CTA/CT perfusion or diffusion-weighted MRI for imaging-based selection. Of the 98 in the intervention arm, 60% achieved a favorable outcome, compared with 36% of the controls, for an absolute difference of 24% ($P<.001$).

The REVASCAT trial was the last to reports results, halting enrollment after only 206 of an intended 690 patients owing to loss of equipoise after the release of the preceding trials' data.[88] The NIHSS cutoff was 6 and patients were included up to 8 hours from symptom onset. The absolute difference between treatment groups in terms of a good outcome at 90 days was 16% favoring EVT (44% vs 28%; $P<.001$).

Clearly there now exists robust evidence supporting the use of EVT in patients with ELVO on baseline vessel imaging. The timeframe for initiation of EVT ranged from 6 to 12 hours in these studies, but evidence suggests that the effectiveness decreases over time.[86,90] Of note, the trials with the fastest time to recanalization showed the largest treatment effect (EXTEND-IA, SWIFT PRIME, and ESCAPE). Furthermore, the "picture-to-puncture" times (ie, the time from first vascular image to groin puncture) was less than 60 minutes in ESCAPE and SWIFT PRIME, which would be nearly impossible to replicate without optimally efficient ED and neurointerventionalist activation processes.[91] In the short time since publication of the 5 positive EVT trials, supporting guidelines from the AHA/ASA and Society of Neurointerventional Surgeons have already followed suit.[92,93] EVT should be considered the standard of care for patients with ELVO, within 6 hours of symptom onset, and regional systems-of-care initiatives should focus on ensuring timely access to this treatment for as many patients as possible.

Processes to improve the availability and speed of access to endovascular therapies should be regional and institution specific. Some examples include the administration of t-PA in the CT scanner bay during dedicated vessel image acquisition, as well as EMS destination protocols based on prehospital stroke severity scale use to improve the proportion of ELVOs triaged to endovascular capable stroke centers. Mobile stroke units, ambulances equipped with a portable CT scanner, point-of-care laboratory capabilities, and access to stroke expertise are becoming increasingly common, have CT angiography capabilities, and have been shown to reduce time to EVT.[94]

TREATMENT OF POSTERIOR CIRCULATION STROKE

Although 15% to 20% of all ischemic strokes are attributed to the posterior circulation, only 1% to 4% are from basilar artery occlusions (BAO). None of the aforementioned EVT trials included BAO and there remains a paucity of outcome data regarding treatment of from BAO.[95] The Basilar Artery International Cooperation Study (BASICS) registry remains the largest prospective, observational registry of consecutive patients comparing 1-month outcomes after IV t-PA, EVT, and conservative management.[96]

Of 592 patients receiving treatment in the registry, 402 (68%) had a poor outcome. Patients with mild to moderate clinical deficits (n = 245) had similar outcomes regardless of treatment strategy. However, patients with severe deficits (n = 347) seemed to benefit from IV t-PA or EVT compared with antithrombotic therapy alone, although the 2 treatment strategies led to similar outcomes when compared with one another (adjusted relative risk, 1.06; 95% CI, 0.91–1.22).

Without aggressive intervention the mortality and morbidity rate in BAO is estimated to be between 80% and 90%, leading to off-label compassionate use of IV and IA therapies beyond their established therapeutic windows.[97] It has been postulated that the brainstem and posterior fossa may be more resilient to longer periods of hypoperfusion given the preponderance of white matter and better collateral flow preserving penumbral tissue for longer periods of time.[98] However, when patients in the BASICS registry were stratified by time to recanalization, the proportion with poor functional outcome (mRS 4–6) increased with progressive 3-hour intervals of time (62% at <3 hours, 67% at 3–6 hours, 77% at 6–9 hours, and 85% beyond 9 hours).[98]

The necessity of recanalization to achieve a good functional outcome in BAO remains unresolved. In a systematic review of published case series of BAO, 38% of patients who were recanalized had a good outcome, compared with only 2% with a good outcome if recanalization was not established.[99] However, more recently the ENDO-STROKE (International Multicenter Registry for Mechanical Recanalization Procedures in Acute Stroke) study involving 148 BAO patients, most treated with the latest generation stent-retriever devices found 34% of patients had a good functional outcome, which was not predicted by recanalization.[100] The ENDOSTROKE study was conducted across 11 academic medical centers and did observe a lower than expected overall mortality rate of 35%.

The ongoing BASICS randomized controlled trial, which is planned to enroll through 2017, aims to answer the unresolved questions regarding efficacy of EVT in addition to IV t-PA in acute BAO. Until then, the approach to the suspected acute posterior circulation ischemic stroke patient should be similar to that of an anterior circulation infarct. One needs to be mindful that posterior circulation strokes often present atypically and the deficits are not reflected accurately on the NIHSS.[101] The severity of deficits should be assessed as well and providers should have a low threshold to obtain baseline vessel imaging to determine if EVT could be performed to increase the likelihood of recanalization. IV t-PA should be considered for symptoms up to 4.5 hours duration, although the oft ill-defined and atypical symptoms of posterior circulation strokes make it difficult to treat within this time window.[97]

APPROACH TO ILL-DEFINED STROKE ONSET

In approximately 25% of all ischemic strokes, patients awaken from sleep with symptoms and the exact time of onset is unknown.[102,103] Commonly, the time last known well exceeds 4.5 hours in wake up strokes; therefore, these patients are excluded from consideration of thrombolytic therapy. In an effort to safely maximize the inclusion of patients for reperfusion therapies, several imaging factors are being explored as surrogates of time and are the subject of multiple ongoing clinical trials. Much of the work to date has focused on a mismatch between diffusion-weighted imaging and either fluid-attenuated inversion recovery signal or perfusion abnormalities.[104,105] The WAKE-UP, EXTEND, and MR WITNESS trials are ongoing to explore IV thrombolysis and the DEFUSE (Endovascular Therapy Following Imaging Evaluation for Ischemic Stroke) 3 trial will soon be enrolling to investigate EVT.

TREATMENT OF MINOR, ISOLATED, AND IMPROVING SYMPTOMS

The most common reason for t-PA exclusion among patients presenting within the therapeutic window is the provider determining that stroke symptoms are minor or improving.[106,107] This has been supported as a relative contraindication to thrombolysis in prior guidelines.[108] Unfortunately, the definition of "minor" is subjective and a consensus definition is lacking.[109] In a cohort of 51 academic stroke clinicians surveyed, 80% reported not using a lower limit cutoff on the NIHSS, below which to exclude patients from treatment.[32] Aphasia is a good example of a stroke symptom that many would consider disabling unto itself, but is ascribed relatively few points on the NIHSS. In fact, aphasia has been found to be a strong and independent predictor of unfavorable outcome in patients with mild stroke.[110] Several case series have reported poor outcomes in roughly one-third of patients excluded from t-PA for minor symptoms.[106,111–114] This is particularly concerning because the efficacy of t-PA is thought to be greater in smaller, more distal occlusions.[115] Indeed, multiple small studies have shown increased proportions of minor stroke patients with favorable outcomes after thrombolytic treatment.[116–119] However, these patients were largely excluded from the landmark t-PA trials with the exception of IST-3, which showed a nonsignificant trend toward harm.[34,120] Moreover, a recent retrospective analysis of Get With The Guidelines data found that among 5910 stroke patients with a NIHSS of less than 6 treated with t-PA, 30% were not independently ambulatory at discharge.[121] So, although it seems that t-PA is still beneficial in this population, data up to this point are inconsistent. The ongoing PRISMS (A Study of the Efficacy and Safety of Activase [Alteplase] in Patients With Mild Stroke) trial will attempt to resolve any remaining uncertainty.[122]

NEUROPROTECTION

Numerous strategies that attempt to slow the conversion of ischemic penumbral tissue into infarcted core and halt the ischemic cascade have shown promise in animal models, but to date there has yet to be successful translation to the bedside.[123] Therapeutic hypothermia has demonstrated efficacy in animal models, but early clinical trials have not shown a definitive benefit.[124] Large-scale clinical trials of whole body and local endovascular cooling are ongoing.[125] Early magnesium administration has been explored given its function as a cerebral vasodilator and inhibitor of excitatory amino acids, but despite promising preliminary data, the recently completed FASTMAG (Field Administration of Stroke Therapy – Magnesium) trial of 1700 patients randomized to prehospital magnesium or placebo failed to show improved 90-day functional outcomes.[126] This trial was remarkable, however, in proving the feasibility of an ambulance-initiated trial of a neuroprotectant in AIS. Uric acid, an endogenous antioxidant and free radical scavenger, seems to be involved in a number of physiologic responses to stroke.[127] The URICOICTUS (Efficacy Study of Combined Treatment With Uric Acid and rtPA in Acute Ischemic Stroke) phase IIb/3 trial investigated the safety and efficacy of uric acid in combination with t-PA in AIS patients within 4.5 hours of symptom onset. An ordinal reduction of the mRS at 3 months was seen in the uric acid group (OR, 1.4; 95% CI, 0.99–1.98; $P = .05$) and treatment effect was even more pronounced in those presenting with hyperglycemia, which will be the subject of further study.[128,129] Hyperoxygenation is another area of research, but has not been shown to be therapeutic to date.[12]

SONOTHROMBOLYSIS

Augmented fibrinolysis through ultrasound-induced mechanical agitation has been an exciting area of research for more than a decade. Continuous 2-MHz transcranial

Doppler performed concurrently with t-PA administration seems to generate mechanical pressure waves and promote fluid motion around a thrombus, thereby weakening fibrin cross-links and increasing lytic concentration within the clot.[130,131] The CLOTBUST (Combined Lysis of Thrombus in Brain Ischemia With Transcranial Ultrasound and Systemic T-PA) trial randomized 126 patients with middle cerebral artery occlusions receiving t-PA to 2 hours of continuous transcranial Doppler versus placebo and showed significantly increased rates of complete recanalization in patients receiving sonolysis (49% vs 30%; $P = .03$).[132] Unfortunately, the augmented rates of recanalization were not associated with improved clinical outcomes. A hands-free transcranial Doppler device was developed to correct for operator dependence and was found to be safe and easily tolerable.[133] This led to a recent multicenter, international phase III efficacy trial, which was unfortunately terminated prematurely (Cerevast Therapeutics, unpublished data, 2015). Three metaanalyses have been performed and all concluded that sonolysis increases the rate of recanalization and reduces death and disability at 3 months without increasing the risk of ICH.[134–136] The addition of IV gaseous microspheres or "microbubbles" may further augment clot disruption and remains an area of research.[137,138]

MANAGEMENT OF HEMORRHAGIC TRANSFORMATION AND TISSUE PLASMINOGEN ACTIVATOR–RELATED BLEEDING

Most ICH occurs within 24 hours of reperfusion therapies and most fatal hemorrhages occur within the first 12 hours.[12] All stroke-ready hospitals should have institutional guidelines for the reversal of t-PA–associated bleeding and often involve the administration of cryoprecipitate to restore depleted fibrinogen levels in addition to immediate cessation of the t-PA infusion.

MANAGEMENT OF CEREBRAL EDEMA

Hypertonic saline and mannitol are reasonable considerations to lower increased intracranial pressure in patients with significant cerebral edema after large territory infarction. Decompressive hemicraniectomy may be life saving in hemispheric infarction with substantial edema. Mortality in these cases has been shown to be reduced from 80% to 20% with surgical decompression.[12] Clinical deterioration is often rapid, however, and waiting for signs of brainstem compression may be too late. The decision for surgery should be made on a case-by-case basis by neurointensivists and neurosurgeons whenever possible. Patients with malignant middle cerebral artery territory infarctions wanting aggressive treatment should, therefore, be considered for interfacility transfer to comprehensive stroke centers whenever feasible.

SECONDARY PREVENTION

For survivors of a completed ischemic stroke, prevention of a recurrent event is paramount. Optimal treatment strategies are largely based on the underlying stroke etiology. For example, large artery atherosclerosis should be considered for endarterectomy, whereas cardioembolic causes should be maintained on anticoagulation. In general, all stroke etiologies other than cardioembolism should be maintained on an antiplatelet agent. The use of aspirin (325 mg) is generally recommended, and should be initiated within 24 to 48 after stroke onset in those for whom t-PA was not administered (AHA/ASA class I; level A).[12] Other options, such as the combination of aspirin and dipyridamole, and clopidogrel monotherapy are also reasonable considerations. The early initiation of combined aspirin and clopidogrel was associated with an absolute risk reduction of 3.5% (hazard ratio, 0.68; 95% CI, 0.57–0.81; P<.001) compared with aspirin alone in a recent trial of more than 5000 minor stroke and transient ischemic attack patients in China.[139] The POINT (Platelet-Oriented Inhibition in New TIA and Minor Ischemic Stroke) trial is ongoing in the United States and may add additional support to combined aspirin and clopidogrel use to reduce recurrent stroke risk.

Lipid modification with the use of statins should be ubiquitous, as well as lifestyle modification and risk factor control interventions. Physical activity should be promoted with a focus on decreasing sedentary behaviors. Further discussion of specific secondary prevention strategies is beyond the scope of this article, but is discussed elsewhere in this issue.

SUMMARY

Presently, we are in an exciting time for acute stroke intervention. Projects are underway investigating ways to safely expand the window for reperfusion therapies, to slow the ischemic cascade and offer life-saving interventions to the most severe stroke population in whom mortality was previously thought certain. Although still imperfect, systemic reperfusion therapies offer the best chance for a meaningful recovery and emergency medicine providers should be as facile with the management of acute ischemic cerebrovascular syndromes as with any other life-threatening emergency. Endovascular therapies have revolutionized care to patients with ischemic stroke secondary to ELVO and better regionalized systems are needed to maximize the potential of this intervention to the population as a whole. The ED is the most efficient and effective place for the acute stroke patient to be managed and substantial progress has been made to expedite the diagnosis and shorten treatment times in recent years. Stroke remains a major cause of death and disability in the United States and worldwide, yet is decreasing, thanks in large part to progressive and evidence-based emergency care.

REFERENCES

1. Siket MS, Silver B. The 10-second stroke: a case report. J Stroke Cerebrovasc Dis 2015;24(6):e133–4.
2. Saver JL. Time is brain — quantified. Stroke 2006;37(1):263–6.
3. Meretoja A, Keshtkaran M, Saver JL, et al. Stroke thrombolysis: save a minute, save a day. Stroke 2014;45(4):1053–8.
4. Go AS, Mozaffarian D, Roger VL, et al. Heart disease and stroke statistics–2014 update: a report from the American Heart Association. Circulation 2014;129(3): 399–410.
5. Brandler ES, Sharma M, Sinert RH, et al. Prehospital stroke scales in urban environments: a systematic review. Neurology 2014;82(24):2241–9.
6. Purrucker JC, Hametner C, Engelbrecht A, et al. Comparison of stroke recognition and stroke severity scores for stroke detection in a single cohort. J Neurol Neurosurg Psychiatry 2015;86(9):1021–8.
7. McTaggart RA, Ansari SA, Goyal M, et al. Initial hospital management of patients with emergent large vessel occlusion (ELVO): report of the standards and guidelines committee of the Society of NeuroInterventional Surgery. J Neurointerv Surg 2015. http://dx.doi.org/10.1136/neurintsurg-2015-011984.
8. Perez de la Ossa N, Carrera D, Gorchs M, et al. Design and validation of a prehospital stroke scale to predict large arterial occlusion: the rapid arterial occlusion evaluation scale. Stroke 2014;45(1):87–91.

9. Katz BS, McMullan JT, Sucharew H, et al. Design and validation of a prehospital scale to predict stroke severity. Stroke 2015;46(6):1508–12.

10. Teleb MS, Ver Hage A, Carter J, et al. Stroke vision, aphasia, neglect (VAN) assessment-a novel emergent large vessel occlusion screening tool: pilot study and comparison with current clinical severity indices. J Neurointerv Surg 2016. http://dx.doi.org/10.1136/neurintsurg-2015-012131.

11. Harrison JK, Mcarthur KS, Quinn TJ. Assessment scales in stroke: clinimetric and clinical considerations. Clin Interv Aging 2013;8:201–11.

12. Jauch EC, Saver JL, Adams HP, et al. Guidelines for the early management of patients with acute ischemic stroke: a guideline for healthcare professionals from the American Heart Association/American Stroke Association. Stroke 2013;44(3):870–947.

13. Middleton S, McElduff P, Ward J, et al. Implementation of evidence-based treatment protocols to manage fever, hyperglycaemia, and swallowing dysfunction in acute stroke (QASC): a cluster randomised controlled trial. Lancet 2011; 378(9804):1699–706.

14. Röther J, Ford GA, Thijs VN. Thrombolytics in acute ischaemic stroke: historical perspective and future opportunities. Cerebrovasc Dis 2013;35(4):313–9.

15. Meyer JS, Gilroy J, Barnhart MI, et al. Therapeutic thrombolysis in cerebral thromboembolism. Double-blind evaluation of intravenous plasmin therapy in carotid and middle cerebral arterial occlusion. Neurology 1963;13:927–37.

16. Meyer JS, Gilroy J, Barnhart MI, et al. Anticoagulants plus streptokinase therapy in progressive stroke. JAMA 1964;189:373.

17. The Multicenter Acute Stroke Trial-Italy (MAST-I) Study Group. Randomised controlled trial of streptokinase, aspirin, and combination of both in treatment of acute ischaemic stroke. Lancet 1995;346(8989):1509–14.

18. The Multicenter Acute Stroke Trial-Europe (MAST-E) Study Group. Thrombolytic therapy with streptokinase in acute ischemic stroke. N Engl J Med 1996;18(3): 145–50.

19. The GUSTO Investigators. An international randomized trial comparing four thrombolytic strategies for acute myocardial infarction. N Engl J Med 1993; 329(10):673–82.

20. The National Institute of Neurological Disorders and Stroke rt-PA Stroke Study Group. Tissue plasminogen activator for ischemic stroke. N Engl J Med 1995; 333(24):1581–7.

21. Hacke W, Kaste M, Fieschi C, et al. Intravenous thrombolysis with recombinant tissue plasminogen activator for acute hemispheric stroke. the European Cooperative Acute Stroke Study (ECASS). JAMA 1995;274:1017–25.

22. Hoffman JR, Schriger DL. A graphic reanalysis of the NINDS Trial. Ann Emerg Med 2009;54(3):329–36.

23. Lees KR, Bluhmki E, von Kummer R, et al. Time to treatment with intravenous alteplase and outcome in stroke: an updated pooled analysis of ECASS, ATLANTIS, NINDS, and EPITHET trials. Lancet 2010;375(9727):1695–703.

24. Ingall TJ, O'Fallon WM, Asplund K, et al. Findings from the reanalysis of the NINDS tissue plasminogen activator for acute ischemic stroke treatment trial. Stroke 2004;35(10):2418–24.

25. Kwiatkowski T, Libman R, Tilley BC, et al. The impact of imbalances in baseline stroke severity on outcome in the national institute of neurological disorders and stroke recombinant tissue plasminogen activator stroke study. Ann Emerg Med 2005;45(4):377–84.

26. Hacke W, Kaste M, Fieschi C, et al. Randomised double-blind placebo-controlled trial of thrombolytic therapy with intravenous alteplase in acute ischaemic stroke (ECASS II). Second European-Australasian Acute Stroke Study Investigators. Lancet 1998;352(9136):1245–51.

27. Clark WM, Wissman S, Albers GW, et al. Recombinant tissue-type plasminogen activator (alteplase) for ischemic stroke 3 to 5 hours after symptom onset. The Atlantis study: a randomized controlled trial. alteplase thrombolysis for acute noninterventional therapy in ischemic stroke. JAMA 1999;282(21):2019–26.

28. Clark WM, Albers GW, Madden KP, et al. The rtPA (alteplase) 0- to 6-hour acute stroke trial, part A (A0276g): results of a double-blind, placebo-controlled, multi-center study. Thromblytic therapy in acute ischemic stroke study investigators. Stroke 2000;31:811–6.

29. Hacke W, Kaste M, Bluhmki E, et al. Thrombolysis with alteplase 3 to 4.5 hours after acute ischemic stroke. N Engl J Med 2008;359:1317–29.

30. Davis SM, Donnan GA, Parsons MW, et al. Effects of alteplase beyond 3 h after stroke in the Echoplanar Imaging Thrombolytic Evaluation Trial (EPITHET): a placebo-controlled randomised trial. Lancet Neurol 2008;7(4):299–309.

31. Lansberg MG, Bluhmki E, Thijs VN. Efficacy and safety of tissue plasminogen activator 3 to 4.5 hours after acute ischemic stroke: a metaanalysis. Stroke 2009;40(7):2438–41.

32. del Zoppo GJ, Saver JL, Jauch EC, et al. Expansion of the time window for treatment of acute ischemic stroke with intravenous tissue plasminogen activator. A science advisory from the American Heart Association/American Stroke Association. Stroke 2009;40:2945–8.

33. Edlow JA, Smith EE, Stead LG, et al. Clinical policy: use of intravenous tPA for the management of acute ischemic stroke in the emergency department. Ann Emerg Med 2013;61(2):225–43.

34. Sandercock P, Wardlaw JM, Lindley RI, et al. The benefits and harms of intravenous thrombolysis with recombinant tissue plasminogen activator within 6 h of acute ischaemic stroke (the third international stroke trial [IST-3]): a randomised controlled trial. Lancet 2012;379(9834):2352–63.

35. Miller JB, Heitsch L, Siket MS, et al. The emergency medicine debate on tPA for stroke: what is best for our patients? efficacy in the first three hours. Acad Emerg Med 2015;22(7):852–5.

36. Sandercock P, Wardlaw JM, Dennis M, et al. Effect of thrombolysis with alteplase within 6 h of acute ischaemic stroke on long-term outcomes (the Third International Stroke Trial [IST-3]): 18-month follow-up of a randomised controlled trial. Lancet Neurol 2013;12(8):768–76.

37. Hoffman JR, Cooper RJ. How is more negative evidence being used to support claims of benefit: the curious case of the Third International Stroke Trial (IST-3). Emerg Med Australas 2012;24(5):473–6.

38. Wardlaw JM, Murray V, Berge E, et al. Thrombolysis for acute ischaemic stroke. Cochrane Database Syst Rev 2014;(7):CD000213.

39. Jauch EC, Holmstedt C. Intravenous thrombolytic therapy for acute ischemic stroke: results of large, randomized clinical trials. In: Lyden PD, editor. Thrombolytic therapy for acute stroke. 3rd edition. (Switzerland): Springer; 2015. p. 95–111.

40. Alper BS, Malone-Moses M, McLellan JS, et al. Thrombolysis in acute ischaemic stroke: time for a rethink? BMJ 2015;350:h1075.

41. Wardlaw J, Berge E. Cochrane reviewers' response to Alper and colleagues' analysis of thrombolysis in acute ischaemic stroke. BMJ 2015;350:h1790.

42. Emberson J, Lees KR, Lyden P, et al. Effect of treatment delay, age, and stroke severity on the effects of intravenous thrombolysis with alteplase for acute ischaemic stroke: a meta-analysis of individual patient data from randomised trials. Lancet 2014;384(9958):1929–35.

43. Harris D, Hall C, Lobay K, et al. Canadian Association of Emergency Physicians position statement on acute ischemic stroke. CJEM 2015;17(2):217–26.

44. Saver JL, Fonarow GC, Smith EE, et al. Time to treatment with intravenous tissue plasminogen activator and outcome from acute ischemic stroke. JAMA 2013; 309(23):2480–8.

45. Siket MS, Baruch JM. Principles of neurologic ethics. In: Scientific American emergency medicine. Decker Intellectual Properties; 2015.

46. Ciccone A, Bonito V. Thrombolysis for acute ischemic stroke: the problem of consent. Neurol Sci 2001;22(5):339–51.

47. Chiong W, Kim AS, Huang IA, et al. Testing the presumption of consent to emergency treatment for acute ischemic stroke. JAMA 2014;311(16):1689.

48. Gadhia J, Starkman S, Ovbiagele B, et al. Assessment and improvement of figures to visually convey benefit and risk of stroke thrombolysis. Stroke 2010; 41(2):300–6.

49. Schwamm LH. Acute stroke: shifting from informed consent to informed refusal of intravenous tissue-type plasminogen activator. Circ Cardiovasc Qual Outcomes 2015;8:S69–72.

50. Decker C, Chhatriwalla E, Gialde E, et al. Qualitative study of patients ' and providers ' perspectives. Circ Cardiovasc Qual Outcomes 2015;8:S109–16.

51. Tsivgoulis G, Zand R, Katsanos AH, et al. Safety of intravenous thrombolysis in stroke mimics: prospective 5-year study and comprehensive meta-analysis. Stroke 2015;46(5):1281–7.

52. Bhatt A, Safdar A, Chaudhari D, et al. Medicolegal considerations with intravenous tissue plasminogen activator in stroke: a systematic review. Stroke Res Treat 2013;2013:562564.

53. Micieli G, Marcheselli S, Tosi PA. Safety and efficacy of alteplase in the treatment of acute ischemic stroke. Vasc Health Risk Manag 2009;5(1):397–409.

54. Niego B, Freeman R, Puschmann TB, et al. t-PA-specific modulation of a human blood-brain barrier model involves plasmin-mediated activation of the Rho kinase pathway in astrocytes. Blood 2012;119(20):4752–61.

55. Tanswell P, Modi N, Combs D, et al. Pharmacokinetics and pharmacodynamics of tenecteplase in fibrinolytic therapy of acute myocardial infarction. Clin Pharmacokinet 2002;41(15):1229–45.

56. Marshall RS. Progress in intravenous thrombolytic therapy for acute stroke. JAMA Neurol 2015;72(8):1–7.

57. O'Gara PT, Kushner FG, Ascheim DD, et al. 2013 ACCF/AHA Guideline for the management of ST-elevation myocardial infarction: a report of the American College of Cardiology Foundation/American Heart Association task force on practice guidelines. Circulation 2013;127(4):e362–425.

58. Matosevic B, Knoflach M, Werner P, et al. Fibrinogen degradation coagulopathy and bleeding complications after stroke thrombolysis. Neurology 2013;80(13): 1216–24.

59. Huang X, Moreton FC, Kalladka D, et al. Coagulation and fibrinolytic activity of tenecteplase and alteplase in acute ischemic stroke. Stroke 2015;46(12): 3543–6.

60. Parsons M, Spratt N, Bivard A, et al. A randomized trial of tenecteplase versus alteplase for acute ischemic stroke. N Engl J Med 2012;366(12):1099–107.

61. Huang X, Cheripelli BK, Lloyd SM, et al. Alteplase versus tenecteplase for thrombolysis after ischaemic stroke (ATTEST): a phase 2, randomised, open-label, blinded endpoint study. Lancet Neurol 2015;14(4):368–76.

62. Haley EC, Thompson JLP, Grotta JC, et al. Phase IIB/III trial of tenecteplase in acute ischemic stroke: results of a prematurely terminated randomized clinical trial. Stroke 2010;41(4):707–11.

63. Logallo N, Kvistad CE, Nacu A, et al. The Norwegian Tenecteplase Stroke Trial (NOR-TEST): randomised controlled trial of tenecteplase vs. alteplase in acute ischaemic stroke. BMC Neurol 2014;14(1):106.

64. Coutts SB, Dubuc V, Mandzia J, et al. Tenecteplase-tissue-type plasminogen activator evaluation for minor ischemic stroke with proven occlusion. Stroke 2015;46(3):769–74.

65. Bringmann P, Gruber D, Liese A, et al. Structural features mediating fibrin selectivity of vampire bat plasminogen activators. J Biol Chem 1995;270(43):25596–603.

66. Hacke W, Furlan AJ, Al-Rawi Y, et al. Intravenous desmoteplase in patients with acute ischaemic stroke selected by MRI perfusion-diffusion weighted imaging or perfusion CT (DIAS-2): a prospective, randomised, double-blind, placebo-controlled study. Lancet Neurol 2009;8(2):141–50.

67. Hacke W, Albers G, Al-Rawi Y, et al. The Desmoteplase in Acute Ischemic Stroke Trial (DIAS): a phase II MRI-based 9-hour window acute stroke thrombolysis trial with intravenous desmoteplase. Stroke 2005;36(1):66–73.

68. Furlan AJ, Eyding D, Albers GW, et al. Dose Escalation of Desmoteplase for Acute Ischemic Stroke (DEDAS): evidence of safety and efficacy 3 to 9 hours after stroke onset. Stroke 2006;37(5):1227–31.

69. Albers GW, von Kummer R, Truelsen T, et al. Safety and efficacy of desmoteplase given 3–9 h after ischaemic stroke in patients with occlusion or high-grade stenosis in major cerebral arteries (DIAS-3): a double-blind, randomised, placebo-controlled phase 3 trial. Lancet Neurol 2015;14(6):575–84.

70. Levine SR, Faraz KS, Piran P, et al. The march of thrombolytic therapy for acute ischemic stroke to clinical trials: pre-clinical thrombolysis and adjuncts to thrombolysis research. In: Lyden PD, editor. Thrombolytic therapy for acute stroke. 3rd edition. (Switzerland): Springer; 2015. p. 27–64.

71. Furlan A, Higashida R, Wechsler L, et al. Intra-arterial Prourokinase for Acute Ischemic Stroke: the PROACT II study: a randomized controlled trial. JAMA 1999;282(21):2003–11.

72. Nogueira RG, Schwamm LH, Hirsch JA. Endovascular approaches to acute stroke, part 1: drugs, devices, and data. AJNR Am J Neuroradiol 2009;30(4):649–61.

73. Molina CA, Saver JL. Extending reperfusion therapy for acute ischemic stroke: emerging pharmacological, mechanical, and imaging strategies. Stroke 2005;36(10):2311–20.

74. Gobin YP, Starkman S, Duckwiler GR, et al. MERCI 1: a phase 1 study of mechanical embolus removal in cerebral ischemia. Stroke 2004;35(12):2848–54.

75. Przybylowski CJ, Ding D, Starke RM, et al. Evolution of endovascular mechanical thrombectomy for acute ischemic stroke. World J Clin Cases 2014;2(11):614–22.

76. Clark W, Lutsep H, Barnwell S, et al. The penumbra pivotal stroke trial: safety and effectiveness of a new generation of mechanical devices for clot removal in intracranial large vessel occlusive disease. Stroke 2009;40(8):2761–8.

77. Ciccone A, Valvassori L, Nichelatti M, et al. Endovascular treatment for acute ischemic stroke. N Engl J Med 2013;368(10):904–13.
78. Kidwell CS, Jahan R, Gornbein J, et al. A trial of imaging selection and endovascular treatment for ischemic stroke. N Engl J Med 2013;368(10):914–23.
79. Broderick JP, Palesch YY, Demchuk AM, et al. Endovascular therapy after intravenous t-PA versus t-PA alone for stroke. N Engl J Med 2013;368(10):893–903.
80. Demchuk AM, Goyal M, Yeatts SD, et al. Recanalization and clinical outcome of occlusion sites at baseline CT angiography in the interventional management of stroke III trial. Radiology 2014;273(1):202–10.
81. Chimowitz MI. Endovascular treatment for acute ischemic stroke - still unproven. N Engl J Med 2013;368(10):952–5.
82. Nogueira RG, Lutsep HI, Gupta R, et al. Trevo versus MERCI retrievers for thrombectomy revascularisation of large vessel occlusions in acute ischaemic stroke (TREVO 2): a randomised trial. Lancet 2012;380(9849):1231–40.
83. Saver JL, Jahan R, Levy EI, et al. Solitaire flow restoration device versus the merci retriever in patients with acute ischaemic stroke (SWIFT): a randomised, parallel-group, non-inferiority trial. Lancet 2012;380(9849):1241–9.
84. Goyal M, Demchuk AM, Menon BK, et al. Randomized assessment of rapid endovascular treatment of ischemic stroke. N Engl J Med 2015;372(11):1019–30.
85. Saver JL, Goyal M, Bonafe A, et al. Stent-retriever thrombectomy after intravenous t-PA vs. t-PA alone in stroke. N Engl J Med 2015;372(24):2285–95.
86. Khatri P, Hacke W, Fiehler J, et al. State of acute endovascular therapy: report from the 12th thrombolysis, thrombectomy, and acute stroke therapy conference. Stroke 2015;46(6):1727–34.
87. Berkherner OA, Fransen PS, Beumer D, et al. A randomized trial of intraarterial treatment for acute ischemic stroke. N Engl J Med 2015;372(1):11–20.
88. Jovin TG, Chamorro A, Cobo E, et al. Thrombectomy within 8 hours after symptom onset in ischemic stroke. N Engl J Med 2015;372(24):2296–306.
89. Campbell BC, Mitchell PJ, Kleinig TJ, et al. Endovascular therapy for ischemic stroke with perfusion-imaging selection. N Engl J Med 2015;372(11):1009–18.
90. Smith EE, Schwamm LH. Endovascular clot retrieval therapy: implications for the organization of stroke systems of care in North America. Stroke 2015;46(6):1462–7.
91. Menon BK, Campbell BC, Levi C, et al. Role of imaging in current acute ischemic stroke workflow for endovascular therapy. Stroke 2015;46(6):1453–61.
92. Powers WJ, Derdeyn CP, Biller J, et al. 2015 AHA/ASA focused update of the 2013 guidelines for the early management of patients with acute ischemic stroke regarding endovascular treatment. Stroke 2015;46(10):3020–35.
93. Jayaraman MV, Hussain MS, Abruzzo T, et al. Embolectomy for stroke with emergent large vessel occlusion (ELVO): report of the standards and guidelines committee of the society of neurointerventional surgery. J Neurointerv Surg 2015;7(5):316–21.
94. John S, Stock S, Masaryk T, et al. Performance of CT angiography on a mobile stroke treatment unit: implications for triage. J Neuroimaging 2016;26(4):391–4.
95. Demel SL, Broderick JP. Basilar occlusion syndromes: an update. Neurohospitalist 2015;5(3):142–50.
96. Schonewille WJ, Wijman CA, Michel P, et al. Treatment and outcomes of acute basilar artery occlusion in the basilar artery international cooperation study (BASICS): a prospective registry study. Lancet Neurol 2009;8(8):724–30.
97. Yeung JT, Matouk CC, Bulsara KR, et al. Endovascular revascularization for basilar artery occlusion. Interv Neurol 2015;3(1):31–40.

98. Vergouwen MDI, Algra A, Pfefferkorn T, et al. Time is brain(stem) in basilar artery occlusion. Stroke 2012;43(11):3003–6.
99. Lindsberg PJ, Mattle HP. Therapy of basilar artery occlusion: a systematic analysis comparing intra-arterial and intravenous thrombolysis. Stroke 2006;37(3): 922–8.
100. Singer OC, Berkefeld J, Nolte CH, et al. Mechanical recanalization in basilar artery occlusion: the ENDOSTROKE study. Ann Neurol 2015;77(3):415–24.
101. Edlow JA, Selim MH. Atypical presentations of acute cerebrovascular syndromes. Lancet Neurol 2011;10(6):550–60.
102. Costa R, Pinho J, Alves JN, et al. Wake-up stroke and stroke within the therapeutic window for thrombolysis have similar clinical severity, imaging characteristics, and outcome. J Stroke Cerebrovasc Dis 2016;25(3):511–4.
103. Fink JN, Kumar S, Horkan C, et al. The stroke patient who woke up: clinical and radiological features, including diffusion and perfusion MRI. Stroke 2002;33(4): 988–93.
104. Song SS, Latour LL, Ritter CH, et al. A pragmatic approach using magnetic resonance imaging to treat ischemic strokes of unknown onset time in a thrombolytic trial. Stroke 2012;43(9):2331–5.
105. Marks MP, Lansberg MG, Mlynash M, et al. Angiographic outcome of endovascular stroke therapy correlated with MR findings, infarct growth, and clinical outcome in the DEFUSE 2 trial. Int J Stroke 2014;9(7):860–5.
106. Fink JN, Selim MH, Kumar S, et al. Why are stroke patients excluded from tPA therapy? An analysis of patient eligibility. Neurology 2001;57(9):1739–40.
107. Kleindorfer D, Kissela B, Schneider A, et al. Eligibility for recombinant tissue plasminogen activator in acute ischemic stroke: a population-based study. Stroke 2004;35(2):e27–9.
108. Adams HP, del Zoppo G, Alberts MJ, et al. Guidelines for the early management of adults with ischemic stroke: a guideline from the American Heart Association/ American Stroke Association stroke council, clinical cardiology council, cardiovascular radiology and intervention council, and the atheros. Stroke 2007;38(5): 1655–711.
109. Fischer U, Baumgartner A, Arnold M, et al. What is a minor stroke? Stroke 2010; 41(4):661–6.
110. Nesi M, Lucente G, Nencini P, et al. Aphasia predicts unfavorable outcome in mild ischemic stroke patients and prompts thrombolytic treatment. J Stroke Cerebrovasc Dis 2014;23(2):204–8.
111. Khatri P, Conaway MR, Johnston KC, et al. Ninety-day outcome rates of a prospective cohort of sonsecutive patients with mild ischemic stroke. Stroke 2012; 43(2):560–2.
112. Hills NK, Johnston SC. Why are eligible thrombolysis candidates left untreated? Am J Prev Med 2006;31(6 Suppl 2):S210–6.
113. van den Berg JS, de Jong G. Why ischemic stroke patients do not receive thrombolytic treatment: results from a general hospital. Acta Neurol Scand 2009;120(3):157–60.
114. Smith EE, Abdullah AR, Petkovska I, et al. Poor outcomes in patients who do not receive intravenous tissue plasminogen activator because of mild or improving ischemic stroke. Stroke 2005;36(11):2497–9.
115. del Zoppo GJ, Poeck K, Pessin MS, et al. Recombinant tissue plasminogen activator in acute thrombotic and embolic stroke. Ann Neurol 1992;32(1):78–86.
116. Kohrmann M, Nowe T, Huttner HB, et al. Safety and outcome after thrombolysis in stroke patients with mild symptoms. Cerebrovasc Dis 2009;27(2):160–6.

117. The National Institute of Neurological Disorders Stroke rt-PA Stroke Study Group. Recombinant tissue plasminogen activator for minor strokes: the national institute of neurological disorders and stroke rt-PA stroke study experience. Ann Emerg Med 2005;46(3):243–52.

118. Wendt M, Tütüncü S, Fiebach JB, et al. Preclusion of ischemic stroke patients from intravenous tissue plasminogen activator treatment for mild symptoms should not be based on low National Institutes of Health Stroke Scale scores. J Stroke Cerebrovasc Dis 2013;22(4):550–3.

119. Hassan AE, Zacharatos H, Hassanzadeh B, et al. Does mild deficit for patients with stroke justify the use of intravenous tissue plasminogen activator? J Stroke Cerebrovasc Dis 2010;19(2):116–20.

120. Khatri P, Kleindorfer DO, Yeatts SD, et al. Strokes with minor symptoms: an exploratory analysis of the national institute of neurological disorders and stroke recombinant tissue plasminogen activator trials. Stroke 2010;41(11):2581–6.

121. Romano JG, Smith EE, Liang L, et al. Outcomes in mild acute ischemic stroke treated with intravenous thrombolysis a retrospective analysis of the get with the guidelines–stroke registry. JAMA Neurol 2015;72(4):423–31.

122. Khatri P, Tayama D, Cohen G, et al. Effect of intravenous recombinant tissue-type plasminogen activator in patients with mild stroke in the third international stroke trial-3. Stroke 2015;46(8):2325–7.

123. Fisher M, Saver JL. Future directions of acute ischaemic stroke therapy. Lancet Neurol 2015;14(7):758–67.

124. Han Z, Liu X, Luo Y, et al. Therapeutic hypothermia for stroke: where to go? Exp Neurol 2015;272:67–77.

125. Wu T-C, Grotta JC. Hypothermia for acute ischaemic stroke. Lancet Neurol 2013;12(3):275–84.

126. Saver JL, Starkman S, Eckstein M, et al. Prehospital use of magnesium sulfate as neuroprotection in acute stroke. N Engl J Med 2015;372(6):528–36.

127. Li R, Huang C, Chen J, et al. The role of uric acid as a potential neuroprotectant in acute ischemic stroke: a review of literature. Neurol Sci 2015;36(7):1097–103.

128. Llull L, Amaro S, Chamorro Á. Administration of uric acid in the emergency treatment of acute ischemic stroke. Curr Neurol Neurosci Rep 2016;16(1):4.

129. Chamorro A, Amaro S, Castellanos M, et al. Safety and efficacy of uric acid in patients with acute stroke (URICO-ICTUS): a randomised, double-blind phase 2b/3 trial. Lancet Neurol 2014;13(5):453–60.

130. Nacu A, Kvistad CE, Logallo N, et al. A pragmatic approach to sonothrombolysis in acute ischaemic stroke: the Norwegian randomised controlled sonothrombolysis in acute stroke study (NOR-SASS). BMC Neurol 2015;15:110.

131. Tsivgoulis G, Katsanos AH, Alexandrov AV. Reperfusion therapies of acute ischemic stroke: potentials and failures. Front Neurol 2014;5:215.

132. Alexandrov AV, Molina CA, Grotta JC, et al. Ultrasound-enhanced systemic thrombolysis for acute ischemic stroke. N Engl J Med 2004;351(21):2170–8.

133. Barreto AD, Alexandrov AV, Shen L, et al. CLOTBUST-hands free: pilot safety study of a novel operator-independent ultrasound device in patients with acute ischemic stroke. Stroke 2013;44(12):3376–81.

134. Saqqur M, Tsivgoulis G, Nicoli F, et al. The role of sonolysis and sonothrombolysis in acute ischemic stroke: a systematic review and meta-analysis of randomized controlled trials and case-control studies. J Neuroimaging 2014;24(3):209–20.

135. Tsivgoulis G, Eggers J, Ribo M, et al. Safety and efficacy of ultrasound-enhanced thrombolysis: a comprehensive review and meta-analysis of randomized and nonrandomized studies. Stroke 2010;41(2):280–7.
136. Ricci S, Dinia L, Del Sette M, et al. Sonothrombolysis for acute ischaemic stroke. Cochrane Database Syst Rev 2012;(10):CD008348.
137. Molina CA, Barreto AD, Tsivgoulis G, et al. Transcranial ultrasound in clinical sonothrombolysis (TUCSON) trial. Ann Neurol 2009;66(1):28–38.
138. Zhou Y, Ramaswami R. Comparison of sonothrombolysis efficiencies of different ultrasound systems. J Stroke Cerebrovasc Dis 2014;23(10):2730–5.
139. Wang Y, Wang Y, Zhao X, et al. Clopidogrel with aspirin in acute minor stroke or transient ischemic attack. N Engl J Med 2013;369(1):11–9.

Diagnosis and Management of Acute Intracerebral Hemorrhage

Andrea Morotti, MD[a], Joshua N. Goldstein, MD, PhD[a,b],*

KEYWORDS

- Intracerebral hemorrhage • Hemorrhagic stroke • Neurocritical care
- Blood pressure • Coagulopathy • Hematoma expansion

KEY POINTS

- Intracerebral hemorrhage (ICH) is a dynamic disease and up to one-third of the patients experience early clinical deterioration caused by hematoma expansion.
- Intensive blood pressure reduction is safe and might improve neurologic outcome.
- Rapid correction of coagulopathy may minimize the risk of ongoing bleeding.
- Surgical evacuation of the hematoma should be considered for patients with clinical deterioration caused by cerebellar ICH.
- Patients with ICH should be admitted to a neuroscience intensive care unit or stroke unit.

INTRODUCTION AND EPIDEMIOLOGY

Intracerebral hemorrhage (ICH) refers to primary, spontaneous, nontraumatic bleeding occurring in the brain parenchyma. ICH accounts for 10% to 20% of all cerebrovascular events in the United States[1] and is the deadliest type of stroke, with 30-day mortality up to 40% and severe disability in most survivors.[2] Older age, hypertension, cerebral amyloid angiopathy (CAA), and oral anticoagulant treatment (OAT) are the most important risk factors for ICH.[1,3,4] Other ICH risk factors are summarized in **Box 1**.

PATHOPHYSIOLOGY

ICH represents an acute manifestation of an underlying progressive small vessel disease. Primary brain damage in the acute phase of ICH is caused by mechanical

---

Funding Sources: NINDS award 5R01NS073344.

Conflicts of Interest: None.

[a] J. P. Kistler Stroke Research Center, Massachusetts General Hospital, Harvard Medical School, 175 Cambridge Street, Suite 300, Boston, MA 02114, USA; [b] Department of Emergency Medicine, Massachusetts General Hospital, Harvard Medical School, Zero Emerson Place, Suite 3B, Boston, MA 02114, USA

* Corresponding author.

E-mail address: jgoldstein@partners.org

Emerg Med Clin N Am 34 (2016) 883–899

http://dx.doi.org/10.1016/j.emc.2016.06.010
emed.theclinics.com

Box 1
Risk factors for ICH

- Hypertension is the most important modifiable risk factor for ICH.[1] Poor control of blood pressure values is also associated with increased risk of recurrent ICH.[85]

- CAA accounts for up to 20% of all spontaneous ICH cases.[4] CAA-related bleeding typically arises from corticosubcortical brain regions and frequently affects elderly patients.[4]

- Alcohol intake: this relationship seems to be dose dependent.[1]

- Smoking: current smoking increases the risk of ICH.[1,3]

- Cholesterol levels and statin use: in contrast with ischemic stroke, hypercholesterolemia has a protective effect against the risk of ICH.[1] The association between statins and ICH risk is still unclear.[86]

- Diabetes: a meta-analysis including almost 70.000 subjects provided evidence in favor of diabetes as a risk factor for ICH.[87]

- Genetics: the gene most strongly associated with ICH is the apolipoprotein E (APOE) gene and its ε2 and ε4 alleles.[1]

- Ethnicity: ICH incidence is higher in Asian populations.[1,2]

- Drug abuse: illicit drug consumption, such as cocaine and methamphetamine, is an important risk factor for ICH, especially in young adults.[88]

---

mass effect of the hematoma, leading to increased intracranial pressure (ICP) and consequent reduced cerebral perfusion and possible herniation.[5] Intraventricular extension of the hemorrhage (intraventricular hemorrhage [IVH]) occurs in up to 40% of ICH cases and is another important determinant of clinical deterioration and an independent predictor of mortality.[6]

CLINICAL PRESENTATION AND DIAGNOSIS

The clinical presentations of ICH and ischemic stroke are similar, typically consisting of abrupt onset of a focal neurologic deficit. Decreased level of consciousness, vomiting, headache, seizures, and very high blood pressure (BP) might suggest the presence of ICH. However, none of these symptoms/signs is specific enough to distinguish hemorrhagic from ischemic stroke and therefore the diagnosis of ICH must always rely on neuroimaging.[7] A significant proportion of patients with ICH manifest a loss of at least 2 points on the Glasgow Coma Scale (GCS) during acute evaluation[7] and coma can be the presenting symptom of posterior fossa hemorrhages.[5]

Clinical Assessment

Vital signs measurement and general physical examination should be performed in all patients. The American Heart Association (AHA) and American Stroke Association (ASA) recommend routine application of a neurologic baseline severity score, and the National Institutes of Health Stroke Scale score seems to be useful in patients with ICH.[7] The GCS is a widely known, rapid, and reproducible tool for consciousness evaluation. The ICH score is a reliable and validated scale for rapid assessment of ICH severity.[8]

Blood Tests

In patients with ICH, complete blood count, electrolytes and creatinine, glucose, and coagulation studies should be obtained.

Neuroimaging

Noncontrast computed tomography

Noncontrast computed tomography (NCCT) is a fast technique with excellent sensitivity for identifying acute ICH, and given its wide availability is considered the gold standard for the diagnosis of ICH in the emergency department (ED).[7,9] Beyond the diagnosis of ICH, NCCT can provide useful elements such as ICH location, intraventricular extension, hydrocephalus, presence and degree of edema, and midline shift or brainstem compression secondary to the mass effect from the hematoma. Furthermore, ICH volume is a strong predictor of ICH outcome[10] and can be rapidly estimated in the ED with the ABC/2 technique (**Fig. 1**).

Computed tomography angiography

Computed tomography angiography (CTA) is a useful diagnostic tool in the acute setting of ICH.[11] It is the most widely available noninvasive technique for the detection of vascular abnormalities as secondary causes of ICH. The presence of lobar ICH, significant IVH, young age, and absence of traditional cerebrovascular risk factors should trigger the suspicion of ICH secondary to vascular malformation or other intracranial disorder.[7,11] Prompt detection of these lesions is crucial and has a significant impact on patient management. Although CTA is an excellent noninvasive screening tool, digital subtraction angiography remains the gold standard investigation for diagnosis, and frequently endovascular treatment, of cerebral vascular malformations.[9]

Presence of contrast extravasation within the hematoma on CTA images, also termed spot sign, is an independent predictor of hematoma expansion and poor outcome in patients with supratentorial ICH[12,13] (**Fig. 2**). Furthermore, CTA spot sign is associated with active bleeding during surgical evacuation, and may help indicate which patients may benefit from surgery.[14] The main drawback of CTA is cost and the additional radiation exposure.[11] Although some clinicians are concerned about the risk of contrast-induced nephropathy, there is debate in the literature about whether this entity exists, and there is no evidence that CTA increases the risk of nephropathy in patients with ICH.[15–17]

MRI

MRI sensitivity for the diagnosis of ICH is equivalent to that of NCCT. MRI can be a useful technique to detect underlying secondary causes of ICH, such as neoplastic

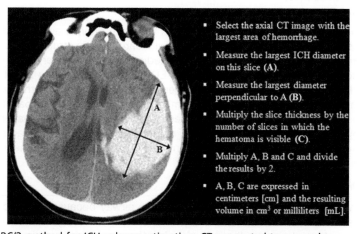

- Select the axial CT image with the largest area of hemorrhage.
- Measure the largest ICH diameter on this slice (**A**).
- Measure the largest diameter perpendicular to A (**B**).
- Multiply the slice thickness by the number of slices in which the hematoma is visible (**C**).
- Multiply A, B and C and divide the results by 2.
- A, B, C are expressed in centimeters [cm] and the resulting volume in cm³ or milliliters [mL].

Fig. 1. ABC/2 method for ICH volume estimation. CT, computed tomography.

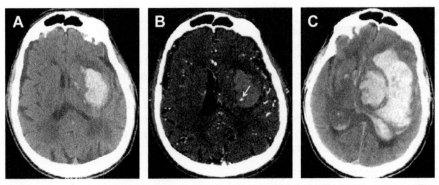

Fig. 2. Spot sign and hematoma expansion. (*A*) Left deep ICH on NCCT, with baseline volume of 45 mL; (*B*) CTA showing presence of spot sign (*arrow*); (*C*) follow-up NCCT at 19 hours showed significant hematoma growth to a volume of 192 mL with severe midline shift and massive intraventricular extension.

lesions or hemorrhagic transformation of ischemic stroke.[9] In addition, in patients with poor kidney function, contrast allergies, or other contraindications to CTA, brain vessel imaging can be achieved without contrast through magnetic resonance angiography. Given the cost, duration of the examination, and poor tolerability for some patients, MRI is rarely used in the ED work-up of ICH.[7]

Natural History and Clinical Evolution

Even though ICH was traditionally viewed as a monophasic disease, growing evidence suggests that ICH is a dynamic disease, characterized by early significant expansion in up to one-third of patients.[18] Early imaging after symptom onset, large baseline hematoma volume, anticoagulant therapy, and presence of CTA spot sign are consistently the most powerful predictors of significant hematoma growth.[13] Other factors associated with clinical deterioration include perihematomal edema, intraventricular extension of the ICH, hydrocephalus, seizures, fever, and infections.[19]

ACUTE MANAGEMENT
Prehospital Care

The main goal of prehospital management of ICH is to provide airway and cardiovascular support to unstable patients, along with careful reconstruction of symptom onset timing, medical history, and current medications.[7] Moreover, early notification reduces the time to NCCT scan in the ED and therefore allows a faster diagnosis of ICH.[7] Mobile stroke units have been developed to reduce the time from symptom onset to intravenous (IV) thrombolysis administration in patients with ischemic stroke.[20] This approach also seems potentially useful for patients with ICH, allowing the possibility of early BP management, reversal of coagulopathy, and delivery of patients to tertiary care centers with neurosurgical and neurocritical care facilities.[21]

Airway Protection

Patients with ICH are often unable to protect the airway because of reduced consciousness. Endotracheal intubation may therefore be necessary, but this decision should be balanced against the risk of losing the neurologic examination. Rapid sequence intubation is typically the preferred approach in the acute setting. Pretreatment with lidocaine may be preferred because it may blunt an increase in ICP associated with intubation.[22]

Blood Pressure Management

Most patients with ICH present with increased BP in the acute phase. BP increase is associated with higher risk of hematoma growth and poor outcome[5] and is therefore an appealing target for ICH treatment. The most robust data on BP management come from the INTERACT2 (Intensive Blood Pressure Reduction in Acute Cerebral Hemorrhage Trial 2) study, a large clinical trial randomizing patients to one of 2 different BP control strategies (systolic BP [SBP] <140 mm Hg vs SBP <180 mm Hg for the first 24 hours). The study failed to meet its primary end point, and did not definitively show improved outcome with intensive BP treatment (SBP target <140 mm Hg).[23] However, intensive BP reduction seemed safe, and numerous secondary measures of outcome seemed to be superior with the intensive strategy. As a result, some clinicians argue that the weight of evidence is now in favor of maintaining SBP less than 140 mm Hg in the acute phase. However, this study had numerous limitations, including the disproportionate inclusion of patients with small ICH, difficulty achieving target BP quickly, and the use of a heterogeneous range of pharmacologic agents.[24,25] The current AHA/ASA guidelines indicate that intensive BP treatment is safe and might be associated with better outcome in patients presenting with SBP between 150 and 220 mm Hg. Increased BP should be treated with agents with short half-lives, such as labetalol or nicardipine, to avoid overshoot hypotension. Hydralazine and nitroprusside should be avoided given their possible association with increased ICP.[24]

Hemostatic Treatment

Platelet function

The utility and safety of platelet transfusion in patients with ICH taking antiplatelet medications remains unclarified and there is not enough evidence to support routine application of a reversal strategy to improve platelet function.[7] Platelet transfusion is indicated in patients with severe thrombocytopenia, with suggested thresholds between 50,000 and 100,000 platelets per microliter.[26,27]

Warfarin-associated coagulopathy

OAT is associated with higher baseline ICH volume, increased risk of hematoma expansion, and poor outcome.[28] Coagulopathy correction is designed to prevent continued bleeding. Warfarin discontinuation and IV administration of vitamin K are the first therapeutic steps. Vitamin K should be infused slowly (over 10 minutes), at a dose of 10 mg with close monitoring of vital signs given the rare but not negligible risk of anaphylaxis (1 in 10,000).[28] Given its slow onset of action (6–24 hours), emergent factor repletion is typically also provided. Fresh frozen plasma (FFP) and prothrombin complex concentrates (PCCs) are commonly used. According to the AHA/ASA guidelines, PCCs may be preferred to FFP because of more rapid action.[7] Two randomized controlled trials of PCC versus FFP showed that PCCs restore coagulation factors and reverse the International Normalized Ratio (INR) more rapidly than FFP, with no clear difference in thromboembolic risk.[29–31] Although these trials failed to show improved clinical outcome in patients with ICH, some observational studies have suggested improved outcome from more rapid INR reversal.[32–34] The optimal INR target is still debated and proposed target values range from 1.3 to 1.5.[35,36] Although it is not clear whether INR values less than 1.7 represent clinically

Table 1
Comparison between FFP and PCCs for warfarin reversal in ICH

FFP	PCCs
• Low cost and widely available	• More expensive than FFP
• Contains all coagulation factors	• Three-factor PCCs: contain factors II, IX, X, with small amounts of factor VII
• Large-volume infusion is required	
• Prolonged time to infuse in routine clinical practice	• Four-factor PCCs: contain factors II, VII, IX, X, and small amounts of proteins C and S
• Contents of vitamin K–dependent factors in each unit of FFP can vary considerably	• Can be rapidly infused (<20 min) with small volumes
• Compatibility testing and thawing are necessary	• Small risk of allergic reaction
• Small risk of allergic reaction	• Small risk of infectious agent transmission
• Small risks of infectious agent transmission	
• Small risk of transfusion-related acute lung injury	

relevant coagulation abnormalities, 1 observational study found that achievement of an INR value less than 1.3 within 4 hours from admission was associated with reduced risk of hematoma expansion.[37] The European Stroke Organization guidelines do not provide a specific recommendation about the warfarin reversal strategy,[38] whereas the Neurocritical Care Society recommends warfarin reversal with either PCCs or FFP with a target INR less than 1.5.[39] Characteristics of FFP and PCCs and 1 reasonable reversal strategy for warfarin-associated ICH are shown in **Table 1** and **Box 2**.

Heparin-associated coagulopathy
If ICH occurs during IV heparin or low-molecular-weight heparin treatment, protamine sulfate administration can be used for coagulopathy reversal, at the dose of 1 mg per 100 units of heparin.[7,28] The maximum dose should be 50 mg and the infusion must be slow (maximum infusion speed: 5 mg/min) with vital signs monitoring given the significant risk of hypotension.[28]

Direct oral anticoagulants
Alternatives to warfarin are now available, and the most commonly used are the factor Xa inhibitors apixaban, rivaroxaban, and edoxaban, and the direct thrombin inhibitor dabigatran.[40] These agents were traditionally termed novel oral anticoagulants but

Box 2
Reversal strategy for warfarin-associated ICH

- Discontinue warfarin treatment

- Obtain complete blood count and INR

- Administer 10 mg of vitamin K intravenously (infuse over 10 minutes)

- Administer 4-factor PCC in weight-based and INR-based dosing:
  ○ PCC: 20 IU/kg if INR less than 2.0
  ○ PCC: 30 IU/kg if INR 2.0 to 3.0
  ○ PCC: 50 IU/kg if INR greater than 3.0

- If PCCs are not available or desired, administer FFP 10 to 20 mL/kg

- Repeat INR after infusion

the International Society of Thrombosis and Hemostasis has recommended the term direct oral anticoagulants (DOACs); this article uses this new terminology.[41] Unlike warfarin, there is no specific commercially available laboratory test to assess level of DOAC function; however, some traditional and novel blood tests may assist clinical providers in estimation of anticoagulant effect. These tests are listed in **Table 2**. Compared with warfarin, DOACs have shorter half-lives and their blood concentrations typically follow a peak-trough format.[42] Therefore, timing of last intake and renal function should always take into consideration whether the patient is still, at the time of presentation, coagulopathic.[43,44] Current evidence for DOACs reversal is limited and comes from in-vitro and animal models or studies on healthy volunteers.[45] For

Table 2
Effect of DOACs on blood tests

	Dabigatran	Rivaroxaban	Apixaban	Edoxaban
aPTT	• Abnormal only at moderate/high levels of drug. • Provides only qualitative indication	• Low sensitivity • Possible paradoxic response	• Low sensitivity • Possible paradoxic response	• Low sensitivity
PT/INR	• High interindividual variability • Mild effect (INR 0.9–1.2)	• Provides qualitative indication only with specific reagents	• Unaffected	• Linear dose-dependent association but low sensitivity at lower therapeutic drug levels
dTT	• Already prolonged at low drug concentration • Normal dTT can rule out anticoagulant activity • Needs calibration	—	—	—
ECT	• Sensitive indicator • Not widely available • Time consuming	—	—	—
Anti-Xa activity	—	• Sensitive indicator • Normal value rules out anticoagulant activity • Not widely available • Needs calibration	• Sensitive indicator • Normal value rules out anticoagulant activity • Not widely available • Needs calibration	• Sensitive indicator • Normal value rules out anticoagulant activity • Not widely available • Needs calibration
Specific test system	Hemoclot: dabigatran-calibrated dTT	Rivaroxaban-calibrated anti-Xa activity	Apixaban-calibrated anti-Xa activity	Edoxaban-calibrated anti-Xa activity

Abbreviations: aPTT, activated partial thromboplastin time; dTT, diluted thrombin time; ECT, ecarin clotting time; PT, prothrombin time.
Data from Refs.[79–81]

dabigatran reversal, a specific antagonist is now available that addresses coagulopathy but has not yet been shown to reduce expansion.[46,47] For reversal of other agents, it may be that no currently available product is effective for this purpose, although more specific reversal agents are under investigation (ClinicalTrials.gov identifiers NCT02329327 and NCT02220725). Patients taking DOACs are not deficient in vitamin K–dependent factors, so vitamin K administration is not likely to be of value. Some authorities use activated PCCs for this purpose, to provide excess coagulation factor activity.[48–51] Activated charcoal can be considered if administered within 2 to 3 hours from the last drug intake.[42,48,49]

Recombinant tissue plasminogen activator–associated coagulopathy

Symptomatic ICH (sICH) is the most dangerous complication of recombinant tissue plasminogen activator (rtPA) administration in patients with ischemic stroke, occurring in about 6% of patients and leading to increased morbidity and mortality.[52] Older age, stroke severity, longer time from onset to treatment, prestroke antiplatelet therapy, and significant increase of BP are among the most important predictors of sICH.[53] Preventive strategies include strict control of BP (target 180/105 mm Hg), and avoidance of any antithrombotic medication in the first 24 hours following the infusion of rtPA.[52] However, once ICH occurs, it is unclear how best to treat it. Given the short half-life of rtPA, by the time sICH is diagnosed, the agent may no longer be present at meaningful levels. As a result, there is great heterogeneity in clinical practice.[52,54] One concern is that rtPA can induce a relative hypofibrinogenemia that is present long after rtPA, and, if so, this can be treated. As a result, the AHA/ASA guidelines recommend immediate discontinuation of rtPA and administration of cryoprecipitate.[55] The optimal dosage of cryoprecipitate is unclear and some clinicians suggest empiric treatment with 10 U of cryoprecipitate, followed by further administration until normalization of fibrinogen level.[56] Other options can include the antifibrinolytic aminocaproic acid (Amicar) as a 5-g IV bolus over 15 to 30 minutes. Although other therapeutic approaches, including vitamin K, FFP, PCC, platelet transfusion, or recombinant activated factor VII, have been used, there is no clear biological reason or evidence to support them.[52] In addition, decompressive craniotomy or surgical hematoma evacuation may be considered for large hemorrhages with severe mass effect and intracranial hypertension.[52,55]

Intracranial Pressure Management

The most common causes of increased ICP in patients with ICH are mass effect from the hematoma and surrounding edema and IVH with secondary hydrocephalus. The indications for ICP monitoring in ICH are mainly derived from traumatic brain injury studies. Current AHA/ASA guidelines suggest ICP monitoring in patients with coma, significant IVH with hydrocephalus, and evidence of transtentorial herniation, with a cerebral perfusion pressure target of 50 to 70 mm Hg.[7] ICP can be measured with parenchymal or ventricular devices. The latter (an external ventricular drain [EVD]) might be preferred in hydrocephalus because it allows cerebrospinal fluid (CSF) drainage. Elevation of the head to 30°, adequate sedation, and avoidance of hyponatremia are mainstays of therapy; hyperosmolar therapy with mannitol or hypertonic saline can be considered in patients at risk of transtentorial herniation.[7]

Seizures and Antiepileptic Treatment

Up to 14% of patients with ICH experience seizures in the early course of the disease.[57] The main risk factors for development of early seizures are cortical location of the ICH and occurrence of medical complications.[57,58] However, it is not clear that prophylactic antiepileptic (antiepileptic drug [AED]) therapy provides benefit to patients, and some data suggest that phenytoin may worsen outcomes in this population.[59] Therefore, prophylactic administration of AED therapy is not recommended and only patients with clinical or electroencephalography (EEG) evidence of seizures should receive antiepileptic drugs.[7] Continuous EEG monitoring should be considered in patients with impaired mental status that is disproportionate to the degree of brain damage.[7]

Blood Glucose Management

Hyperglycemia has been shown to be associated with poor outcome in ICH[60] and declining values of glucose seem to be associated with lower risk of hematoma expansion.[61] Some data suggest that careful glucose control (with sliding-scale insulin) may improve neurologic outcome.[62] However, it is not clear that continuous insulin infusion improves outcomes in this population.[63,64] The AHA/ASA guidelines suggest the avoidance of both hyperglycemia and hypoglycemia, although a specific blood glucose target level is not provided.[7]

Temperature Management

The presence of fever is a common finding in patients with ICH, especially in those with extensive IVH, and seems to be independently associated with poor outcome.[62] Treatment of fever therefore seems reasonable but the optimal temperature management is still unclear.[7] Therapeutic normothermia failed to improve outcome in 1 trial,[65] although treatment of fever did improve outcome in another.[62] It seems reasonable to minimize fever, and the role of targeted temperature management in ICH is still under investigation in a randomized clinical trial.[66]

Surgical Treatment

Intraventricular hemorrhage management

IVH occurs in nearly half of patients with ICH, particularly in those with deep hematomas, and is an independent predictor of poor outcome.[6] EVD placement is recommended for patients with hydrocephalus, coma, and significant IVH, in order to drain blood and CSF and avoid significant increase of ICP.[7] Several other approaches have been proposed for IVH treatment.[67] A recent meta-analysis showed that EVD placement in conjunction with thrombolytic drugs is associated with reduced mortality and better outcomes.[68] However, intraventricular fibrinolysis for IVH treatment is still considered investigational[7] and further insights will be provided by the ongoing CLEAR III (Clot Lysis Evaluation of Accelerated Resolution of Intraventricular Hemorrhage III) trial.[69]

Surgical hematoma evacuation

Two large randomized controlled trials, the Surgical Trial in Intracerebral Haemorrhage (STICH) I and STICH II trials, investigated the role of surgical hematoma evacuation, compared with conservative treatment in patients with supratentorial ICH.[70,71] Neither trial showed a statistically significant benefit of surgery compared with best medical management. As a result, the role of surgical therapy remains controversial and surgical evacuation of supratentorial hematomas should be considered only as a lifesaving measure in deteriorating patients.[7] The only condition in which there is consensus in favor of surgical intervention is in cerebellar hematomas with clinical or imaging signs of hydrocephalus and/or brainstem compression.[7] In these cases, surgical decompression and hematoma evacuation should probably be performed as soon as possible.

Decompressive craniotomy with or without hematoma evacuation

Decompressive craniotomy seems an appropriate and safe procedure and may be associated with better outcome in a subset of patients with supratentorial ICH.[72,73] This subset includes those with coma, large hematoma with significant midline shift, or increased ICP not controlled by optimal medical therapy.[7]

Minimally invasive surgery

Although open surgical evacuation has failed to definitively show benefit, it may be that minimally invasive surgery (MIS) can still offer benefit. The development of less invasive techniques might allow hematoma evacuation with less damage to viable brain tissue and reduce the rate of secondary complications compared with traditional craniotomy.[67,74] Another potential advantage of MIS compared with conventional surgery is faster access to the hematoma, with reduction of surgical and anesthesia duration in patients with clinical deterioration and increased ICP.[75] Several MIS techniques have been proposed, ranging from endoscopic treatment of IVH to parenchymal hematoma evacuation with or without combined administration of rtPA.[74,75] The clinical efficacy of all these MIS approaches is still uncertain and clinical trials are ongoing.

ADMISSION TO STROKE UNIT OR NEUROSCIENCE INTENSIVE CARE UNIT

Following diagnosis of ICH, patients should be admitted to a dedicated stroke or neuroscience intensive care unit. Management of ICH in a dedicated stroke unit is associated with reduced mortality and better functional outcome compared with treatment in a general neurology ward.[76]

PROGNOSIS PREDICTION

Despite progress in primary prevention and acute treatment, ICH is still a disease with high morbidity and mortality. Outcome estimation, palliative care, and withdrawal of support are therefore important aspects of care in patients with ICH. The ICH score predicts 1-month mortality risk, whereas the FUNC score predicts 3-month functional independence (**Tables 3** and **4**).[8,77] However, none of these tools should be used as a singular indicator of outcome or guide the decision of medical support withdrawal.[7] Early limitation of care is an independent predictor of poor prognosis[78] and the AHA/ASA guidelines recommend full medical support for all patients with ICH at least until the second day of admission, apart from those with preexisting specific directives.[7]

FUTURE PERSPECTIVES

Acute treatment of ICH is an active area of research. Hematoma expansion is an appealing target and identification of patients with the higher likelihood to benefit from antiexpansion therapy will be an important challenge. Aggressive BP treatment, hemostatic therapy, neuroprotection, reduction of secondary injury and perihematomal edema development, and MIS are some of the therapeutic strategies under investigation. Some ongoing clinical trials in acute ICH management are listed in **Table 5**.

Table 3
ICH score for prediction of 30-day mortality

Component	ICH Score
GCS	
3–4	2
5–12	1
13–15	0
ICH Volume (mL)	
≥30	1
<30	0
IVH Presence	
Yes	1
No	0
Infratentorial ICH	
Yes	1
No	0
Age (y)	
≥80	1
<80	0
Total score	0–6

The mortality increases linearly with the ICH score. A total score of 3 is associated with a 30-day fatality rate around 70%. A total score greater than or equal to 4 confers a 30-day mortality risk close to 100%.

Table 4
FUNC score for prediction of 90-day functional independence

Component	FUNC Score
GCS	
≥9	2
3–8	0
ICH Volume (mL)	
<30	4
30–60	2
>60	0
ICH Location	
Lobar	2
Deep	1
Infratentorial	0
Age (y)	
<70	2
70–79	1
≥80	0
Pre-ICH Cognitive Impairment	
No	1
Yes	0
Total score	0–11

The probability of reaching functional independence at 3 months increases steadily with the total score. Total scores greater than or equal to 7 are associated with a functional independence probability of more than 70%.

Table 5	
Some ongoing clinical trials in acute ICH management	
Trial	**Intervention**
SCORE-IT[82,83]	Investigate whether CTA spot sign or other imaging markers identify patients with high likelihood to benefit from BP reduction
TICH II Tich-2.org	Administration of intravenous tranexamic acid
STOP-AUST ClinicalTrials.gov, NCT01702636	Administration of intravenous tranexamic acid to patients with ICH with CTA spot sign
STOP-IT ClinicalTrials.gov, NCT00810888	Administration of rFVIIa to patients with ICH with CTA spot sign
SPOTLIGHT ClinicalTrials.gov, NCT01359202	Administration of rFVIIa to patients with ICH with CTA spot sign
iDEF ClinicalTrials.gov, NCT02175225	Iron chelation with administration of intravenous deferoxamine
SHRINC ClinicalTrials.gov, NCT00827892	Enhancing hematoma reabsorption with administration of pioglitazone
MISTIE III ClinicalTrials.gov, NCT01827046	MIS plus rtPA for parenchymal hematoma evacuation
CLEAR III[69] ClinicalTrials.gov, NCT00784134	EVD placement combined with intraventricular administration of rtPA for IVH treatment
MISTICH[84]	MIS for evacuation of supratentorial hematomas
SATIH ClinicalTrials.gov, NCT00752024	Stereotactic hematoma aspiration combined with thrombolysis
SWITCH ClinicalTrials.gov, NCT02258919	Decompressive craniectomy plus best medical therapy

Abbreviations: CLEAR III, The Clot Lysis Evaluation of Accelerated Resolution of Intraventricular Hemorrhage; iDEF, Intracerebral Hemorrhage Deferoxamine Trial; MISTICH, Minimally invasive surgery treatment for the patients with spontaneous supratentorial intracerebral hemorrhage; MISTIE III, Minimally Invasive Surgery Plus Rt-PA for ICH Evacuation Phase III; rFVIIa, recombinant activated factor VII; SATIH, Stereotactic Aspiration and Thrombolysis of Intracerebral Hemorrhage; SCORE-IT, the spot sign score in restricting ICH growth; SHRINC, The Safety of Pioglitazone for Hematoma Resolution in IntraCerebral Hemorrhage; SPOTLIGHT, "Spot Sign" Selection of Intracerebral Hemorrhage to Guide Hemostatic Therapy; STOP-AUST, The spot sign and tranexamic acid on preventing ICH growth—AUStralasia Trial; STOP-IT, The Spot Sign for Predicting and Treating ICH Growth Study (STOP-IT); SWITCH, Decompressive Hemicraniectomy in Intracerebral Hemorrhage (SWITCH); TICH II, Tranexamic acid for IntraCerebral Haemorrhage 2.

REFERENCES

1. Ikram MA, Wieberdink RG, Koudstaal PJ. International epidemiology of intracerebral hemorrhage. Curr Atheroscler Rep 2012;14(4):300–6.

2. Van Asch CJ, Luitse MJ, Rinkel GJ, et al. Incidence, case fatality, and functional outcome of intracerebral haemorrhage over time, according to age, sex, and ethnic origin: a systematic review and meta-analysis. Lancet Neurol 2010;9(2):167–76.

3. O'Donnell MJ, Denis X, Liu L, et al. Risk factors for ischaemic and intracerebral haemorrhagic stroke in 22 countries (the INTERSTROKE study): a case-control study. Lancet 2010;376(9735):112–23.

4. Charidimou A, Gang Q, Werring DJ. Sporadic cerebral amyloid angiopathy revisited: recent insights into pathophysiology and clinical spectrum. J Neurol Neurosurg Psychiatry 2012;83(2):124–37.

5. Qureshi AI, Mendelow AD, Hanley DF. Intracerebral haemorrhage. Lancet 2009; 373(9675):1632–44.

6. Hallevi H, Albright KC, Aronowski J, et al. Intraventricular hemorrhage: anatomic relationships and clinical implications. Neurology 2008;70(11):848–52.

7. Hemphill JC, Greenberg SM, Anderson CS. Guidelines for the management of spontaneous intracerebral hemorrhage: a guideline for healthcare professionals from the American Heart Association/American Stroke Association. Stroke 2015;46(7):2032–60.

8. Hemphill JC, Bonovich DC, Besmertis L, et al. The ICH score: a simple, reliable grading scale for intracerebral hemorrhage. Stroke 2001;32(4):891–7.

9. Macellari F, Paciaroni M, Agnelli G, et al. Neuroimaging in intracerebral hemorrhage. Stroke 2014;45(3):903–8.

10. Broderick JP, Brott TG, Duldner JE, et al. Volume of intracerebral hemorrhage. A powerful and easy-to-use predictor of 30-day mortality. Stroke 1993;24(7): 987–93.

11. Khosravani H, Mayer SA, Demchuk A, et al. Emergency noninvasive angiography for acute intracerebral hemorrhage. Am J Neuroradiol 2013;34(8):1481–7.

12. Demchuk AM, Dowlatshahi D, Rodriguez-Luna D, et al. Prediction of haematoma growth and outcome in patients with intracerebral haemorrhage using the CT-angiography spot sign (PREDICT): a prospective observational study. Lancet Neurol 2012;11(4):307–14.

13. Brouwers HB, Chang Y, Falcone GJ, et al. Predicting hematoma expansion after primary intracerebral hemorrhage. JAMA Neurol 2014;71(2):158–64.

14. Brouwers HB, Raffeld MR, van Nieuwenhuizen KM, et al. CT angiography spot sign in intracerebral hemorrhage predicts active bleeding during surgery. Neurology 2014;83(10):883–9.

15. Oleinik A, Romero JM, Schwab K, et al. CT angiography for intracerebral hemorrhage does not increase risk of acute nephropathy. Stroke 2009;40(7): 2393–7.

16. Sinert R, Brandler E, Subramanian RA, et al. Does the current definition of contrast-induced acute kidney injury reflect a true clinical entity? Acad Emerg Med 2012;19(11):1261–7.

17. Sinert R, Brandler E. Contrast-induced acute kidney injury: time for a step backward. Acad Emerg Med 2014;21(6):701–3.

18. Brouwers HB, Greenberg SM. Hematoma expansion following acute intracerebral hemorrhage. Cerebrovasc Dis 2013;35(3):195–201.

19. Lord AS, Gilmore E, Choi HA, et al. Time course and predictors of neurological deterioration after intracerebral hemorrhage. Stroke 2015;46(3):647–52.

20. Ebinger M, Kunz A, Wendt M, et al. Effects of golden hour thrombolysis: a Prehospital Acute Neurological Treatment and Optimization of Medical Care in Stroke (PHANTOM-S) substudy. JAMA Neurol 2015;72(1):25–30.

21. Gomes JA, Ahrens CL, Hussain MS, et al. Prehospital reversal of warfarin-related coagulopathy in intracerebral hemorrhage in a mobile stroke treatment unit result of initial pilot implementation. Stroke 2015;46:e118–20.

22. Salhi B, Stettner E. In defense of the use of lidocaine in rapid sequence intubation. Ann Emerg Med 2007;49(1):84–6.

23. Anderson CS, Heeley E, Huang Y, et al. Rapid blood-pressure lowering in patients with acute intracerebral hemorrhage. N Engl J Med 2013;368(25): 2355–65.

24. Qureshi AI, Palesch YY, Martin R, et al. Interpretation and Implementation of Intensive Blood Pressure Reduction in Acute Cerebral Hemorrhage Trial (INTERACT II). J Vasc Interv Neurol 2014;7(2):34–40.

25. Anderson CS, Qureshi AI. Implications of INTERACT2 and other clinical trials: blood pressure management in acute intracerebral hemorrhage. Stroke 2014; 46(1):291–5.

26. Slichter SJ. Evidence-based platelet transfusion guidelines. Hematology Am Soc Hematol Educ Program 2007;172–8.

27. Hunt BJ. Bleeding and coagulopathies in critical care. N Engl J Med 2014;370(9): 847–59.

28. Aguilar MI, Freeman WD. Treatment of coagulopathy in intracranial hemorrhage. Curr Treat Options Neurol 2010;12(2):113–28.

29. Milling TJ, Refaai MA, Goldstein JN, et al. thromboembolic events after vitamin K antagonist reversal with 4-factor prothrombin complex concentrate: exploratory analyses of two randomized, plasma-controlled studies. Ann Emerg Med 2016; 67(1):96–105.e5.

30. Goldstein JN, Refaai MA, Milling TJ Jr, et al. Four-factor prothrombin complex concentrate versus plasma for rapid vitamin K antagonist reversal in patients needing urgent surgical or invasive interventions: a phase 3b, open-label, non-inferiority, randomised trial. Lancet 2015;6736(14):1–11.

31. Sarode R, Milling TJ, Refaai MA, et al. Efficacy and safety of a 4-factor prothrombin complex concentrate in patients on vitamin K antagonists presenting with major bleeding: a randomized, plasma-controlled, phase IIIb study. Circulation 2013;128(11):1234–43.

32. Frontera JA, Gordon E, Zach V, et al. Reversal of coagulopathy using prothrombin complex concentrates is associated with improved outcome compared to fresh frozen plasma in warfarin-associated intracranial hemorrhage. Neurocrit Care 2014;21(3):397–406.

33. Huhtakangas J, Tetri S, Juvela S, et al. Improved survival of patients with warfarin-associated intracerebral haemorrhage: a retrospective longitudinal population-based study. Int J Stroke 2015;10(6):876–81.

34. Hickey M, Gatien M, Taljaard M, et al. Outcomes of urgent warfarin reversal with frozen plasma versus prothrombin complex concentrate in the emergency department. Circulation 2013;128(4):360–4.

35. Marietta M, Pedrazzi P, Girardis M, et al. Intracerebral haemorrhage: an often neglected medical emergency. Intern Emerg Med 2007;2(1):38–45.

36. Morgenstern LB, Hemphill JC, Anderson C, et al. Guidelines for the management of spontaneous intracerebral hemorrhage: a guideline for healthcare professionals from the American Heart Association/American Stroke Association. Stroke 2010;41(9):2108–29.

37. Kuramatsu JB, Gerner ST, Schellinger PD, et al. Anticoagulant reversal, blood pressure levels, and anticoagulant resumption in patients with anticoagulation-related intracerebral hemorrhage. JAMA 2015;313(8):824–36.

38. Steiner T, Al-Shahi Salman R, Beer R, et al. European Stroke Organisation (ESO) guidelines for the management of spontaneous intracerebral hemorrhage. Int J Stroke 2014;9:840–55.

39. Andrews CM, Jauch EC, Hemphill JC, et al. Emergency neurological life support: intracerebral hemorrhage. Neurocrit Care 2012;17(Suppl 1):S37–46.

40. Camm JA, Lip GY, De Caterina R, et al. 2012 focused update of the ESC guidelines for the management of atrial fibrillation: an update of the 2010 ESC guidelines for

the management of atrial fibrillation. Developed with the special contribution of the European Heart Rhythm Association. Eur Heart J 2012;33(21):2719–47.

41. Barnes GD, Ageno W, Ansell J, et al. Recommendation on the nomenclature for oral anticoagulants: communication from the SSC of the ISTH. J Thromb Haemost 2015;13(6):1154–6.

42. Siegal DM, Garcia DA, Crowther MA, et al. How I treat target-specific oral anticoagulant-associated bleeding. Blood 2014;123(8):1152–8.

43. Miller MP, Trujillo TC, Nordenholz KE. Practical considerations in emergency management of bleeding in the setting of target-specific oral anticoagulants. Am J Emerg Med 2014;32(4):375–82.

44. Liew A, Eikelboom JW, O'Donnell M, et al. Assessment of anticoagulation intensity and management of bleeding with old and new oral anticoagulants. Can J Cardiol 2013;29(Suppl 7):S34–44.

45. Siegal DM. Managing target-specific oral anticoagulant associated bleeding including an update on pharmacological reversal agents. J Thromb Thrombolysis 2015;39(3):395–402.

46. Pollack CV, Reilly PA, Eikelboom J, et al. Idarucizumab for dabigatran reversal. N Engl J Med 2015;373(6):511–20.

47. Glund S, Stangier J, Schmohl M, et al. Safety, tolerability, and efficacy of idarucizumab for the reversal of the anticoagulant effect of dabigatran in healthy male volunteers: a randomised, placebo-controlled, double-blind phase 1 trial. Lancet 2015;386(9994):680–90.

48. Kaatz S, Kouides PA, Garcia DA, et al. Guidance on the emergent reversal of oral thrombin and factor Xa inhibitors. Am J Hematol 2012;87(Suppl 1):141–5.

49. Steiner T, Böhm M, Dichgans M, et al. Recommendations for the emergency management of complications associated with the new direct oral anticoagulants (DOACs), apixaban, dabigatran and rivaroxaban. Clin Res Cardiol 2013;102(6): 399–412.

50. Levine M, Goldstein JN. Emergency reversal of anticoagulation: novel agents. Curr Neurol Neurosci Rep 2014;14(8):471.

51. Baumann Kreuziger LM, Reding MT. Management of bleeding associated with dabigatran and rivaroxaban: a survey of current practices. Thromb Res 2013; 132(2):161–3.

52. Yaghi S, Eisenberger A, Willey JZ. Symptomatic intracerebral hemorrhage in acute ischemic stroke after thrombolysis with intravenous recombinant tissue plasminogen activator: a review of natural history and treatment. JAMA Neurol 2014;71(9):1181–5.

53. Mazya M, Egido JA, Ford GA, et al. Predicting the risk of symptomatic intracerebral hemorrhage in ischemic stroke treated with intravenous alteplase: Safe Implementation of Treatments in Stroke (SITS) symptomatic intracerebral hemorrhage risk score. Stroke 2012;43(6):1524–31.

54. Goldstein JN, Marrero M, Masrur S, et al. Management of thrombolysis-associated symptomatic intracerebral hemorrhage. Arch Neurol 2010;67(8): 965–9.

55. Jauch EC, Saver JL, Adams HP, et al. Guidelines for the early management of patients with acute ischemic stroke: a guideline for healthcare professionals from the American Heart Association/American Stroke Association. Stroke 2013; 44(3):870–947.

56. Yaghi S, Boehme AK, Dibu J, et al. Treatment and outcome of thrombolysis-related hemorrhage: a multicenter retrospective study. JAMA Neurol 2015; 72(12):1451–7.

57. De Herdt V, Dumont F, Hénon H, et al. Early seizures in intracerebral hemorrhage: incidence, associated factors and outcome. Neurology 2011;77(20):1794–800.
58. Pezzini A, Grassi M, Del Zotto E, et al. Complications of acute stroke and the occurrence of early seizures. Cerebrovasc Dis 2013;35(5):444–50.
59. Naidech AM, Garg RK, Liebling S, et al. Anticonvulsant use and outcomes after intracerebral hemorrhage. Stroke 2009;40(12):3810–5.
60. Stead LG, Jain A, Bellolio MF, et al. Emergency department hyperglycemia as a predictor of early mortality and worse functional outcome after intracerebral hemorrhage. Neurocrit Care 2010;13(1):67–74.
61. Qureshi AI, Palesch YY, Martin R, et al. Association of serum glucose concentrations during acute hospitalization with hematoma expansion, perihematomal edema, and three month outcome among patients with intracerebral hemorrhage. Neurocrit Care 2011;15(3):428–35.
62. Middleton S, McElduff P, Ward J, et al. Implementation of evidence-based treatment protocols to manage fever, hyperglycaemia, and swallowing dysfunction in acute stroke (QASC): a cluster randomised controlled trial. Lancet 2011; 378(9804):1699–706.
63. Finfer S, Chittock DR, Su SY, et al. Intensive versus conventional glucose control in critically ill patients. N Engl J Med 2009;360(13):1283–97.
64. Gray CS, Hildreth AJ, Sandercock PA, et al. Glucose-potassium-insulin infusions in the management of post-stroke hyperglycaemia: the UK Glucose Insulin in Stroke Trial (GIST-UK). Lancet Neurol 2007;6(5):397–406.
65. Lord AS, Karinja S, Lantigua H, et al. Therapeutic temperature modulation for fever after intracerebral hemorrhage. Neurocrit Care 2014;21(2):200–6.
66. Rincon F, Friedman DP, Bell R, et al. Targeted temperature management after intracerebral hemorrhage (TTM-ICH): methodology of a prospective randomized clinical trial. Int J Stroke 2014;9(5):646–51.
67. Dey M, Stadnik A, Awad IA. Spontaneous intracerebral and intraventricular hemorrhage: advances in minimally invasive surgery and thrombolytic evacuation, and lessons learned in recent trials. Neurosurgery 2014;74(Suppl 1):S142–50.
68. Khan NR, Tsivgoulis G, Lee SL, et al. Fibrinolysis for intraventricular hemorrhage: an updated meta-analysis and systematic review of the literature. Stroke 2014; 45(9):2662–9.
69. Ziai WC, Tuhrim S, Lane K, et al. A multicenter, randomized, double-blinded, placebo-controlled phase III study of Clot Lysis Evaluation of Accelerated Resolution of Intraventricular Hemorrhage (CLEAR III). Int J Stroke 2014;9(4):536–42.
70. Mendelow AD, Gregson BA, Fernandes HM, et al. Early surgery versus initial conservative treatment in patients with spontaneous supratentorial intracerebral haematomas in the International Surgical Trial in Intracerebral Haemorrhage (STICH): a randomised trial A. Lancet 2005;365:387–97.
71. Mendelow AD, Gregson BA, Rowan EN, et al. Early surgery versus initial conservative treatment in patients with spontaneous supratentorial lobar intracerebral haematomas (STICH II): A randomised trial. Lancet 2013;382(9890):397–408.
72. Fung C, Murek M, Z'Graggen WJ, et al. Decompressive hemicraniectomy in patients with supratentorial intracerebral hemorrhage. Stroke 2012;43(12):3207–11.
73. Hayes SB, Benveniste RJ, Morcos JJ, et al. Retrospective comparison of craniotomy and decompressive craniectomy for surgical evacuation of nontraumatic, supratentorial intracerebral hemorrhage. Neurosurg Focus 2013;34(5):E3.
74. Barnes B, Hanley DF, Carhuapoma JR. Minimally invasive surgery for intracerebral haemorrhage. Curr Opin Crit Care 2014;20(2):148–52.

75. Beynon C, Schiebel P, Bösel J, et al. Minimally invasive endoscopic surgery for treatment of spontaneous intracerebral haematomas. Neurosurg Rev 2015; 38(3):421–8.
76. Langhorne P, Fearon P, Ronning OM, et al. Stroke unit care benefits patients with intracerebral hemorrhage: systematic review and meta-analysis. Stroke 2013; 44(11):3044–9.
77. Rost NS, Smith EE, Chang Y, et al. Prediction of functional outcome in patients with primary intracerebral hemorrhage: The FUNC score. Stroke 2008;39(8): 2304–9.
78. Zahuranec DB, Brown DL, Lisabeth LD, et al. Early care limitations independently predict mortality after intracerebral hemorrhage. Neurology 2007;68(20):1651–7.
79. Diener HC, Foerch C, Riess H, et al. Treatment of acute ischaemic stroke with thrombolysis or thrombectomy in patients receiving anti-thrombotic treatment. Lancet Neurol 2013;12(7):677–88.
80. Veltkamp R, Horstmann S. Treatment of intracerebral hemorrhage associated with new oral anticoagulant use: the neurologist's view. Clin Lab Med 2014;34(3): 587–94.
81. Cuker A, Husseinzadeh H. Laboratory measurement of the anticoagulant activity of edoxaban: a systematic review. J Thromb Thrombolysis 2015;39:288–94.
82. Almandoz JED, Yoo AJ, Stone MJ, et al. The spot sign score in primary intracerebral hemorrhage identifies patients at highest risk of in-hospital mortality and poor outcome among survivors. Stroke 2010;41(1):54–60.
83. Goldstein JN, Brouwers HB, Romero J, et al. SCORE-IT: the Spot Sign score in restricting ICH growth–an Atach-II ancillary study. J Vasc Interv Neurol 2012; 5(Supp):20–5.
84. Zheng J, Li H, Guo R, et al. Minimally Invasive Surgery Treatment for the Patients with Spontaneous Supratentorial Intracerebral Hemorrhage (MISTICH): protocol of a multi-center randomized controlled trial. BMC Neurol 2014;14:206.
85. Biffi A, Anderson CD, Battey TWK, et al. Association between blood pressure control and risk of recurrent intracerebral hemorrhage. JAMA 2015;314(9):904.
86. Lauer A, Greenberg SM, Gurol ME. Statins in intracerebral hemorrhage. Curr Atheroscler Rep 2015;17(8):46.
87. The Emerging Risk Factors Collaboration. Diabetes mellitus, fasting blood glucose concentration, and risk of vascular disease: a collaborative meta-analysis of 102 prospective studies. Lancet 2010;375(9733):2215–22.
88. Martin-Schild S, Albright KC, Hallevi H, et al. Intracerebral hemorrhage in cocaine users. Stroke 2010;41(4):680–4.

Subarachnoid Hemorrhage

Michael K. Abraham, MD, MS, Wan-Tsu Wendy Chang, MD*

KEYWORDS

- Subarachnoid hemorrhage • Aneurysm • CT • Lumbar puncture
- Clinical decision rules • Grading scales • Delayed cerebral ischemia
- Cerebral vasospasm

KEY POINTS

- All patients with acute thunderclap headache should be evaluated for subarachnoid hemorrhage.
- Noncontrast computed tomography scanning, the first diagnostic test, is extremely sensitive early after the hemorrhage, but the sensitivity decreases with time.
- Once the diagnosis of subarachnoid hemorrhage has been established, the next steps, which should be coordinated with a neurosurgeon or cerebrovascular specialist, include imaging to define the vascular lesion and identification and prevention of complications such as rebleeding and vasospasm.

INTRODUCTION

Subarachnoid hemorrhage (SAH) is simply defined as the extravasation of blood into the subarachnoid space **Fig. 1**. Overwhelmingly, the most common cause of SAH is traumatic injury to the brain. Most of the remainder of cases are caused by spontaneous rupture of a blood vessel. The cause of spontaneous SAH can be classified into aneurysmal, nonaneurysmal, and perimesencephalic causes. Because the preponderance of morbidity and mortality related to SAH is from the aneurysmal type, the article focuses on this entity.

Aneurysmal SAH is associated with a 30-day mortality of approximately 45% and 30% of the survivors have significant disabilities.[1] There are few diseases that cause as much difficulty as SAH for emergency physicians. Debate over the recommended diagnostic algorithms exists in the specialties of emergency medicine, neurology, and neurosurgery. Current advances in imaging modalities, fear of invasive diagnostic testing, and a possible debilitating outcome for patients who are misdiagnosed fuel this fervent debate. The low incidence of the disease also complicates matters, because the diagnosis can easily be missed. However, once diagnosed, management of this

Disclosures: None.
Department of Emergency Medicine, University of Maryland School of Medicine, 110 South Paca Street, 6th Floor, Suite 200, Baltimore, MD 21201, USA
* Corresponding author.
E-mail address: wchang@em.umaryland.edu

Emerg Med Clin N Am 34 (2016) 901–916
http://dx.doi.org/10.1016/j.emc.2016.06.011
0733-8627/16/© 2016 Elsevier Inc. All rights reserved.

emed.theclinics.com

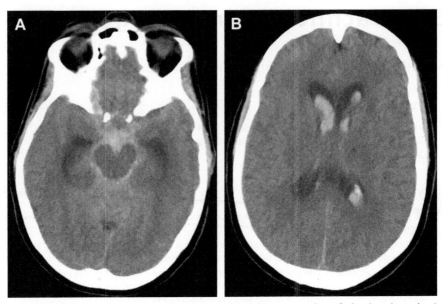

Fig. 1. (*A* and *B*) Noncontrast enhanced computed tomography of the head; a classic example of subarachnoid hemorrhage with intraventricular extension. Note the starfish appearance of the hyperdensity caused by the blood in the subarachnoid space. (*Courtesy of* Michael Abraham MD, MS, Baltimore, MD.)

neurosurgical emergency is less debatable. This article discusses the epidemiology, diagnosis, and management of aneurysmal SAH in the emergency department (ED).

Causes and Incidence

Approximately 80% of nontraumatic SAHs are from a ruptured aneurysm. Other causes of nontraumatic SAH include arteriovenous malformations, moyamoya disease, vasculitis, and amyloid angiopathy. The initial identification of the cause can be important, because the treatments of traumatic SAH and spontaneous nontraumatic SAH can be different. However, this distinction can also be difficult, because the rupture of the aneurysm may have led to the traumatic incident.

The incidence of spontaneous SAH worldwide ranges from 2 to 20 per 100,000 people, with the United States at approximately 10 per 100,000 people or roughly 30,000 patients annually, making it an uncommon disease. SAH is associated with both modifiable and nonmodifiable risk factors (**Table 1**). Smoking and hypertension are the

Table 1 Risk factors for subarachnoid hemorrhage	
Modifiable Risk Factors	**Nonmodifiable Risk Factors**
Hypertension	Female gender
Smoking history	First-degree family member with SAH
Alcohol abuse	Autosomal dominant PCKD
Cocaine use	Sickle cell disease
Caffeine consumption	Alpha1-antitrypsin deficiency

Abbreviation: PCKD, polycystic kidney disease.

most widely studied and reported risk factors; however, alcohol abuse (especially recent binge drinking), cocaine use, and caffeine consumption may also play a role. As for nonmodifiable risk factors, female patients and patients with a family history of SAH in a first-degree relative are at increased risk. Some genetic disorders, such as sickle cell disease, alpha1-antitrypsin deficiency, and polycystic kidney disease, can carry an increased risk as well.

Symptoms and Clinical Presentation

The classic presentation for SAH is an abrupt onset of severe headache.[2] This single symptom has been reported to be present in up to 97% of people with the diagnosis of SAH. The descriptive terms of abrupt, thunderclap, and worst of life should all elicit concern in emergency physicians when determining the probability of the presence of SAH. Sudden or near-sudden onset, described as maximal pain within minutes, is typical of the headache from SAH.

Depending on the time from headache onset to presentation, the pain may be resolving or even resolved if the initial hemorrhage is small. This so-called sentinel hemorrhage is simply a small leak from an aneurysm. These sentinel hemorrhages can occur 5 to 20 days before the full presentation of the SAH and are reported to be present in 10% to 40% of patients with aneurysmal SAH.[3] Other symptoms of SAH include seizures, loss of consciousness, vomiting, meningismus, or even sudden death. Recent studies report that both seizures and loss of consciousness at the outset of the hemorrhage are associated with a worse prognosis. These patients had a 2.8-fold increase in death or severe disability based on the modified Rankin Scale at 1 year, even when controlling for age, severity at presentation, and aneurysm size.[4,5]

It is important to recall that the headache, although almost always present, is sometimes overshadowed by other symptoms and this results in misdiagnosis.[6,7] Prior migraine, present in 12% of the general population, may lead to migraine as an incorrect diagnosis. Facial pain may lead to a misdiagnosis of sinusitis, whereas neck pain may lead to a misdiagnosis of neck strain. Patients with prominent vomiting have been incorrectly diagnosed with gastroenteritis. Increased blood pressure or electrocardiographic abnormalities has resulted in the incorrect diagnosis of hypertensive emergency and resulting fall or trauma can lead the physician to misdiagnose a traumatic SAH. Not working up patients because their headache has responded to various analgesics, including triptans, is another reason for misdiagnosis.[8]

Clinical Decision Rules and Differential Diagnosis

The differential diagnosis for headache, which is one of the most common complaints encountered in the ED, is long (see Ramin R. Tabatabai and Stuart P. Swadron article, "Headache in the Emergency Department Avoiding Misdiagnosis of Dangerous Secondary Causes," in this issue). The description of the headache can be instrumental in the process of determining the next steps in the evaluation of the patient. Like many other chief complaints in the ED, the use of some simple questioning can help to narrow the differential diagnosis and need for further testing. There should always be documentation of the onset, character, severity, and any associated symptoms or findings that accompany the headache. One common mistake is to overlook patients with a chronic headache history who present with a different or more severe headache than the previous headache episodes. In these patients, the history should focus on how well established the chronic headache diagnosis is, and how similar or different the current headache is compared with prior ones.

Historically, the diagnosis of SAH was missed on initial presentation in 20% to 25% of patients. Even recent data specific to the ED suggest that it is missed on the initial presentation about 5% of the time, and this is especially true when the patients are triaged to a lower acuity or seen at a nonacademic hospital.[6,9] Although SAH should be prioritized on the differential diagnosis of thunderclap headache, other diseases can also present with thunderclap headache, including cerebral or cervical arterial dissection, cerebral venous sinus thrombosis (CVST), and reversible cerebral vaso-constriction syndrome (RCVS) (**Table 2**).

Based on the presence, or absence, of certain clinical features, emergency physicians must decide who needs further evaluation for SAH. As stated previously, the incidence of SAH is low and the diagnostic testing can be invasive, leading to some trepidation on the part of emergency physicians to entertain the full work-up. Recent clinical decision rules have been developed and validated to assist in the decision to begin the work-up based on certain clinical features. The most widely studied is the Ottawa SAH Rule (**Box 1**). Using classic clinical presentations of SAH and follow-up diagnostic testing, the investigators were able to develop a clinical decision rule that was 100% sensitive and 15% specific. The subjects in this study were adult patients greater than 15 years old with no new neurologic deficits, previous history of aneurysm, or recurrent headaches. The presence of any 1 of the following variables (age >40 years, neck stiffness with limited mobility on examination, witnessed loss of consciousness, onset during exertion, and the history of headache with instantly peaking pain) were 100% sensitive for the presence of SAH.[10]

This rule suggests that all patients with thunderclap headache should undergo work-up for SAH. However, there is no 100% sensitive and specific decision rule to prevent unnecessary diagnostic work-ups, and ultimately the decision to proceed with a diagnostic work-up relies on the clinical gestalt of the treating clinicians.

Clinical Severity Grading Scales

Once the diagnosis of SAH has been confirmed, there are several clinical severity grading scales in use. The most widely used and clinically accepted is the Hunt and Hess Scale[11] (**Box 2**). Based on characteristics on presentation, this scale is a predictor of mortality to guide surgical risk. The World Federation of Neurological Surgeons

Table 2
Differential diagnosis for severe headache

Cause	History and Clinical Features
Cervical or cerebral artery dissection	Neck pain, abrupt-onset neurologic findings
CVST	Hypercoagulable, female gender
Meningitis	Fevers, meningismus
Acute narrow-angle-closure glaucoma	Painful eye, mid-dilated pupil
RCVS	Multiple thunderclap headaches over days, with or without stroke or hemorrhage
Hypertensive encephalopathy/Posterior reversible encephalopathy syndrome	Altered mental status with accelerated hypertension, papilledema, or retinal hemorrhages
Idiopathic intracranial hypertension	Obesity, papilledema, female gender
Pituitary apoplexy	Known pituitary lesion, visual field abnormalities

Adapted from Aisiku I, Abraham JA, Goldstein J, et al. An evidence-based approach to diagnosis and management of subarachnoid hemorrhage in the emergency department. Emerg Med Pract 2014;16(10):1–24.

Box 1
Ottawa SAH Rule

- For alert patients older than 15 years with new severe nontraumatic headache reaching maximum intensity within 1 hour

- Not for patients with new neurologic deficits, previous aneurysms, SAH, brain tumors, or history of recurrent headaches (≥3 episodes over the course of ≥6 months)

- Investigate if 1 or more high-risk variables present:
  - Age greater than or equal to 40 years
  - Neck pain or stiffness
  - Witnessed loss of consciousness
  - Onset during exertion
  - Thunderclap headache (instantly peaking pain)
  - Limited neck flexion on examination

From Perry JJ, Stiell IG, Sivilotti MA, et al. Clinical decision rules to rule out subarachnoid hemorrhage for acute headache. JAMA 2013;310(12):1248–55.

---

has also developed a scale to grade clinical severity of SAH (**Table 3**).[12] Although this scale also correlates with mortality, it is used more for research purposes and less for clinical outcomes.[13]

DIAGNOSTIC EVALUATION

Neuroimaging

In a patient with a concerning history and physical examination suggestive of SAH, the first step is to confirm the presence of bleeding with noncontrast head computed tomography (CT). Location of the blood on CT is important. Blood from an aneurysmal SAH is general localized to the basal cisterns, whereas traumatic SAH is generally found in frontal and temporal regions where there is deceleration of brain against the skull. In the absence of trauma, high-convexity SAH suggests RCVS in younger patients and amyloid angiopathy in elderly patients. There are varying rates of sensitivity and specificity for head CT reported in the literature. This variability can be attributed to many factors, including, but not limited to, type of CT scanner and experience of the radiologist interpreting the images. One critical point is that although noncontrast CT scanning can be very sensitive and specific, the reliability of the CT findings decreases with time.

Box 2
Hunt and Hess Scale

- Grade 1: asymptomatic, mild headache

- Grade 2: moderate to severe headache, nuchal rigidity, no focal deficit other than cranial nerve palsy

- Grade 3: mild mental status change (drowsy or confused), mild focal neurologic deficit

- Grade 4: stupor or moderate to severe hemiparesis

- Grade 5: comatose or decerebrate rigidity

Based on initial neurologic examination.
From Hunt WE, Hess RM. Surgical risk as related to time of intervention in the repair of intracranial aneurysms. J Neurosurg 1968;28(1):14–20.

Table 3 World Federation of Neurologic Surgeons scale		
Grade	Glasgow Coma Scale	Motor Deficit
1	15	Absent
2	13–14	Absent
3	13–14	Present
4	7–12	Present or absent
5	3–6	Present or absent

Based on initial neurologic examination.

From Teasdale GM, Drake CG, Hunt W, et al. A universal subarachnoid hemorrhage scale: Report of a committee of the world federation of neurosurgical societies. J Neurol Neurosurg Psychiatry 1988;51(11):1457.

Studies have shown that the sensitivity of noncontrast CT can be less than 80% and 60% on days 2 and 5 respectively.[14] Older data show that CT done within 24 hours of the onset of headache is highly, but not 100%, sensitive.[15–17] This is especially true in patients who are neurologically intact and using modern CT scanners.[18] More recently, studies have found that the sensitivity and specificity of third-generation CT scanners read by attending-level radiologists and performed within the first 6 hours of symptom onset approaches 100%.[19–21]

A recent meta-analysis of these newer data suggests that, in a worst-case scenario, 1 patient in 700 might be missed if lumbar puncture (LP) is not done.[22] This worst-case scenario includes patients who had negative angiography, and also patients with vascular lesions, which may have been incidental. Note that this incidence only applies to neurologically intact patients without meningismus whose CT was performed on a modern scanner within 6 hours of headache onset, and that the scan must be technically adequate and interpreted by an attending-level radiologist. Although it is not known whether the communication to the radiologist makes a difference, it makes sense to specifically inform the radiologist that SAH is the suspected diagnosis, because in several of the studies mentioned earlier CT scans that read as negative had SAH visible on review of the scan. Given the very low risk of SAH in these early-presenting patients with negative CT scans, emergency physicians may consider shared decision making with these patients.

In addition to the scanner, the radiologist, and the time since rupture, other factors can influence the sensitivity and specificity of noncontrast head CT. These factors include the size of the hemorrhage, the patient's hematocrit (<30%), and the presence of motion or bone artifact.[14,17,23,24] Another important factor is the slice thickness of the CT. Experts recommend using very thin slices such as 2.5 mm through the base of the brain and 5 mm higher up. These factors should all be considered in patients with a high clinical suspicion for SAH and head CT that is reported as negative.

Because of the high sensitivity and specificity of CT scans, there is debate whether advanced neuroimaging techniques add to the diagnostic yield in SAH. In addition to noncontrast CT, CT angiography (CTA) and MRI with or without angiography have been used to aid in the diagnosis of SAH. As discussed later, LP is an integral part of the diagnosis of SAH. However, there are data that, despite a worrisome history and negative CT, LP is not pursued by some practitioners.[25–27] Some centers use CTA or magnetic resonance angiography (MRA) if the noncontrast CT is negative with the reasoning that, if there is no appreciable aneurysm, then the patient can be categorized as low risk and possibly discharged. Although CTA and MRA can identify aneurysms as small as 3 mm with reasonable sensitivity,[28] the limitation to this approach is that CTA and MRA do not identify whether the aneurysm has bled, and between 2% and 5% of the population have aneurysms.

In this scenario the patient may be subjected to more invasive tests, because the aneurysm may be incidental and not responsible for the patient's symptoms. There have been studies that prospectively evaluated the usage of CTA to assess for SAH and aneurysmal rupture. In 1 study all participants received noncontrast CT followed by CTA and LP if the noncontrast CT was negative. This single-center study found that 6 out of 116 patients had aneurysms.[29] However, although the investigators suggested that only 1 of the 6 was a false-positive CTA, the data presented do not show whether the other 5 aneurysms were symptomatic or not. There have also been attempts to form mathematical models that evaluate the diagnostic accuracy of the CT/CTA approach, and these have reported a less than 1% miss rate using computed models.[30] However, there are numerous negative downstream implications of switching to a CT followed by CTA paradigm, including radiation exposure, adverse events from intravenous contrast use, unnecessary procedures on asymptomatic aneurysms, patient anxiety, and ambiguity about incidental findings.[31] Although CTA may become a viable option in the diagnostic evaluation of SAH, at this time the gold standard remains noncontrast CT followed by LP.

MRI can be used for primary diagnosis of SAH. MRI is fairly sensitive for acute blood and has the additional advantage of being much more sensitive than CT for more chronic bleeding. If available, MRI, which should include fluid-attenuated inversion recovery sequences, could be used as an alternative to CT. Importantly, if the MRI is negative, an LP should still be performed, as after a negative CT.[32] However, there are specific time and resource conditions that may be difficult to overcome depending on the practice setting and the patient's clinical stability, and these limit the widespread utility of MRI/MRA.

One point to remember is that the earlier discussion refers to SAH only. If other diagnostic competitors, such as arterial dissection, CVST, or RCVS, are considered, further testing is indicated.[33] Occasionally, an unruptured aneurysm that has acutely expanded, dissected, or thrombosed can present with thunderclap headache.[7] It is worth noting that in neurologically intact patients with thunderclap headache with negative CT and LP, outcomes are excellent and guidelines do not recommend obtaining CTA in these patients.[34,35]

Lumbar Puncture

The 2008 American College of Emergency Physicians and 2012 American Heart Association guidelines, both recommend the use of LP after negative CT to adequately rule out SAH.[35,36] The main concern with the use of LP is the invasive and time-consuming nature of the procedure, coupled with the possibility of an inconclusive or uninterpretable result, which introduces diagnostic ambiguity. Classically, an LP is considered positive if the cerebrospinal fluid (CSF) is positive for erythrocytes in tubes 1 and 4 that are equal in number or if there is xanthochromia. Although xanthochromia is the most meaningful finding, it may not be present early in the disease course because it is produced as a breakdown product of hemoglobin. The accuracy of xanthochromia by visual inspection has been debated.[37,38] Although spectrophotometry is very sensitive, it is not very specific.[39] In addition, there are few centers in North America that have the capability to perform spectroscopy on CSF.[40]

One of the most fervent debates in emergency medicine has been over the necessity to perform an LP after a negative CT scan in appropriate patients. Owing to the dislike of patients and providers in performing the LP procedure, the utility of LP after negative

CT has been well studied. Recent studies report a very low diagnostic yield of LP in patients who present with headaches typical for SAH and negative CT. The largest retrospective observational study, by Sayer and colleagues,[41] evaluated 2248 patients who presented to the ED and in whom the physician was considering SAH. In this study, 92 of 2248 patients had a positive LP after a negative CT, and, of these, 9% had a vascular abnormality that could be attributed to the LP results. In another much smaller case series of CT-negative LP-positive patients, the likelihood of finding an aneurysm was higher, although still low, in patients presenting after 3 days from headache onset.[42] Although patients may defer the LP, it can be beneficial not only in identifying SAH but may also incidentally diagnose other causes of headache, including idiopathic intracranial hypertension (pseudotumor cerebri), spontaneous intracranial hypotension, encephalitis, or meningitis.[43] However, this presumes that the opening pressure is measured when doing the LP.

Although the LP continues to have benefit in the diagnostic work-up of SAH, the utility is greatly debated. With a low diagnostic yield, a serious discussion with the patient about the risks and benefits of the procedure needs to occur, and the patient needs to be an informed participant in the decision to proceed. With more studies and increasing sensitivity of CT scanners, especially if done in the first 6 hours after headache onset, the performance of LP in these patients may become unnecessary in the near future.

MANAGEMENT

Once the patient has been diagnosed with an SAH, treatment should focus on limiting secondary neurologic injuries to improve the patient's functional outcome. Resuscitation of a patient with SAH should follow all established protocols with immediate attention to airway and circulatory support. After stabilization of the airway and circulation, treatments specific to SAH can begin. The patient should ultimately be cared for at an institution with expertise in neurovascular emergencies, and transfer should be established as soon as the patient is stable to transfer. The emergency physician should discuss implementation of the following treatments with the accepting cerebrovascular specialist.

Pharmacologic Treatments

Antiepileptic drugs

In patients with a suspected ruptured aneurysm, seizures can lead to aneurysmal rebleeding and result in intracranial hypertension and herniation. Seizures have been described in up to 26% of patients with SAH, most occurring before hospital presentation.[5,44–46] The risk of seizures is highest in patients with poor Hunt and Hess grade and those with thick subarachnoid blood.[47] Early seizures at onset of SAH symptoms are often a sign of rebleeding and a predictor of poor outcomes.[5,47]

Routine prophylactic antiepileptic drug use in patients with SAH is a common practice despite limited evidence. No randomized controlled trials have investigated the safety and effectiveness of antiepileptic drugs in SAH.[48] In one study, adverse drug effects such as drug eruption, fever, thrombocytopenia, and toxic hepatitis were reported with routine antiepileptic drugs use in 23% of patients.[47] Phenytoin has been found to be independently associated with worse cognitive outcomes after SAH.[49] The American Stroke Association (ASA) guideline recommends consideration of short-term prophylactic antiepileptic drug use in the immediate posthemorrhage period.[36]

Nimodipine

Delayed cerebral ischemia (DCI) is one of the most serious complications associated with aneurysmal SAH. DCI occurs in one-third of patients surviving the initial hemorrhage and results in poor outcome in half of the patients with this complication.[50] Although DCI can occur in conjunction with angiographic evidence of cerebral vasospasm, each may occur independently of the other. Nimodipine is a calcium antagonist that is thought to reduce the rate of cerebral vasospasm by reducing the influx of calcium into the vascular smooth muscle cells. However, it likely has other neuroprotective properties, because similar effects are not seen with other calcium antagonists and its neuroprotective effects are not associated with decrease in angiographically apparent vasospasm. A Cochrane Review that includes a large randomized controlled trial shows a reduced risk of poor outcome with a corresponding number needed to treat of 19.[51,52] The administration of nimodipine to reduce the risk of poor outcome and DCI is the only level IA evidence recommended by the ASA.[36]

Blood pressure management

There is general consensus that hypertension should be controlled after SAH and until the ruptured aneurysm is secured. However, specific parameters for blood pressure have not been defined and data are sparse. Early retrospective studies suggest a higher rate of rebleeding with SBP greater than 160 mm Hg and severity of initial hemorrhage.[53] Therefore, the ASA and Neurocritical Care Society recommend maintaining SBP less than 160 mm Hg and mean arterial pressure less than 110 mm Hg before the ruptured aneurysm is secured to reduce the risk of rebleeding.[36,54] Many practicing neurosurgeons and endovascular specialists use a lower target of SBP less than 140 mm Hg.

The ideal antihypertensive to use in SAH would be a parenteral agent that produces a rapid and reproducible dose response while concurrently minimizing adverse cerebral effects. Classic agents used for hypertensive emergencies, such as sodium nitroprusside, hydralazine, and enalaprilat, are less desirable in acute SAH because of adverse effects on cerebral blood flow (CBF) and intracranial pressure (ICP), as well as unpredictable and prolonged antihypertensive effects.[55] Labetalol, nicardipine, and clevidipine are agents recommended by the ASA.[36]

Antifibrinolytics

When early definitive treatment of the ruptured aneurysm is not possible, antifibrinolytic therapies such as aminoepsilon caproic acid or tranexamic acid can be considered to reduce the risk of early aneurysmal rebleeding. Early studies showed a reduction in rebleeding but an increase in cerebral ischemia with prolonged use of antifibrinolytics.[56] Studies on early and short-term use of antifibrinolytics showed a reduction in rebleeding but no significant effect on outcomes.[57,58] Neither aminocaproic acid or tranexamic acid is approved by the US Food and Drug Administration for prevention of aneurysmal rebleeding, thus the use of antifibrinolytic therapies should be discussed with neurosurgical consultants on a case-by-case basis.

Nonpharmacologic Treatments

Fever management

Fever is the most common medical complication of SAH. Even a single occurrence of fever in SAH is associated with worse outcomes.[59,60] Fever induces cerebral metabolism, whereas induced normothermia reduces episodes of cerebral metabolic crises.[61] Strong predictors of fever are poor Hunt and Hess grade and presence of intraventricular hemorrhage.[62]

Antipyretics, although traditionally first-line therapy, are less effective in brain-injured patients because of impaired thermoregulatory mechanisms. Infusion of 4°C normal saline is a rapid, safe, and effective method for induction of fever control.

Surface and endovascular cooling devices are more effective than evaporative cooling methods. Although stepwise, escalating fever management is conventional, prophylactic normothermia may be most effective in reducing fever burden and may improve outcome.[63,64]

Aggressive fever control is often limited by shivering, which is associated with significant metabolic demand and thus can eliminate any benefit of fever control. Therefore, shivering control is an essential component to inducing and maintaining normothermia. Techniques in controlling shivering include surface counterwarming, intravenous magnesium, and buspirone.[65]

Surgical and Endovascular Treatments

External ventricular drainage

Acute hydrocephalus is common in patients with SAH and is a common cause of early neurologic decline.[66–68] Treatment of symptomatic hydrocephalus often requires placement of an external ventricular drain, which allows ICP monitoring as well as CSF drainage. Untreated hydrocephalus can lead to intracranial hypertension and cerebral ischemia with potential cerebral herniation. Identification of the presence of hydrocephalus on CT and communication of this finding with neurosurgical consultants are key steps in the management of SAH.

Microsurgical clipping versus endovascular coiling

Definitive treatment of SAH is early microsurgical clipping or endovascular coiling of the ruptured aneurysm to prevent rebleeding and its associated complications. Choice of treatment modality depends on aneurysm size, characteristics, and location, as well as the patient's clinical grade and comorbidities.[50,69,70] Patient outcomes are improved when treated at a high-volume SAH center with experienced cerebrovascular surgeons, endovascular specialists, and neurointensivists.[71–74]

COMPLICATIONS

Various complications of SAH can occur, even very early while the patient is still in the ED. Acute decompensation of a patient should prompt cardiopulmonary reassessment and repeat noncontrast CT to distinguish the cause. Hypotension may occur from neurogenic stress cardiomyopathy, whereas hypoxia may be the result of an aspiration event. Neurologic deterioration may be the result of aneurysmal rebleeding, development of hydrocephalus, or cerebral herniation, each of which suggests its own next steps.

Rebleeding

Rebleeding can occur before the ruptured aneurysm is secured, and is associated with significant mortality and poor prognosis for functional recovery. Rebleeding is most common within the first 24 hours, with some studies reporting peak time of rebleeding within 2 hours.[53,75] Factors associated with rebleeding include longer time to aneurysm treatment, worse neurologic status on presentation, initial loss of consciousness, previous sentinel headaches, larger aneurysm size, and possibly SBP greater than 160 mm Hg.[76,77] Although early definitive treatment of ruptured aneurysms can reduce the risk of rebleeding, approximately 12% to 15% of patients die before reaching the hospital.[35,77]

Cerebral Edema

Up to 20% of patients with SAH develop global cerebral edema.[78] Early global cerebral edema results from ictal intracranial circulatory arrest, in which an acute increase

---

Box 3
Fisher Scale

- Grade 1: no blood
- Grade 2: diffuse deposits of SAH blood, no clots, no layers of blood thicker than 1 mm
- Grade 3: localized clots or vertical layers of blood greater than or equal to 1 mm thickness
- Grade 4: SAH of any thickness with intracerebral or intraventricular extension

Based on initial CT scan.
From Fisher C, Kistler J, Davis J. Relation of cerebral vasospasm to subarachnoid hemorrhage visualized by computerized tomographic scanning. Neurosurgery 1980;6(1):1–9.

---

in ICP at the time of aneurysm rupture causes global cerebral hypoperfusion. This condition is associated with the clinical presentation of loss of consciousness at onset. Delayed cerebral edema can result from cytotoxic effects of blood products, microvascular ischemia, and autoregulation dysfunction.[79] CT evidence of global cerebral edema on presentation is an independent predictor of mortality and poor outcome.[78]

Vasospasm and Cerebral Ischemia

Vasospasm of the cerebral arteries after SAH is common, occurring most frequently 7 to 10 days after aneurysm rupture. The Fisher Scale can be used to estimate risk of symptomatic vasospasm (**Box 3**).[80] Although radiographic vasospasm can be seen in 30% to 70% of patients, about half are clinically symptomatic.[81] Development of cerebral ischemia is likely multifactorial, including microcirculatory failure and poor collateral anatomy.[82] Treatment of symptomatic vasospasm and cerebral ischemia is directed at improving cerebral perfusion. Avoiding hypovolemia is important, although there is no evidence that hypervolemia is more beneficial than euvolemia.[83,84] Hemodynamic augmentation is another strategy in improving CBF; however, this technique is limited in patients with unsecured aneurysms. Endovascular administration of vasodilators and angioplasty can be considered in selected patients in consultation with neurosurgery and interventional neuroradiology. Although vasospasm and associated cerebral ischemia are less commonly seen in the ED because of the natural time course of the disease process, it should be considered in patients with delayed presentations of SAH.

SUMMARY

Aneurysmal SAH is a neurologic emergency with high risk of neurologic decline and death. Although the presentation of a thunderclap headache or the worst headache of a patient's life easily triggers the evaluation for SAH, subtler presentations are still missed. The gold standard for diagnostic evaluation of SAH remains noncontrast head CT followed by LP if the CT is negative for SAH. Management of patients with SAH follows standard resuscitation of critically ill patients with the emphasis on reducing risks of rebleeding and avoiding secondary brain injuries.

REFERENCES

1. Hop JW, Rinkel GJ, Algra A, et al. Case-fatality rates and functional outcome after subarachnoid hemorrhage: a systematic review. Stroke 1997;28(3):660–4.
2. Fine B, Singh N, Aviv R, et al. Decisions: does a patient with a thunderclap headache need a lumbar puncture? CMAJ 2012;184(5):555–6.

3. Polmear A. Sentinel headaches in aneurysmal subarachnoid haemorrhage: what is the true incidence? A systematic review. Cephalalgia 2003;23(10):935–41.
4. Suwatcharangkoon S, Meyers E, Falo C, et al. Loss of consciousness at onset of subarachnoid hemorrhage as an important marker of early brain injury. JAMA Neurol 2015;73(1):28–35.
5. Butzkueven H, Evans AH, Pitman A, et al. Onset seizures independently predict poor outcome after subarachnoid hemorrhage. Neurology 2000;55(9):1315–20.
6. Edlow JA, Caplan LR. Avoiding pitfalls in the diagnosis of subarachnoid hemorrhage. N Engl J Med 2000;342(1):29–36.
7. Edlow JA, Malek AM, Ogilvy CS. Aneurysmal subarachnoid hemorrhage: update for emergency physicians. J Emerg Med 2008;34(3):237–51.
8. Pope JV, Edlow JA. Favorable response to analgesics does not predict a benign etiology of headache. Headache 2008;48(6):944–50.
9. Vermeulen MJ, Schull MJ. Missed diagnosis of subarachnoid hemorrhage in the emergency department. Stroke 2007;38(4):1216–21.
10. Perry JJ, Stiell IG, Sivilotti MA, et al. Clinical decision rules to rule out subarachnoid hemorrhage for acute headache. JAMA 2013;310(12):1248–55.
11. Hunt WE, Hess RM. Surgical risk as related to time of intervention in the repair of intracranial aneurysms. J Neurosurg 1968;28(1):14–20.
12. Teasdale GM, Drake CG, Hunt W, et al. A universal subarachnoid hemorrhage scale: report of a committee of the world federation of neurosurgical societies. J Neurol Neurosurg Psychiatry 1988;51(11):1457.
13. Degen LA, Dorhout Mees SM, Algra A, et al. Interobserver variability of grading scales for aneurysmal subarachnoid hemorrhage. Stroke 2011;42(6):1546–9.
14. Kassell NF, Torner JC, Haley EC Jr, et al. The international cooperative study on the timing of aneurysm surgery. Part 1: overall management results. J Neurosurg 1990;73(1):18–36.
15. Sames TA, Storrow AB, Finkelstein JA, et al. Sensitivity of new-generation computed tomography in subarachnoid hemorrhage. Acad Emerg Med 1996;3: 16–20.
16. Sidman R, Connolly E, Lemke T. Subarachnoid hemorrhage diagnosis: lumbar puncture is still needed when the computed tomography scan is normal. Acad Emerg Med 1996;3:827–31.
17. van der Wee N, Rinkel GJ, Hasan D, et al. Detection of subarachnoid haemorrhage on early CT: is lumbar puncture still needed after a negative scan? J Neurol Neurosurg Psychiatry 1995;58(3):357–9.
18. Byyny RL, Mower WR, Shum N, et al. Sensitivity of noncontrast cranial computed tomography for the emergency department diagnosis of subarachnoid hemorrhage. Ann Emerg Med 2008;51:697–703.
19. Backes D, Rinkel GJ, Kemperman H, et al. Time-dependent test characteristics of head computed tomography in patients suspected of nontraumatic subarachnoid hemorrhage. Stroke 2012;43(8):2115–9.
20. Perry JJ, Spacek A, Forbes M, et al. Is the combination of negative computed tomography result and negative lumbar puncture result sufficient to rule out subarachnoid hemorrhage? Ann Emerg Med 2008;51(6):707–13.
21. Blok KM, Rinkel GJ, Majoie CB, et al. CT within 6 hours of headache onset to rule out subarachnoid hemorrhage in nonacademic hospitals. Neurology 2015; 84(19):1927–32.
22. Dubosh NM, Bellolio MF, Rabinstein AA, et al. Sensitivity of early brain computed tomography to exclude aneurysmal subarachnoid hemorrhage: a systematic review and meta-analysis. Stroke 2016;47(3):750–5.

23. Leblanc R. The minor leak preceding subarachnoid hemorrhage. J Neurosurg 1987;66(1):35–9.
24. Schriger DL, Kalafut M, Starkman S, et al. Cranial computed tomography interpretation in acute stroke: physician accuracy in determining eligibility for thrombolytic therapy. JAMA 1998;279(16):1293–7.
25. O'Neill J, McLaggan S, Gibson R. Acute headache and subarachnoid haemorrhage: a retrospective review of CT and lumbar puncture findings. Scott Med J 2005;50(4):151–3.
26. Perry JJ, Stiell I, Wells G, et al. Diagnostic test utilization in the emergency department for alert headache patients with possible subarachnoid hemorrhage. CJEM 2002;4(5):333–7.
27. Morgenstern LB, Luna-Gonzales H, Huber J, et al. Worst headache and subarachnoid hemorrhage: prospective, modern computed tomography and spinal fluid analysis. Ann Emerg Med 1998;32:297–304.
28. Li MH, Cheng YS, Li YD, et al. Large-cohort comparison between three-dimensional time-of-flight magnetic resonance and rotational digital subtraction angiographies in intracranial aneurysm detection. Stroke 2009;40(9):3127–9.
29. Carstairs SD, Tanen DA, Duncan TD, et al. Computed tomographic angiography for the evaluation of aneurysmal subarachnoid hemorrhage. Acad Emerg Med 2006;13(5):486–92.
30. McCormack RF, Hutson A. Can computed tomography angiography of the brain replace lumbar puncture in the evaluation of acute-onset headache after a negative noncontrast cranial computed tomography scan? Acad Emerg Med 2010; 17(4):444–51.
31. Edlow JA. What are the unintended consequences of changing the diagnostic paradigm for subarachnoid hemorrhage after brain computed tomography to computed tomographic angiography in place of lumbar puncture? Acad Emerg Med 2010;17:991–5 [discussion: 996–7].
32. Edlow JA, Figaji A, Samuels O. Emergency neurological life support: subarachnoid hemorrhage. Neurocrit Care 2015;23(Suppl 2):S103–9.
33. Ducros A, Bousser MG. Thunderclap headache. BMJ 2013;346:e8557.
34. Savitz SI, Levitan EB, Wears R, et al. Pooled analysis of patients with thunderclap headache evaluated by CT and LP: is angiography necessary in patients with negative evaluations? J Neurol Sci 2009;276:123–5.
35. Edlow JA, Panagos PD, Godwin SA, et al, American College of Emergency Physicians. Clinical policy: critical issues in the evaluation and management of adult patients presenting to the emergency department with acute headache. Ann Emerg Med 2008;52:407–36.
36. Connolly ES Jr, Rabinstein AA, Carhuapoma JR, et al. Guidelines for the management of aneurysmal subarachnoid hemorrhage: a guideline for healthcare professionals from the American Heart Association/American Stroke Association. Stroke 2012;43(6):1711–37.
37. Sidman R, Spitalnic S, Demelis M, et al. Xanthrochromia? By what method? A comparison of visual and spectrophotometric xanthrochromia. Ann Emerg Med 2005;46(1):51–5.
38. Linn FH, Voorbij HA, Rinkel GJ, et al. Visual inspection versus spectrophotometry in detecting bilirubin in cerebrospinal fluid. J Neurol Neurosurg Psychiatry 2005; 76:1452–4.
39. Perry JJ, Sivilotti ML, Stiell IG, et al. Should spectrophotometry be used to identify xanthochromia in the cerebrospinal fluid of alert patients suspected of having subarachnoid hemorrhage? Stroke 2006;37:2467–72.

40. Edlow JA, Bruner KS, Horowitz GL. Xanthochromia - a survey of laboratory methodology and its clinical implications. Arch Pathol Lab Med 2002;126:413–5.
41. Sayer D, Bloom B, Fernando K, et al. An observational study of 2,248 patients presenting with headache, suggestive of subarachnoid hemorrhage, who received lumbar punctures following normal computed tomography of the head. Acad Emerg Med 2015;22(11):1267–73.
42. Horstman P, Linn FH, Voorbij HA, et al. Chance of aneurysm in patients suspected of SAH who have a 'negative' CT scan but a 'positive' lumbar puncture. J Neurol 2012;259:649–52.
43. Brunell A, Ridefelt P, Zelano J. Differential diagnostic yield of lumbar puncture in investigation of suspected subarachnoid haemorrhage: a retrospective study. J Neurol 2013;260:1631–6.
44. Hart R, Byer J, Slaughter J, et al. Occurrence and implications of seizures in subarachnoid hemorrhage due to ruptured intracranial aneurysms. Neurosurgery 1981;8(4):417–21.
45. Pinto A, Canhao P, Ferro J. Seizures at the onset of subarachnoid haemorrhage. J Neurol 1996;243(2):161–4.
46. Rhoney D, Tipps L, Murry K, et al. Anticonvulsant prophylaxis and timing of seizures after aneurysmal subarachnoid hemorrhage. Neurology 2000;55(2):258–65.
47. Choi K, Chun H, Yi K, et al. Seizure and epilepsy following aneurysmal subarachnoid hemorrhage: incidence and risk factors. J Korean Neurosurg Soc 2009;46:93–8.
48. Lanzino G, D'Urso PI, Suarez J, Participants in the International Multi-Disciplinary Consensus Conference on the Critical Care Management of Subarachnoid, Hemorrhage. Seizures and anticonvulsants after aneurysmal subarachnoid hemorrhage. Neurocrit Care 2011;15(2):247–56.
49. Naidech AM, Kreiter KT, Janjua N, et al. Phenytoin exposure is associated with functional and cognitive disability after subarachnoid hemorrhage. Stroke 2005;36(3):583–7.
50. Brilstra EH, Rinkel GJ, van der Graaf Y, et al. Treatment of intracranial aneurysms by embolization with coils - a systematic review. Stroke 1999;30:470–6.
51. Dorhout MS, Rinkel GJ, Feigin VL, et al. Calcium antagonists for aneurysmal subarachnoid haemorrhage. Cochrane Database Syst Rev 2007;(3):CD000277.
52. Allen G, Ahn H, Preziosi T, et al. Cerebral arterial spasm - a controlled trial of nimodipine in patients with subarachnoid hemorrhage. N Engl J Med 1983;308(11):619–24.
53. Ohkuma H, Tsurutani H, Suzuki S. Incidence and significance of early aneurysmal rebleeding before neurosurgical or neurological management. Stroke 2001;32(5):1176–80.
54. Diringer MN, Bleck TP, Claude Hemphill J 3rd, et al. Critical care management of patients following aneurysmal subarachnoid hemorrhage: Recommendations from the neurocritical care society's multidisciplinary consensus conference. Neurocrit Care 2011;15(2):211–40.
55. Rose JC, Mayer SA. Optimizing blood pressure in neurological emergencies. Neurocrit Care 2004;1(3):287–99.
56. Baharoglu MI, Germans MR, Rinkel GJ, et al. Antifibrinolytic therapy for aneurysmal subarachnoid haemorrhage. Cochrane Database Syst Rev 2013;(8):CD001245.
57. Hillman J, Fridriksson S, Nilsson O, et al. Immediate administration of tranexamic acid and reduced incidence of early rebleeding after aneurysmal subarachnoid hemorrhage: A prospective randomized study. J Neurosurg 2002;97(4):771–8.

58. Starke RM, Kim GH, Fernandez A, et al. Impact of a protocol for acute antifibri-nolytic therapy on aneurysm rebleeding after subarachnoid hemorrhage. Stroke 2008;39(9):2617–21.

59. Diringer MN, Reaven NL, Funk SE, et al. Elevated body temperature indepen-dently contributes to increased length of stay in neurologic intensive care unit pa-tients. Crit Care Med 2004;32(7):1489–95.

60. Todd MM, Hindman BJ, Clarke WR, et al. Perioperative fever and outcome in sur-gical patients with aneurysmal subarachnoid hemorrhage. Neurosurgery 2009; 64(5):897–908.

61. Oddo M, Frangos S, Milby A, et al. Induced normothermia attenuates cerebral metabolic distress in patients with aneurysmal subarachnoid hemorrhage and re-fractory fever. Stroke 2009;40(5):1913–6.

62. Commichau C, Scarmeas N, Mayer SA. Risk factors for fever in the neurologic intensive care unit. Neurology 2003;60(5):837–41.

63. Broessner G, Lackner P, Fischer M, et al. Influence of prophylactic, endovascu-larly based normothermia on inflammation in patients with severe cerebrovascu-lar disease: a prospective, randomized trial. Stroke 2010;41(12):2969–72.

64. Badjatia N, Fernandez L, Schmidt JM, et al. Impact of induced normothermia on outcome after subarachnoid hemorrhage: a case-control study. Neurosurgery 2010;66(4):696–700.

65. Scaravilli V, Tinchero G, Citerio G, Participants in the International Multi-Disciplinary Consensus Conference on the Critical Care Management of Sub-arachnoid, Hemorrhage. Fever management in SAH. Neurocrit Care 2011; 15(2):287–94.

66. Milhorat TH. Acute hydrocephalus after aneurysmal subarachnoid hemorrhage. Neurosurgery 1987;20(1):15–20.

67. Hasan D, Vermeulen M, Wijdicks EF, et al. Management problems in acute hydro-cephalus after subarachnoid hemorrhage. Stroke 1989;20(6):747–53.

68. Rajshekhar V, Harbaugh R. Results of routine ventriculostomy with external ven-tricular drainage for acute hydrocephalus following subarachnoid haemorrhage. Acta Neurochir (Wien) 1992;115(1–2):8–14.

69. Murayama Y, Nien YL, Duckwiler G, et al. Guglielmi detachable coil embolization of cerebral aneurysms: 11 years' experience. J Neurosurg 2003;98:959–66.

70. Ioannidis I, Lalloo S, Corkill R, et al. Endovascular treatment of very small intracra-nial aneurysms. J Neurosurg 2010;112(3):551–6.

71. Bardach NS, Zhao S, Gress DR, et al. Association between subarachnoid hem-orrhage outcomes and number of cases treated at California hospitals. Stroke 2002;33(7):1851–6.

72. Boogaarts HD, van Amerongen MJ, de Vries J, et al. Caseload as a factor for outcome in aneurysmal subarachnoid hemorrhage: a systematic review and meta-analysis. J Neurosurg 2014;120(3):605–11.

73. Varelas PN, Schultz L, Conti M, et al. The impact of a neuro-intensivist on patients with stroke admitted to a neurosciences intensive care unit. Neurocrit Care 2008; 9(3):293–9.

74. Cross DT, Tirschwell DL, Clark MA, et al. Mortality rates after subarachnoid hem-orrhage: variations according to hospital case volume in 18 states. J Neurosurg 2003;99:810–7.

75. Cha KC, Kim JH, Kang HI, et al. Aneurysmal rebleeding - factors associated with clinical outcome in the rebleeding patients. J Korean Neurosurg Soc 2010;47(2): 119–23.

76. Starke RM, Connolly ES Jr, Participants in the International Multi-Disciplinary Consensus Conference on the Critical Care Management of Subarachnoid, Hemorrhage. Rebleeding after aneurysmal subarachnoid hemorrhage. Neurocrit Care 2011;15(2):241–6.

77. Schievink W, Wijdicks E, Parisi J, et al. Sudden death from aneurysmal subarachnoid hemorrhage. Neurology 1995;45(5):871–4.

78. Claassen J, Carhuapoma JR, Kreiter KT, et al. Global cerebral edema after subarachnoid hemorrhage: frequency, predictors, and impact on outcome. Stroke 2002;33(5):1225–32.

79. Mocco J, Prickett CS, Komotar RJ, et al. Potential mechanisms and clinical significance of global cerebral edema following aneurysmal subarachnoid hemorrhage. Neurosurg Focus 2007;22(5):E7.

80. Fisher C, Kistler J, Davis J. Relation of cerebral vasospasm to subarachnoid hemorrhage visualized by computerized tomographic scanning. Neurosurgery 1980; 6(1):1–9.

81. Vergouwen MD, Vermeulen M, van Gijn J, et al. Definition of delayed cerebral ischemia after aneurysmal subarachnoid hemorrhage as an outcome event in clinical trials and observational studies: proposal of a multidisciplinary research group. Stroke 2010;41(10):2391–5.

82. Yundt KD, Grubb RL Jr, Diringer MN, et al. Autoregulatory vasodilation of parenchymal vessels is impaired during cerebral vasospasm. J Cereb Blood Flow Metab 1998;18(4):419–24.

83. Egge A, Waterloo K, Sjoholm H, et al. Prophylactic hyperdynamic postoperative fluid therapy after aneurysmal subarachnoid hemorrhage: a clinical, prospective, randomized, controlled study. Neurosurgery 2001;49(3):593–606.

84. Lennihan L, Mayer SA, Fink ME, et al. Effect of hypervolemic therapy on cerebral blood flow after subarachnoid hemorrhage: a randomized controlled trial. Stroke 2000;31(2):383–91.

Diagnosis and Treatment of Central Nervous System Infections in the Emergency Department

Maia Dorsett, MD, PhD[a], Stephen Y. Liang, MD, MPHS[a,b],*

KEYWORDS

- Meningitis • Encephalitis • Brain abscess • Emergency department • Diagnosis
- Treatment

KEY POINTS

- The classic triad of fever, neck stiffness, and altered mental status is present in only a minority of patients with meningitis.
- Kernig's and Brudzinski's signs are poorly sensitive but relatively specific physical examination maneuvers for identifying meningitis.
- Imaging tests and lumbar puncture should not delay initiation of empiric antibiotic therapy in patients suspected to have bacterial meningitis.
- Although certain cerebrospinal fluid (CSF) profiles are highly suggestive of viral or bacterial meningitis infection, emergency physicians should not be not falsely reassured by a benign CSF fluid profile supporting a viral cause.
- Encephalitis should be considered in any patient presenting with new-onset seizure or focal neurologic deficit accompanied by fever, headache, altered mental status, or behavioral changes.

Disclosures: The authors report no conflicts of interest in this work. S.Y. Liang is the recipient of a KM1 Comparative Effectiveness Research Career Development Award (KM1CA156708-01) and received support through the Clinical and Translational Science Award (CTSA) program (UL1RR024992) of the National Center for Advancing Translational Sciences (NCATS) as well as the Barnes-Jewish Patient Safety & Quality Career Development Program, which is funded by the Foundation for Barnes-Jewish Hospital.
a Division of Emergency Medicine, Washington University School of Medicine, 660 South Euclid Avenue, Campus Box 8072, St Louis, MO 64110, USA; b Division of Infectious Diseases, Washington University School of Medicine, 660 South Euclid Avenue, Campus Box 8051, St Louis, MO 63110, USA
* Corresponding author. Division of Infectious Diseases, Washington University School of Medicine, 660 South Euclid Avenue, Campus Box 8051, St Louis, MO 63110.
E-mail address: sliang@dom.wustl.edu

Emerg Med Clin N Am 34 (2016) 917–942
http://dx.doi.org/10.1016/j.emc.2016.06.013
0733-8627/16/© 2016 Elsevier Inc. All rights reserved.

emed.theclinics.com

INTRODUCTION

A key clinical responsibility of the emergency physician is to consider the "worst case scenario" for a given chief complaint. When it comes to infections of the central nervous system (CNS), the greatest challenge is identifying patients that have a rare life-threatening diagnosis amid the multitude of patients presenting with nonspecific symptoms. Alone or in combination, fever, headache, altered mental status, and behavior changes encompass a broad differential diagnosis. A diagnosis not considered is a diagnosis never made. In this vein, this review discusses the clinical signs and symptoms that should lead emergency physicians to consider CNS infection, paying particular attention to the sensitivity and specificity of different clinical findings at the bedside. Subsequently, the diagnostic workup and management of patients for whom there is high clinical suspicion for CNS infection is discussed.

MENINGITIS

The term "meningitis" applies broadly to inflammation of the meninges. While meningitis can arise from a wide variety of pathologies, infectious and non-infectious, for the purpose of this review we specifically refer to acute infections of the meninges of bacterial, viral, or fungal origin. Bacterial meningitis occurs when organisms gain access to the subarachnoid space either through bacteremia (usually from an upper airway source), contiguous spread from dental or sinus infections, traumatic or congenital communications with the exterior, or a neurosurgical procedure.[1] The severe inflammation associated with bacterial meningitis results in edema of the brain and meninges, and eventually increased intracranial pressure once the compensatory mechanisms for cerebrospinal fluid (CSF) displacement have been overwhelmed.[1] Bacterial meningitis is associated with significant morbidity with mortality rates ranging from 13 to 27%.[2]

In contrast to bacterial infection, meningitis caused by viral infection is usually less severe. The most common causes are enteroviruses (eg, Coxsackie A and B, echovirus). Herpes simplex virus (HSV, types 1 and 2), cytomegalovirus (CMV), Epstein-Barr virus (EBV), varicella zoster virus (VZV), mumps virus, and human immunodeficiency virus (HIV) may also cause viral meningitis.[3] Fungal meningitis is usually secondary to systemic mycoses (eg, *Cryptococcus neoformans*, *Coccidioides immitis*, *Histoplasma capsulatum*) originating elsewhere in the body, usually from a pulmonary focus of infection in an immunocompromised patient.[4] Rare fungal infections have also been associated with contaminated glucocorticoid injections to treat chronic pain.[5]

Meningitis is a poster child for the success of childhood vaccination in reducing the incidence of many life-threatening infectious diseases. Before the introduction of an effective vaccine in 1988, *Haemophilus influenzae type B* (Hib) was the leading cause of bacterial meningitis in the United States. After the recommendation that all infants receive the Hib vaccination starting at age 2 months, the incidence of Hib meningitis among children less than 5 years of age declined by greater than 99%.[6] Similarly, the advent of the pneumococcal seven-valent conjugate vaccine and the meningococcal conjugate vaccine significantly decreased the incidence and mortality of pneumococcal and meningococcal meningitis in the United States.[7] Meningitis due to nosocomial pathogens, including Gram-negative bacteria and *Staphylococcus*, have now surpassed *Neisseria meningitidis* and *H influenzae* in incidence.[7] With changing pathogen demographics, the average age of a patient with meningitis has increased from 15 months of age in 1986 to 35 years in the present day.[8]

Meningitis is a relatively rare diagnosis in US emergency departments (ED). Between 1993 and 2008, approximately 66,000 US ED patients were diagnosed with meningitis annually, with an incidence of 62 per 100,000 visits.[9] With regards to the cause of meningitis, ED diagnoses include unspecified (60%), viral (31%), bacterial (8%), and fungal (1%) causes. Bacterial meningitis is much more prevalent in developing countries, where the average incidence approaches 50 cases per 100,000 and 1 in 250 children are affected within the first year of life.[8]

Clinical Presentation

The number of patients presenting to the ED with symptoms suggestive of meningitis far exceeds the number of patients who actually have the disease. The classic symptom triad of fever, neck stiffness, and altered mental status is present in only a minority of patients.[10] Other associated symptoms may include nausea and vomiting, cranial nerve abnormalities, rash, and seizure. Infants can also present with nonspecific symptoms such as lethargy and irritability. With regards to the accuracy of the clinical history and physical examination in diagnosing meningitis in adults, low sensitivity plagues common complaints and findings, including headache (27%–81%), nausea and vomiting (29%–32%), and neck pain (28%).[11] Sensitivity varies for individual components of the "classic triad" of fever (42%–97%), neck stiffness (15%–92%), and altered mental status (32%–89%). In some cases, 99% to 100% of patients found to have meningitis had at least one component of the classic triad. Therefore, if the patient presenting with acute headache does not have neck stiffness or fever and is mentating normally, it is extremely unlikely that they have meningitis.[12,13] A prospective study of children ages 2 months to 16 years from Israel also demonstrated the nondiscriminatory value of symptoms in diagnosing meningitis.[14]

Classic physical examination maneuvers for the evaluation of meningitis have been taught to generations of physicians. Kernig's sign, first described in 1882, consists of flexing the patient's neck and then extending the patient's knees. It is considered positive when the maneuver elicits pain at an angle of less than 135°.[15] First reported in 1909, Brudzinski's sign, where the neck is passively flexed with the patient in supine position, is considered positive if it results in flexion of the hips and knees. The sensitivities of Kernig's and Brudzinski's signs reported in Brudzinski's original paper were 42% and 97%, respectively. However, most of Kernig's and Brudzinski's patients were children with meningitis due to *Mycobacterium tuberculosis* and *Streptococcus pneumoniae*, both of which are associated with severe meningeal inflammation.[15] Several recent studies have examined the usefulness of these classic signs in contemporary patient populations. These studies collectively demonstrate that these signs have low sensitivity in predicting CSF pleocytosis (**Table 1**).[10,16,17] The absence of these clinical signs, therefore, cannot adequately rule out of the presence of meningitis or obviate the need for a lumbar puncture (LP). However, Kernig's and Brudzinski's signs are quite specific (92%–98%) for predicting CSF pleocytosis, and therefore, their presence should increase clinical suspicion for meningitis.

An additional maneuver to elicit meningeal irritation is the "head-jolt" test. The patient is asked to move their head back and forth in the horizontal plane at a rate of 2 to 3 turns per second. It is considered positive if the patient's headache worsens. It was initially tested in a cohort of patients with both fever and headache and had a reported sensitivity of 97% for CSF pleocytosis.[18] Two subsequent studies in US ED patients and intensive care unit patients in India demonstrated much lower sensitivity (6%–21%), suggesting that the absence of a positive head jolt does not effectively rule out meningitis.[10,16]

Table 1
Sensitivities, specificities, and likelihood ratios for classic meningeal signs in predicting cerebrospinal fluid pleocytosis

	Sensitivity (95% CI)	Specificity (95% CI)	LR+	LR−	Reference
Nuchal rigidity	30	68	0.94	1.02	Thomas et al,[17] 2002
	39.4 (29.7, 49.7)	70.3 (59.8, 79.5)	1.33 (0.89, 1.98)	0.86 (0.7, 1.06)	Waghdhare et al,[10] 2010
	13 (8, 17)	80 (74, 85)	0.6	1.1	Nakao et al,[16] 2014
Kernig's sign	5	95	0.97	1.0	Thomas et al,[17] 2002
	14.1 (7.95, 22.6)	92.3 (84.8, 96.9)	1.84 (0.77, 4.35)	1.0	Waghdhare et al,[10] 2010
	2 (0, 4)	97 (95, 99)	0.8	0.93 (0.84, 1.03)	Nakao et al,[16] 2014
Brudzinski's sign	5	95	0.97	1.0	Thomas et al,[17] 2002
	11.1 (5.68, 19)	93.4 (86.2, 97.5)	1.69 (0.65, 4.35)	1.0	Waghdhare et al,[10] 2010
	2 (0, 4)	98 (96, 100)	1.0	0.95 (0.87, 1.04)	Nakao et al,[16] 2014
Head jolt	6.06 (2.26, 12.7)	98.9 (94, 100)	5.52 (0.67, 44.9)	0.95 (0.89, 1.0)	Waghdhare et al,[10] 2010
	21 (15, 27)	82 (76, 87)	1.2	1.0	Nakao et al,[16] 2014

Abbreviation: LR, likelihood ratio.

Given the poor performance of clinical signs and the physical examination in ruling out meningitis, overall clinical gestalt remains an important part of making the diagnosis. In a prospective cohort, Nakao and colleagues[16] found that physician suspicion had a sensitivity of only 44% in predicting pleocytosis. However, in 3 patients where the CSF culture grew an infective organism (*N meningitidis, C. neoformans,* and *Enterovirus*), clinicians suspected bacterial meningitis before performing the LP, suggesting that physician judgment may be the best current diagnostic tool.

Diagnostic Workup

In the absence of clear contraindications, patients suspected of having meningitis should undergo LP. If the clinical suspicion for bacterial meningitis is high, *empiric antibiotics should be started immediately when the LP cannot be performed right away.*[19–21] Although the sensitivity of the CSF culture decreases with antibiotic administration, cultures can remain positive for up to 4 hours afterward.[22]

In patients at risk for an intracranial mass or midline shift, it is recommended that computed tomography (CT) of the head be obtained before LP given the potential for brain herniation.[23] Current guidelines from the Infectious Disease Society of America recommend obtaining a head CT before LP in patients who are immunocompromised, have a history of CNS disease, have had a new-onset seizure within 1 week of presentation, or have examination findings consistent with papilledema, abnormal level of consciousness, or focal neurologic deficit.[24] In patients in whom head CT is thought to be necessary, the correct sequence of actions are first, immediate administration of antibiotics, then CT, followed by LP as soon as possible.

In Sweden, it was found that adoption of guidelines recommending head CT before LP in patients with altered mental status led to increased CT use even in patients who did not meet criteria. Far worse, adherence to guidelines for early empiric antibiotics in suspected bacterial meningitis was poor.[25] This undesirable practice pattern has been replicated in other environments as well.[22] In 2009, moderate-to-severe impairment of mental status and new onset seizures were removed from the list of indications for head CT before LP in the Swedish guidelines, leading to significantly earlier treatment of bacterial meningitis and a decrease in overall mortality.[25]

Once the LP has been completed, ideally with an opening-pressure performed, CSF fluid analysis can help predict a bacterial, viral, or fungal cause for meningitis (**Table 2**).[1,2] In addition to cell count, glucose, and protein, CSF should be sent for culture. Molecular studies such as polymerase chain reaction (PCR) assays for HSV

Table 2				
Typical cerebrospinal fluid profiles for bacterial, viral, and fungal meningitis				
Parameter	Normal	Bacterial	Viral[a]	Fungal[a]
CSF opening pressure	<170 mm	Elevated	Normal	Normal or elevated
Cell count	<5 cells/mm^3	>1000/mm^3	<1000 mm^3	<500/mm^3
Cell predominance	—	Neutrophils	Lymphocytes	Lymphocytes
CSF glucose	>0.66 × serum	Low	Normal	Low
CSF protein	<45 mg/dL	Elevated	Normal	Elevated

[a] CSF consistent with these profiles are not sufficient to rule out bacterial meningitis.

Data from Fitch MT, Abrahamian FM, Moran GJ, et al. Emergency department management of meningitis and encephalitis. Infect Dis Clin North Am 2008;22(1):33–52; and Tintinalli JE, Stapczynski JS. Tintinalli's emergency medicine: a comprehensive study guide. 7th edition. New York: McGraw-Hill; 2011.

should be considered in immunocompetent individuals. Special CSF testing for fungal (eg, cryptococcal antigen, fungal culture) and mycobacterial infection (eg, acid fast bacteria stain and mycobacterial culture) can be sent in cases where there is higher clinical suspicion for an atypical infection, particularly in immunocompromised patients.

Although certain CSF profiles are highly suggestive of viral or bacterial infection, emergency physicians should not be falsely reassured by CSF profiles suggestive that a patient has viral rather than bacterial meningitis. In a prospective study of 696 patients with culture-proven bacterial meningitis, only 88% of patients had one or more CSF findings predictive of bacterial meningitis.[26] A fifth had a negative CSF Gram stain. Two studies have assessed the discriminatory value of CSF laboratory tests in distinguishing viral versus bacterial meningitis in the setting of a negative Gram stain.[27,28] Both studies found low discriminatory value for classic CSF parameters, including significantly elevated neutrophil count, high protein, or low glucose in distinguishing bacterial from viral meningitis.[28] For example, 50% of patients with bacterial meningitis had a neutrophil count less than 440/mm^3 and greater than 10% of the patients with viral meningitis had a neutrophil count of greater than 500/mm^3.

Several studies have assessed the discriminatory value of CSF lactate in distinguishing viral from bacterial meningitis. CSF lactate, produced by bacterial anaerobic metabolism or ischemic brain tissue, is not affected by blood lactate concentration.[29] A meta-analysis assessing the diagnostic accuracy of CSF lactate for differentiating bacterial from viral meningitis found that in both pediatric and adult patients with Gram stain–positive or culture-proven bacterial meningitis, a CSF lactate level of greater than 3.9 mmol/L had a sensitivity of 96% (95% confidence interval [CI] 93%–98%) and specificity of 97% (95% CI 96%–99%) for differentiating bacterial meningitis.[30] The sensitivity of the test dropped dramatically to 29% (95% CI 23%–75%) in the subset of patients pretreated with antibiotics.

Apart from CSF analysis, procalcitonin is a serum marker that has shown promise in distinguishing bacterial from viral meningitis. In general, serum procalcitonin is an inflammatory marker that increases disproportionately in patients with underlying bacterial infection.[31,32] It has been used in a wide variety of clinical settings to assess likelihood of underlying bacterial infection.[32] In the setting of suspected meningitis but a negative CSF Gram stain, a serum procalcitonin level of greater than 0.98 ng/mL was found to have a sensitivity of 87%, specificity of 100%, positive predictive value of 100%, and negative predictive value of 99% for identifying bacterial meningitis.[27]

Generally, in patients with CSF pleocytosis or with moderate-to-high clinical suspicion for bacterial meningitis, empiric antibiotics should be continued pending finalization of CSF cultures and other diagnostic tests when indicated. In the pediatric population, the bacterial meningitis score is a validated clinical prediction tool that identifies children with CSF pleocytosis at very low risk for bacterial meningitis. Patients are considered "very low risk" for bacterial meningitis if they lack all of the following criteria: positive CSF Gram stain, CSF absolute neutrophil count (ANC) of at least 1000 cell/μL, CSF protein of at least 80 mg/dL, peripheral blood ANC of at least 10,000 cells/μL, and a history of seizure before or at time of presentation.[33–35] As the bacterial meningitis score was developed to assist clinicians in deciding which patients warrant admission for parental antibiotics in the presence of CSF pleocytosis, patients warranting admission regardless were excluded from the derivation and validation cohorts. Thus, the score does not apply to patients less than 29 days of age or those with critical illness, a ventricular shunt device, recent neurosurgery, immunosuppression, or other bacterial infection necessitating inpatient antibiotic therapy. Patients who were pretreated with antibiotics were also excluded. In a meta-analysis of 8 independent validation studies, the bacterial meningitis score was 99.3% (95% CI 98.7% to 99.7%) sensitive for bacterial meningitis, with a negative predictive value of 99.7% (95% CI 99.3% to 99.9%). Of 4896 patients with CSF pleocytosis, the bacterial meningitis score misclassified 9 as having aseptic rather than bacterial meningitis. As 7 of these children were either less than 2 months of age or had petechiae or purpura on examination, the authors recommended that the score only be applied to non-ill-appearing children older than 2 months of age who do not have petechiae or purpura on examination and have not been pretreated with antibiotics.

Treatment

Bacterial meningitis

Common pathogens responsible for bacterial meningitis vary with age, degree of immunocompromise, and clinical history (**Table 3**).[8] For example, in neonates, the most common causative organisms in the first week of life, *Streptococcus galactiae*, *Escherichia coli*, and *Listeria monocytogenes*, are replaced by *S pneumoniae* and *N meningitidis* by the sixth week. Antibacterial therapy should be geared toward the most likely pathogen (see **Table 2**).[8] With the exception of the very young, patients who have recently undergone a neurosurgical procedure, or those who have suffered penetrating head trauma, *S pneumoniae* remains the most common bacterial pathogen. Meningitis due to *S pneumoniae* is treated intravenously with a combination of a high-dose third-generation cephalosporin (eg, ceftriaxone) and vancomycin in light of worldwide emergence of resistant *S pneumoniae*.[8]

Table 3
Etiologic and recommended antimicrobial therapy by age and clinical context

Patient Subgroup	Most Common Bacterial Pathogen	Initial Intravenous Therapy
Neonates, <1 wk	*S agalactiae, E coli, L monocytogenes*	Ampicillin (50 mg/kg every 8 h) AND Cefotaxime (50 mg/kg every 8 h)
Neonates, >1 wk and <6 wk	*L monocytogenes, S agalactiae,* Gram-negative bacilli	Ampicillin (50 mg/kg every 6 h) AND Cefotaxime (50 mg/kg every 6 h)
Infants and children	*S pneumoniae, N meningiditis*	Cefriaxone (80–100 mg daily) OR Cefotaxime (75 mg/kg every 6 h) AND Vancomycin (15–20 mg/kg every 8 h)
Adults	*S pneumoniae, N meningiditis*	Ceftriaxone (2 g every 12 h) OR Cefotaxime (3 g every 6 h) AND Vancomycin (15–20 mg/kg every 8 h)
Elderly	*S pneumoniae, N meningiditis, L monocytogenes*	Ceftriaxone (2 g every 12 h) OR Cefotaxime (3 g every 6 h) AND Vancomycin (15–20 mg/kg every 8 h) AND Ampicillin (2 g every 4 h)
Immunocompromised	*S pneumoniae, N meningiditis, H influenzae,* aerobic Gram-negative bacilli	Vancomycin (15–20 mg/kg every 8 h) AND Ceftazidime (2 g every 8 h) OR Cefepime (2 g every 8 h) OR Meropenem (2 g every 8 h) AND Ampicillin (2 g every 4 h)
Nosocomial	*S aureus, S epidermidis,* aerobic Gram-negative bacilli	Vancomycin (15–20 mg/kg every 8 h) AND Ceftazidime (2 g every 8 h) OR Cefepime (2 g every 8 h) OR Meropenem (2 g every 8 h)

In addition to prompt antibiotic therapy, corticosteroids should be considered as adjunctive therapy in some cases of suspected bacterial meningitis. The use of corticosteroids for the treatment of meningitis was prompted by the finding in animal models that meningitis outcomes were worse with increasing severity of the inflammatory process in the subarachnoid space.[36] There have been conflicting results as to their benefit in bacterial meningitis ever since the first clinical trials examining their use were published in the 1960s. A 2013 *Cochrane Review* analyzed 25 randomized control trials spanning patients of all ages and types of bacterial meningitis to determine the benefit of corticosteroids in reducing overall mortality, deafness, and other neurologic sequelae.[37] Overall, there was a nonsignificant reduction in mortality (17.7% vs 19.9%; risk ratio [RR] 0.90, 95% CI 0.80–1.01) with corticosteroid use. However, in subgroup analysis, corticosteroids reduced mortality in patients with bacterial meningitis due to *S pneumoniae* (RR 0.84, 95% CI 0.72–0.98) but not *H influenzae* or *N meningitidis*. There was a significant reduction in hearing loss (RR 0.74, 95% CI 0.63–0.87) and subsequent neurologic sequelae (RR 0.83, 95% CI 0.69–1). There was no benefit found for patients treated with corticosteroids in low-income countries. With regards to the timing of corticosteroid administration, it is traditionally thought that they should be administered before or at the time of antibiotic infusion. However, the results of the *Cochrane Review* suggest that there is no significant difference in mortality reduction if corticosteroids are administered before, with, or after antibiotics are given. There was a slightly more favorable effect on reducing hearing loss and short-term neurologic sequelae if corticosteroids were administered before or with antibiotics.

Viral meningitis

There is no specific antiviral therapy for most viral causes of meningitis, and treatment is largely supportive with spontaneous recovery anticipated in most cases. HSV-1 and HSV-2 cause different CNS diseases in adults. Although HSV-1 is associated with devastating encephalitis, HSV-2 causes a benign viral meningitis with meningeal signs and CSF pleocytosis, usually in the concurrent setting of primary genital infection.[38] If HSV-2 meningitis is suspected or confirmed in an *adult*, treatment with acyclovir can be initiated but is of unclear benefit. In stark contrast, HSV-2 infection in an infant can lead to life-threatening encephalitis.

Fungal meningitis

Fungal meningitis is almost always a disease of the immunocompromised. If the clinical suspicion for fungal meningitis is high, empiric antifungal therapy with amphotericin B is appropriate pending isolation of a specific fungus to tailor antifungal therapy.

ENCEPHALITIS

Encephalitis is inflammation of the brain parenchyma. It is technically a pathologic diagnosis, but the term is commonly used to describe a clinical syndrome of brain inflammation.[39] The differential diagnosis for encephalitis is broad, with infectious (viral, bacterial, or parasitic), postinfectious, and noninfectious (metabolic, toxic, autoimmune, paraneoplastic) causes possible. Viral infections are associated with 2 distinct forms of encephalitis. The first is a direct infection of the brain parenchyma due to viremia (eg, West Nile virus) or viral reactivation in neuronal tissue (eg, HSV, VZV).[40] The second is a postinfectious encephalomyelitis (also known as acute disseminated encephalomyelitis), likely an autoimmune phenomenon more often seen in children and young adults following a disseminated viral illness or vaccination.[40,41] This review focuses on viral encephalitis due to direct infection because it is responsible for the majority of acute encephalitis encountered in emergency care.

In the Western world, encephalitis is an uncommon disorder. The reported incidence of encephalitis from all causes ranges from 0.7 to 12.6 per 100,000 adults and 10.5 to 13.8 per 100,000 children.[39] Worldwide, the causes of encephalitis remain unidentified in up to 85% of cases, due in part to limited diagnostic capabilities as well as emerging pathogens.[42] Even in a British study in which 203 patient samples underwent exhaustive testing for infectious and noninfectious causes of encephalitis, 37% of causes were unknown.[42] HSV encephalitis (HSV-1) remains the most common cause of sporadic viral encephalitis in industrialized nations, accounting for 10% to 15% of cases with an annual incidence of 1 in 250,000 to 500,000, and a bimodal age distribution primarily affecting the very young and the elderly.[43,44] VZV comes in at a close second and is actually more common than HSV in immunocompromised individuals, accounting for 19% to 29% of encephalitis cases.[42,45,46]

Clinical Presentation

The first step in approaching a patient with suspected CNS infection is to determine if bacterial meningitis is present, necessitating emergent empiric antibiotic therapy. However, when there is also evidence of brain parenchymal involvement in the form of focal neurologic findings or seizures, one must consider encephalitis as well. The clinical presentation of encephalitis correlates with the underlying function of the brain parenchyma involved (**Table 4**). For example, because HSV encephalitis is classically associated with the temporal lobes, it can present with personality changes, psychosis, olfactory or gustatory hallucinations, or acute episodes of terror that may initially be misdiagnosed as a psychiatric disorder.[40,47] Inferior frontal and temporal lobe involvement may also present with upper-quadrant visual field deficits, difficulty storing or recalling new information, hemiparesis with greater involvement of the face and arm, or aphasia when the dominant hemisphere is involved.[40] Certain viruses, such as West Nile virus and Eastern equine encephalitis virus, have a predilection for basal ganglia and thalamus and are associated with tremors or other movement disorders.[48–50] Several bacterial and viral causes, including *Bartonella henselae, M tuberculosis*, Enterovirus-71, flaviviruses (eg, West Nile virus, Japanese encephalitis virus), and alphaviruses (eg, Eastern equine encephalitis virus), can cause brainstem encephalitis manifesting as autonomic dysfunction, lower cranial nerve involvement, and respiratory drive disturbance.[39,42] Despite these classic associations, no presenting sign, symptom, or CSF finding alone or in combination with another can accurately distinguish one cause of encephalitis from another.[42]

Diagnosis

Because antibiotic therapy should be initiated rapidly in a patient with suspected CNS infection, the most urgent question to ask when you suspect encephalitis is whether a patient requires antiviral coverage in addition to standard antibiotics. The initial approach to diagnosis parallels that of meningitis (**Fig. 1**). All patients should have an LP, unless there is a clear clinical contraindication such as a coagulation abnormality, local infection at the LP site, or evidence of significant mass effect on imaging studies. Head CT should be performed before LP if the patient has moderate-to-severe impairment of consciousness, focal neurologic deficit, posturing, papilledema, seizures, relative bradycardia with hypertension, or immunocompromise.[39] In addition to a standard laboratory evaluation, all patients with suspected encephalitis should be tested for HIV infection because this may change the scope of subsequent diagnostic testing and empiric treatment. CSF findings in HSV encephalitis vary along a spectrum from normal to lymphocytic pleocytosis to hemorrhagic. However, no general CSF findings can reliably distinguish HSV from

Table 4
Demographics, clinical presentation, and treatment of select causes of viral encephalitis

Pathogen	Demographics	Neurologic Symptoms (in Addition to Headache, Fever, Altered Mental Status)	Non-neurologic Symptoms	Diagnostic Test	Treatment (Adult Dosing)
HSV	Usually young and elderly; no seasonal predilection	Seizures, olfactory/gustatory hallucinations, aphasia, personality changes, hemiparesis (face/arm > leg), upper visual field cut	Rash	HSV-1, HSV-2PCR (CSF)	Acyclovir 10 mg/kg every 8 h (adjust for renal function)
VZV	Most common in immunocompromised	Cranial nerve palsies, cerebellitis	Shingles	VZV PCR (CSF)	Acyclovir 10 mg/kg every 8 h (adjust for renal function)
CMV	Immunocompromised	Behavior changes, coma	Pneumonitis, retinitis, myelitis	CMV PCR (CSF)	Ganciclovir 5 mg/kg every 12 h
Enterovirus	Usually young	Rhombencephalitis (myoclonus, tremors, ataxia, cranial nerve palsies), poliolike acute flaccid paralysis, neurogenic shock	Hand-foot-mouth disease, rash, myocarditis, pericarditis, conjunctivitis, pulmonary edema	Enterovirus PCR (CSF)	Supportive care

Arboviruses	Summer months			IgG and IgM (CSF and serum)	Supportive care
Flaviviridae					
West Nile virus (80% infections asymptomatic)	US, Africa, Europe, Middle East, Asia	Tremors, parkinsonism, asymmetric flaccid paralysis	Insect bite, myalgias, hepatitis, pancreatitis, myocarditis, rhabdomyolysis, orchitis, rash		
St. Louis encephalitis virus	Widespread in US; adults (>50 y)	Vomiting, confusion, disorientation, stupor, coma	Insect bite, malaise, myalgias, syndrome of inappropriate antidiuretic hormone secretion		
Togaviridae					
Eastern equine encephalitis virus	Eastern and gulf coasts of US, Caribbean, and South America; children and adults	Seizures	Myalgias, malaise		
Western equine encephalitis virus	West, Midwest US, and Canada; infants and adults	Seizures	Myalgias, malaise		
Rabies virus	Exposure to infected animal	Agitation, bizarre behavior, coma, stupor	Hydrophobia, fever, malaise, anxiety, pain, or itching at site of the bite wound	Rabies virus RNA by rtPCR (saliva)	Postexposure vaccination; once infected, supportive care but universally fatal

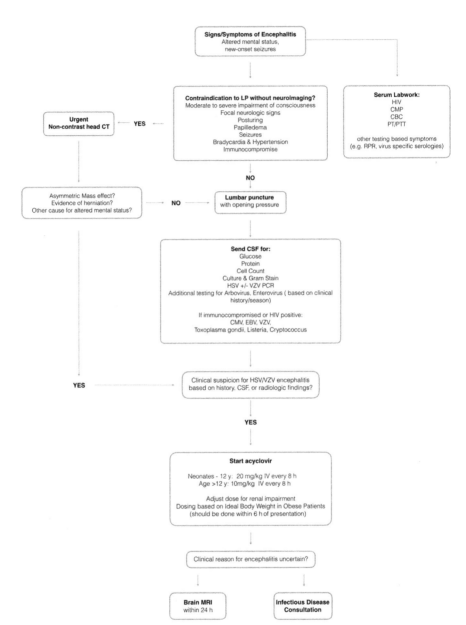

Fig. 1. Algorithm for diagnostic workup of encephalitis in the ED setting blood count. CMP, complete metabolic panel; IV, intravenous; PT/PTT, prothrombin time/partial thromboplastin.

other causes of viral encephalitis.[43,47] As a consequence, molecular (eg, PCR) and serologic testing are important for establishing a specific diagnosis (see **Table 4**). During early infection, initial diagnostic tests may be negative. Approximately 5% to 10% of adults with HSV encephalitis will initially have a normal CSF profile and a negative HSV PCR. In patients in whom the diagnosis is strongly suspected, a repeat LP at 24 to 48 hours is recommended.[39] From the perspective of emergency medicine, treatable causes of viral encephalitis are limited predominantly to HSV and VZV, and it is unlikely that sending a diverse battery of expensive diagnostic molecular tests will influence immediate care. However, it can be helpful to have the microbiology laboratory save CSF so that other clinicians can expand the initial diagnostic workup as needed without repeating the LP.

MRI is significantly more sensitive than CT in detecting early cerebral changes in viral encephalitis. In HSV encephalitis, CT is abnormal in approximately a quarter of patients. MRI is abnormal in approximately 90% of patients, with the most characteristic findings being edematous changes in the orbital surfaces of the frontal lobes and medial temporal lobe.[39] MRI also offers the advantage of identifying alternative causes of encephalitis, and thus, should be performed on all patients with suspected encephalitis in whom the diagnosis remains uncertain.[39,51]

An electroencephalogram (EEG) does not need to be performed routinely in all patients with suspected encephalitis. However, it is a potentially useful adjunct in several situations. First, in patients who are comatose or poorly responsive, EEG may reveal non-convulsive status epilepticus requiring antiepileptic management. In a subset of patients presenting with psychiatric symptoms, an abnormal EEG can point to an organic cause. For instance, HSV encephalitis is associated with characteristic non-specific diffuse high-amplitude slow waves, sometimes with temporal lobe spike-and-wave activity and periodic lateralized epileptiform discharges.[39]

Treatment

The management of encephalitis should be directed toward the underlying cause. Because no clinical sign, symptom, or CSF finding can reliably differentiate HSV from other viral causes of encephalitis, the initiation of empiric treatment with intravenous acyclovir is indicated in any patient suspected to have viral encephalitis until a definitive diagnosis can be achieved. The most significant factor determining outcome in HSV encephalitis is starting antiviral treatment as early as possible, ideally within 6 hours of presentation.[52,53] A multicenter observational study of 93 patients found that the only 2 factors significantly associated with poor outcome were how sick the patient was at presentation (Simplified Acute Physiology score >27) and the initiation of acyclovir more than 2 days after initial presentation.[54]

In the study mentioned above, 41% of patients did not have acyclovir initiated until after 2 days of presentation.[54] This proportion of patients was similar to a second retrospective study of 184 patients in which acyclovir was initiated more than 1 day after hospital admission in 37% of patients eventually diagnosed with HSV encephalitis.[55] These data suggest that HSV encephalitis can be difficult to diagnose and requires a high degree of initial clinical suspicion. In a retrospective study, several patient characteristics were significantly associated with delay of acyclovir initiation, including severe underlying disease (odds ratio [OR] 4.1; 95% CI 1.5–11.7), alcohol abuse (OR 3.4; 95% CI 1.3–8.9), delay of greater than 1 day from admission to first brain imaging (OR 8.4; 95% CI 3.9–18.0), and a finding of less than 10 leukocytes/mm^3 in CSF at admission (OR 2.5; 95% CI 0.7–5.8).

Acyclovir is dosed according to weight and age. The ideal body weight (IBW) should be used to calculate the acyclovir dose (males: IBW [kg] = 50 kg + 2.3 kg for each inch over 5 feet; females: IBW [kg] = 45.5 kg + 2.3 kg for each inch over 5 feet).[56] The dose should be reduced in patients with pre-existing renal impairment because acyclovir is renally excreted. In order to help prevent acyclovir-induced crystalluria and nephrotoxicity, patients should be well hydrated to maintain adequate urine output. Concurrent administration of nephrotoxic drugs should be minimized.

BRAIN ABSCESS

A brain abscess is a collection of purulent material resulting from infection within the brain parenchyma. Focal inflammation and edema (early cerebritis) expand and progress over days to a wider inflammatory response in the white matter, surrounding an increasingly necrotic core (late cerebritis). In the course of a few weeks, a collagenous capsule surrounds and walls off the core, although surrounding inflammation and edema may persist. A predisposing contiguous focus of infection is present in more than half of all cases of bacterial (pyogenic) abscess, with otitis, mastoiditis, sinusitis, meningitis, and odontogenic infections being the most common.[57] Metastatic or hematogenous seeding of the brain parenchyma from a distant source of infection (eg, bacterial endocarditis, congenital heart disease with right-to-left shunt, pulmonary infection) accounts for up to a third of cases. Traumatic inoculation through gunshot wounds and other penetrating injuries can likewise predispose to brain abscess formation, as can open neurosurgical procedures.

Streptococcus and *Staphylococcus* species are implicated in the vast majority of bacterial brain abscesses, although Gram-negative bacteria (*Proteus* spp, *Klebsiella* spp, *E coli*, and *Enterobacteriae*) have been found in up to 15% of cases, particularly in Europe, Asia, and Africa.[57] Nearly a quarter of all brain abscesses are polymicrobial in nature. *Nocardia*, fungal (eg, *Aspergillus* spp, *Candida* spp, *C neoformans*), and parasitic (eg, *Toxoplasma gondii*) brain abscesses are most likely to be encountered in the setting of severe immunocompromise (eg, HIV infection, transplantation).

The reported incidence of brain abscess ranges from 0.4 to 0.9 cases per 100,000 persons, with higher incidence reported in immunocompromised populations.[58,59] Most patients present in the third or fourth decade of life, and brain abscess is more commonly diagnosed in men.[57,59] Mortality from brain abscess has historically run as high as 40%, but has decreased to 10% since 2000, owing much to advances in diagnostic imaging and management strategies.[57]

Clinical Presentation

The classic triad of headache, fever, and focal neurologic deficits associated with brain abscess is present in only 20% of patients.[57] Fever is only present in half of the cases.[57] Onset of neurologic symptoms can be subtle and indolent, spanning days to weeks, manifesting as hemiparesis, cranial nerve palsy, gait disorders, or signs and symptoms of increased intracranial pressure (eg, nausea, vomiting, papilledema, altered mental status).[60] Up to a quarter of cases may be accompanied by focal or generalized seizures.[57] Frontal lobe abscess may present as headache and behavioral changes. An occipital lobe abscess, cerebellar abscess, or abscess with concomitant meningitis or intraventricular rupture can present with neck stiffness. In many cases, headache alone may be the only initial symptom of a brain abscess, particularly in its earliest stages. In the absence of associated neurologic findings, a heightened clinical suspicion for brain abscess, particularly in immunocompromised patients, is necessary to carry the evaluation forward.

Diagnosis

Imaging is paramount to diagnosing brain abscess. Emergent CT with contrast can reveal ring-enhancing lesions characteristic of abscess in the late stages of cerebritis and as the lesion encapsulates.[61] MRI with gadolinium remains the most sensitive modality to look for and characterize the extent of brain abscess, particularly in early cerebritis as well as in the posterior fossa (eg, brainstem) where visualization by CT may be limited. Given the hematogenous nature of many brain abscesses, blood cultures can aid with identifying a causative organism in a quarter of cases.[57] In most cases, the CSF is sterile; however, if there is suspicion for concomitant meningitis or abscess rupture into a ventricle, LP may be useful in obtaining CSF for culture. In this situation, contraindications to LP, including the risk for brain herniation due to mass effect, must be carefully weighed against any potential benefit, particularly if neurosurgical aspiration, drainage, or excision of the abscess is already anticipated.

Treatment

A multidisciplinary approach combining surgical and medical therapy to treat brain abscess optimizes clinical outcomes. Neurosurgical consultation should be sought to determine whether an invasive procedure is necessary to obtain a culture from the abscess to guide antibiotic therapy and definitively drain its contents. Stereotactic needle abscess aspiration under CT or other imaging guidance is preferred in most situations, although surgical excision may be needed in others (eg, patients at high risk for brain herniation due to mass effect or with multiloculated abscess).

If surgical intervention is planned within hours and the patient is clinically stable, empiric antibiotic therapy may be withheld to optimize the yield of bacterial cultures obtained from the abscess, but this decision is best made in conjunction with the neurosurgeon. Empiric broad-spectrum antibiotic therapy targeted against *Staphylococcus*, *Streptococcus*, Gram-negative organisms, and anaerobes can be achieved through a combination of intravenous vancomycin, a third- or fourth-generation cephalosporin (eg, ceftriaxone, cefepime), and metronidazole. Long-term intravenous antibiotic therapy, tailored to causative organisms identified on culture, is favored and traditionally averages 6 to 8 weeks.[57]

SPECIAL SITUATIONS
The Febrile Neonate

In infants less than 48 hours old, CNS infection can present as temperature instability, spells of apnea and bradycardia, feeding difficulty, and irritability alternating with lethargy. At greater than 48 hours of age, infants with CNS infection are more likely to present with neurologic symptoms, including seizures, a bulging anterior fontanel, extensor posturing, focal cerebral signs, or cranial nerve palsies. Although the workup and management of an ill-appearing infant are relatively clear-cut (blood, urine, and CSF cultures accompanied by timely initiation of empiric antibiotics), the more common clinical conundrum encountered is the diagnostic workup and management of the well-appearing febrile infant younger than 90 days. Many febrile infants in this age group will have no focus of infection on physical examination, but ~ 10% will have an underlying serious bacterial infection (SBI).[62] Most of these are urinary tract infections (7%–9% overall), whereas meningitis represents less than 0.5%. The low prevalence of meningitis in this population opens the door to a wide variety of practice patterns when it comes to deciding when it is appropriate to perform an LP.[62–64] As infants less than 28 days are at greater risk for SBI (overall prevalence of 11%–25%), the general consensus favors performing an LP in all cases and admitting to the hospital pending culture results.[62] Well-appearing febrile infants 28 to 90 days old present more of a management dilemma. Several criteria (Rochester, Boston, Philadelphia, and subsequent derivations) have been developed to determine which patients should undergo LP in the first place and who should be admitted for empiric antibiotics pending culture results.[65–67] Only the Rochester criteria do not include a mandatory CSF analysis (**Box 1**). In the original study, 1% of the low-risk infants had an SBI, which included urinary tract infections and one case of *N meningitidis* bacteremia.[67] Procalcitonin is a promising

---

Box 1
The Rochester criteria for identifying the febrile neonate at low risk for serious bacterial infection

Rochester Criteria

- Infant appears generally well

- Infant has been previously healthy
  - Born at $\geq$37 weeks' gestation
  - Did not receive perinatal antimicrobial therapy
  - Was not treated for unexplained hyperbilirubinemia
  - Had not yet received antimicrobial agents
  - Had not been previously hospitalized
  - Had no chronic or underlying illness
  - Was not hospitalized longer than the mother

- No evidence of skin, soft tissue, bone, joint, or ear infection

- Laboratory values
  - WBC between greater than 5000 and less than 15,000/mm^3
  - Absolute band count less than or equal to 1500/mm^3
  - Less than or equal to 10 WBC per high-power field on urine microscopic examination
  - Less than or equal to 5 WBC per high-power field in microscopic examination of stool smear for infants presenting with diarrhea

Abbreviation: WBC, white blood cell.
Data from Pantell RH, Newman TB, Bernzweig J, et al. Management and outcomes of care of fever in early infancy. JAMA 2004;291(10):1203–12.

---

marker of SBI (including meningitis) in the pediatric population, but may not be widely available as a rapid diagnostic test.[68] In general, in low-risk infants less than 90 days of age, empiric antibiotics should not be administered without performing an LP.

In addition to SBI, neonates, especially between days 9 and 17 days of life, are at significant risk for HSV-2 infection. Apart from the typical features of infection in neonates, HSV should be suspected if a neonate presents with seizures, hepatic failure, or characteristic skin lesions (present in 35% of neonates with HSV), or if there is a maternal history of HSV-2 genital infection.[69] Empiric antibiotic coverage for the neonate (see **Table 3**) generally consists of a third-generation cephalosporin in combination with ampicillin. Acyclovir should be added if there is sufficient suspicion for HSV infection.

The Elderly Patient

At the opposite end of life's continuum, clinical signs and symptoms of CNS infection vary, and atypical presentations abound. Fever, headache, and neck stiffness are less common features in older patients with bacterial meningitis than non-specific symptoms such as altered mental status, stupor, or coma.[70–73] Kernig's and Brudzinski's signs are also less likely to be present or reliable. In light of this, performing an LP as part of the evaluation of mental status change, even in the absence of fever, should be strongly considered in this population. In contrast to younger adults where bacterial meningitis due to *N meningitidis* is common, patients 65 years and older are more likely to develop meningitis due to *S pneumoniae*, *L monocytogenes* or gram-negative bacteria, or of an unknown origin.[70,71] Empiric antibiotic therapy in the elderly patient should therefore include expanded coverage for *L monocytogenes* with intravenous ampicillin in addition to vancomycin and a third-generation cephalosporin.

Although the differential diagnoses for mental status change and behavioral changes in the elderly patient can be wide ranging, HSV encephalitis should always be considered. In a Swedish national retrospective study, HSV encephalitis was more commonly seen in those greater than the age of 60 years and was associated with significantly greater mortality in those older than 70 years.[74] If the clinical suspicion for HSV encephalitis is high, an LP should be performed and empiric acyclovir started pending molecular testing of the CSF for HSV.

Patients with Exposure to Arthropod Vectors

Arthropod vectors, including ticks and mosquitoes, can transmit a range of pathogens capable of causing CNS infection. Lyme disease, a tick-borne infection associated predominantly with the spirochete *Borrelia burgdorferi* and the most common vector-borne illness in the United States, can lead to neurologic disease in up to 12% of untreated patients.[75] Lymphocytic meningitis and encephalitis associated with Lyme disease are acute in onset and can be hard to distinguish from viral CNS infections. Lyme meningitis is often associated with cranial neuropathies, particularly involving the seventh cranial nerve (facial nerve palsy) as well as radiculoneuritis leading to pain in peripheral nerve distributions. In patients with suspected CNS infection due to *B burgdorferi*, CSF should be sent to assess for presence of antibodies to this pathogen. Antibiotic therapy should consist of intravenous ceftriaxone, cefotaxime, or penicillin G. Rocky Mountain Spotted Fever (RMSF), an infection caused by *Rickettsia rickettsii*, is classically associated with a constellation of fever, headache, and a diffuse macular and/or petechial rash that is inclusive of the palms and soles. In some cases, a lymphocytic meningitis and encephalitis can also be seen with RMSF. Doxycycline is the preferred antibiotic for treating RMSF. Human monocytic ehrlichiosis (HME) due to *Ehrlichia chaffeensis* and human granulocytic anaplasmosis (HGA) due to *Anaplasma phagocytophilum* are likewise tick-borne and can manifest with CSF lymphocytic pleocytosis; both are also treated with doxycycline. Apart from ticks, mosquito vectors can carry arboviruses (eg, West Nile virus, St. Louis encephalitis virus, Eastern and Western equine encephalitis virus) responsible for causing meningitis and/or encephalitis as already discussed before.

Arthropod-borne infections follow seasonal and geographic patterns centered on the life cycle and distribution of the vectors. Infections generally peak in the warm, summer months (June, July, and August) when vectors are active and patients are most likely to come into contact with them. Vectors such as the *Ixodes* tick that transmits Lyme disease are found primarily in the eastern United States, whereas the *Dermacentor* tick responsible for RMSF has a wider distribution across southeastern and south-central states. Infections associated with these ticks tend to fall along similar geographic lines. The same can be said of HME and HGA. Therefore, knowledge of the geographic distribution of potential arthropod vectors and careful assessment of other epidemiologic risk factors in combination with a recent history of arthropod exposure and/or bite are important when considering the diagnosis of an arthropod-borne CNS infection.

Human Immunodeficiency Virus and Other Immunocompromised States

HIV infection preferentially impairs cell-mediated immunity, predisposing patients to viral, fungal, and parasitic diseases. In addition to the common CNS infections seen in the general population, HIV-related CNS infections are frequently opportunistic, stemming from the reactivation of latent pathogens such as JC virus, EBV, CMV, and *T gondii*.[76,77] Disseminated histoplasmosis with CNS involvement can result from either acute infection or reactivation. Susceptibility to such infections occurs when the CD4$^+$ count falls to less than 200 cells per microliter, and many are considered AIDS-defining illnesses.

Opportunistic CNS infection should always be considered in patients with advanced HIV who present with signs or symptoms of CNS infection, including altered mental status, fever, headache, seizures, or focal neurologic signs. The underlying cause hinges on the overall clinical presentation, time course of disease, CSF analysis, and radiographic features (**Table 5**). Chronic headache with indolent symptoms (eg, low-grade fever) can be characteristic of CNS tuberculosis as well as fungal meningitis due to *C neoformans*, *C immitis*, or *H capsulatum*. Multiple brain abscesses on imaging and a history of a positive *T gondii* serum immunoglobulin G (IgG) should trigger concern for toxoplasmosis. Coinfections may be present in up to 15% of patients.[76] The initial diagnostic workup for patients with HIV infection and presumed CNS opportunistic infection is outlined in **Fig. 2**. Treatment depends on the most likely cause and should be initially broad pending the results of this workup. In addition to empiric antibiotic therapy, treatment may consist of initiating or continuing antiretroviral therapy (ART). Paradoxic worsening of the infection following initiation of ART therapy can occur as a result of immune reconstitution inflammatory syndrome, a consequence of exaggerated activation of the recovering immune system classically encountered in patients with tuberculosis, cryptococcal meningitis, or progressive multifocal leukoencephalopathy.[78]

Although syphilis can cause CNS infections in immunocompetent patients, neurosyphilis has become closely associated with coexisting HIV infection in the post-penicillin era.[79–81] In general, the neurologic manifestations of syphilis are classified as either early or late neurosyphilis. Early symptomatic neurosyphilis (also known as acute syphilitic meningitis) usually occurs within the first 12 months of infection and involves diffuse inflammation of the meninges, resulting in headache, photophobia, nausea, vomiting, and cranial nerve palsies.[79] Ocular findings, most commonly uveitis, can also be observed.[81] Acute syphilitic meningitis, with and without ocular manifestations, has become the most common neurologic infection in HIV patients and can occur even after the patient received initial treatment of primary or secondary syphilis.[81] Late neurosyphilis can take upwards of 15 to 20 years to develop and includes manifestations such as meningovascular syphilis, tabes dorsalis, and CNS gummas. A low CD4$^+$ count (<350 cells/mL) is an independent risk factor for developing neurosyphilis.[80] For patients suspected of having neurosyphilis, a serum nontreponemal test, usually a rapid plasma reagin or Venereal Disease Research Laboratory (VDRL), should be sent but may be nonreactive in late disease. In such cases, a serum treponemal test, such as fluorescent treponemal antibody absorption (FTA-ABS), should also be sent because these tests remain reactive lifelong after infection with syphilis. The diagnosis of neurosyphilis is usually established by the presence of a reactive CSF-VDRL but cannot be excluded if the test is nonreactive.[81] Treatment with penicillin G is the standard for neurosyphilis.

Apart from HIV, other immunocompromised patients, particularly those receiving immunosuppressive therapy for solid organ or hematopoietic stem cell transplantation or those with hematologic malignancy, are not only at increased risk for bacterial CNS infection but opportunistic infections as well.[82–84] Solid-organ transplant recipients are at heightened susceptibility for developing brain abscess due to *Nocardia* as well as fungi (eg, *Aspergillus* spp, *Candida* spp). In addition to empiric antibiotic therapy directed against usual bacteria, appropriate therapy targeted toward these organisms may be warranted. Consultation with an infectious disease specialist can be beneficial in optimizing empiric therapy in these complex patient populations.

Table 5
Clinical presentation, diagnosis, and treatment of opportunistic infections in HIV disease

Infection	Typical CD4$^+$ Cell Count at Presentation (Cells/µL)	Clinical Presentation	Temporal Evolution	Special CSF Tests (Sensitivity/Specificity)	Typical Radiographic Appearance	Treatment = Antiretroviral Therapy AND
CMV encephalitis	<50	Altered mental status, seizures	Days	CMV PCR (>90%/>90%)	Usually normal; may have evidence of ventriculitis with ventriculomegaly and periventricular enhancement on MRI	Ganciclovir
Cryptococcal meningitis	<50 (rarely up to 200)	Fever, headache, altered mental status, vomiting	Days	Elevated opening pressure; cryptococcal antigen	May be normal; "Punched-out" cystic lesions on MRI if cryptococcocomas develop	Amphotericin B and flucytosine
Progressive multifocal leukoencephalopathy	<100	Altered mental status, focal neurologic deficits	Weeks to months	JC virus PCR (50%–90%/ 90%–100%)	Hyperintense areas in white matter on T2-FLAIR imaging	—
CNS lymphoma	<100	Altered mental status, focal neurologic deficits, headache	Weeks to months	EBV PCR (100%/50% specific)	Usually solitary, heterogeneously enhancing lesions with mass effect	—
Toxoplasma encephalitis	<200	Fever, headache, altered mental status	Days	*T gondii* PCR (50%–80%/100%)	Multiple ring-enhancing lesions with mass effect	Pyrimethamine, folinic acid, and sulfadiazine OR trimethoprim-sulfamethoxazole
Tuberculous meningitis	<200	Altered mental status, cranial neuropathies	Days to weeks	Culture and acid-fast bacilli stain (>80%)	Rarely basilar enhancement; possibly abscesses or tuberculomas	Rifampin, isoniazid, pyrazinamide, ethambutol
Acute syphilitic meningitis	<350	Headache, photophobia, emesis. Ocular manifestations (CN palsies, uveitis, optic neuritis) commonly associated	Within 12 mo (chronic neurosyphilis 5–20 y)	CSF VDRL (CSF FTA-ABS more sensitive but less specific)	No pathognomonic findings	Pencillin-G 3–4 million units every 4 h × 10–14 d

Abbreviation: FLAIR, fluid-attenuated inversion recovery.

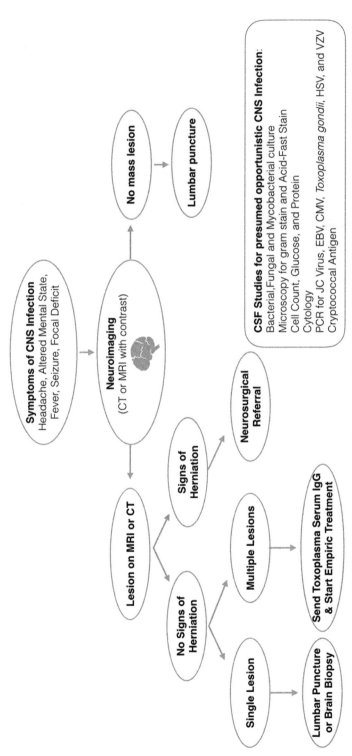

Fig. 2. Workup for presumed CNS infection in a patient with advanced HIV disease. *(Modified from* Tan IL, Smith BR, von Geldern G, et al. HIV-associated opportunistic infections of the CNS. Lancet Neurol 2012;11(7):605–17.)

Cerebrospinal Fluid Shunt Infections

CSF shunt infection can be a cause for shunt failure and manifests with signs of increased intracranial pressure and hydrocephalus (eg, depressed level of consciousness, nausea, vomiting, headache, irritability in young children). It is the most common complication of CSF shunt surgery (>11% in one multicenter prospective study) and most often seen within 6 months of shunt placement due to intraoperative contamination with skin flora.[85,86] As far as clinical presentation, there are several factors that increase the likelihood that shunt infection is the underlying cause of shunt malfunction. These factors include a history of recent shunt revision (adjusted odds ratio [aOR] 2.4; 95% CI 1.3–4.4), presence of fever (aOR 8.4; 95% CI 4.3–16.3), and white blood cell greater than 15,000/μL (aOR 3.2; 95% CI 1.5–6.6).[87,88] For patients with ventriculoperitoneal shunts, abdominal pain and peritonitis are less commonly seen, but are highly predictive of shunt infection.[89] Evaluation of patients with suspected CSF shunt infection includes imaging to evaluate for shunt malfunction with either a head CT (sensitivity of 53%–92%) or rapid cranial MRI (sensitivity of 51%–59%), shunt series radiographs, and sampling of CSF through LP or shunt aspiration, and should involve neurosurgical consultation.[90] Empiric antibiotic therapy should be directed primarily against skin flora and nosocomial pathogens, including *Streptococcus aureus* and *Pseudomonas aeruginosa*.

SUMMARY

Despite the broad range of causative organisms and clinical presentations possible in CNS infection, the initial ED evaluation is fundamentally the same. First, a high index of clinical suspicion is necessary. The diagnosis should be considered in patients presenting with headache, fever, altered mental status, or behavior change, especially in the young, the elderly, or the immunocompromised. Second, the clinical history and physical examination must be viewed as a whole when deciding whether further evaluation for CNS infection is warranted. If a patient has focal neurologic deficits, signs of increased intracranial pressure, a history of neurosurgical procedure or immunocompromise, or is obtunded, neuroimaging should be performed to rule out asymmetric mass effect before LP. As time is of the essence, empiric antibiotic coverage tailored to the patient's age and clinical risk factors should be initiated as soon as possible if bacterial meningitis or HSV encephalitis is suspected. Finally, benign imaging and CSF analysis can be falsely reassuring early on in disease, and an aggressive course of action is always prudent in cases where a strong clinical suspicion for serious CNS infection exists.

REFERENCES

1. Tintinalli JE, Stapczynski JS. Tintinalli's emergency medicine: a comprehensive study guide. 7th edition. New York: McGraw-Hill; 2011.
2. Fitch MT, Abrahamian FM, Moran GJ, et al. Emergency department management of meningitis and encephalitis. Infect Dis Clin North Am 2008;22(1):33–52.
3. Logan SAE, MacMahon E. Viral meningitis. BMJ 2008;336(7634):36–40.
4. Gottfredsson M, Perfect JR. Fungal meningitis. Semin Neurol 2000;20(3):307–22.
5. Smith RM, Schaefer MK, Kainer MA, et al. Fungal infections associated with contaminated methylprednisolone injections. N Engl J Med 2013;369(17): 1598–609.
6. Centers for Disease Control and Prevention (CDC). Progress toward elimination of Haemophilus influenzae type b invasive disease among infants and

children–United States, 1998-2000. MMWR Morb Mortal Wkly Rep 2002;51(11): 234–7.

7. Castelblanco RL, Lee M, Hasbun R. Epidemiology of bacterial meningitis in the USA from 1997 to 2010: a population-based observational study. Lancet Infect Dis 2014;14(9):813–9.

8. Brouwer MC, Tunkel AR, van de Beek D. Epidemiology, diagnosis, and antimicrobial treatment of acute bacterial meningitis. Clin Microbiol Rev 2010;23(3): 467–92.

9. Takhar SS, Ting SA, Camargo CA, et al. U.S. emergency department visits for meningitis, 1993–2008. Acad Emerg Med 2012;19(6):632–9.

10. Waghdhare S, Kalantri A, Joshi R, et al. Accuracy of physical signs for detecting meningitis: a hospital-based diagnostic accuracy study. Clin Neurol Neurosurg 2010;112(9):752–7.

11. Attia J, Hatala R, Cook DJ, et al. The rational clinical examination. Does this adult patient have acute meningitis? JAMA 1999;282(2):175–81.

12. Durand ML, Calderwood SB, Weber DJ, et al. Acute bacterial meningitis in adults. A review of 493 episodes. N Engl J Med 1993;328(1):21–8.

13. Sigurdardóttir B, Björnsson OM, Jónsdóttir KE, et al. Acute bacterial meningitis in adults. A 20-year overview. Arch Intern Med 1997;157(4):425–30.

14. Amarilyo G, Alper A, Ben-Tov A, et al. Diagnostic accuracy of clinical symptoms and signs in children with meningitis. Pediatr Emerg Care 2011;27(3):196–9.

15. Ward MA, Greenwood TM, Kumar DR, et al. Josef Brudzinski and Vladimir Mikhailovich Kernig: signs for diagnosing meningitis. Clin Med Res 2010;8(1):13–7.

16. Nakao JH, Jafri FN, Shah K, et al. Jolt accentuation of headache and other clinical signs: poor predictors of meningitis in adults. Am J Emerg Med 2014;32(1):24–8.

17. Thomas KE, Hasbun R, Jekel J, et al. The diagnostic accuracy of Kernig's sign, Brudzinski's sign, and nuchal rigidity in adults with suspected meningitis. Clin Infect Dis 2002;35(1):46–52.

18. Uchihara T, Tsukagoshi H. Jolt accentuation of headache: the most sensitive sign of CSF pleocytosis. Headache 1991;31(3):167–71.

19. Aronin SI, Peduzzi P, Quagliarello VJ. Community-acquired bacterial meningitis: risk stratification for adverse clinical outcome and effect of antibiotic timing. Ann Intern Med 1998;129(11):862–9.

20. Proulx N, Fréchette D, Toye B, et al. Delays in the administration of antibiotics are associated with mortality from adult acute bacterial meningitis. QJM 2005;98(4): 291–8.

21. Auburtin M, Wolff M, Charpentier J, et al. Detrimental role of delayed antibiotic administration and penicillin-nonsusceptible strains in adult intensive care unit patients with pneumococcal meningitis: the PNEUMOREA prospective multi-center study. Crit Care Med 2006;34(11):2758–65.

22. Michael B, Menezes BF, Cunniffe J, et al. Effect of delayed lumbar punctures on the diagnosis of acute bacterial meningitis in adults. Emerg Med J 2010;27(6): 433–8.

23. van Crevel H, Hijdra A, de Gans J. Lumbar puncture and the risk of herniation: when should we first perform CT? J Neurol 2002;249(2):129–37.

24. Tunkel AR, Hartman BJ, Kaplan SL, et al. Practice guidelines for the management of bacterial meningitis. Clin Infect Dis 2004;39(9):1267–84.

25. Glimaker M, Johansson B, Grindborg O, et al. Adult bacterial meningitis: earlier treatment and improved outcome following guideline revision promoting prompt lumbar puncture. Clin Infect Dis 2015;60(8):1162–9.

26. van de Beek D, de Gans J, Spanjaard L, et al. Clinical features and prognostic factors in adults with bacterial meningitis. N Engl J Med 2004;351(18):1849–59.

27. Ray P, Badarou-Acossi G, Viallon A, et al. Accuracy of the cerebrospinal fluid results to differentiate bacterial from non bacterial meningitis, in case of negative gram-stained smear. Am J Emerg Med 2007;25(2):179–84.

28. Viallon A, Desseigne N, Marjollet O, et al. Meningitis in adult patients with a negative direct cerebrospinal fluid examination: value of cytochemical markers for differential diagnosis. Crit Care 2011;15(3):R136.

29. Posner JB, Plum F. Independence of blood and cerebrospinal fluid lactate. Arch Neurol 1967;16(5):492–6.

30. Sakushima K, Hayashino Y, Kawaguchi T, et al. Diagnostic accuracy of cerebrospinal fluid lactate for differentiating bacterial meningitis from aseptic meningitis: a meta-analysis. J Infect 2011;62(4):255–62.

31. Assicot M, Gendrel D, Carsin H, et al. High serum procalcitonin concentrations in patients with sepsis and infection. Lancet 1993;341(8844):515–8.

32. Schuetz P, Müller B, Christ-Crain M, et al. Procalcitonin to initiate or discontinue antibiotics in acute respiratory tract infections. Evid Based Child Health 2013; 8(4):1297–371.

33. Nigrovic LE, Kuppermann N, Malley R. Development and validation of a multivariable predictive model to distinguish bacterial from aseptic meningitis in children in the post-Haemophilus influenzae era. Pediatrics 2002;110(4):712–9.

34. Nigrovic LE, Kuppermann N, Macias CG, et al. Clinical prediction rule for identifying children with cerebrospinal fluid pleocytosis at very low risk of bacterial meningitis. JAMA 2007;297(1):52–60.

35. Nigrovic LE, Malley R, Kuppermann N. Meta-analysis of bacterial meningitis score validation studies. Arch Dis Child 2012;97(9):799–805.

36. Tauber MG, Khayam-Bashi H, Sande MA. Effects of ampicillin and corticosteroids on brain water content, cerebrospinal fluid pressure, and cerebrospinal fluid lactate levels in experimental pneumococcal meningitis. J Infect Dis 1985; 151(3):528–34.

37. Brouwer MC, McIntyre P, Prasad K, et al. Corticosteroids for acute bacterial meningitis. Cochrane Database Syst Rev 2013;(6):CD004405.

38. Steiner I, Benninger F. Update on herpes virus infections of the nervous system. Curr Neurol Neurosci Rep 2013;13(12):414.

39. Solomon T, Michael BD, Smith PE, et al. Management of suspected viral encephalitis in adults—Association of British Neurologists and British Infection Association National Guidelines. J Infect 2012;64(4):347–73.

40. Johnson RT. Acute encephalitis. Clin Infect Dis 1996;23(2):219–24.

41. Murthy SNK, Faden HS, Cohen ME, et al. Acute disseminated encephalomyelitis in children. Pediatrics 2002;110(2 Pt 1):e21.

42. Granerod J, Ambrose HE, Davies NW, et al. Causes of encephalitis and differences in their clinical presentations in England: a multicentre, population-based prospective study. Lancet Infect Dis 2010;10(12):835–44.

43. Greenlee JE. Encephalitis and postinfectious encephalitis. Continuum (Minneap Minn) 2012;18:1271–89.

44. Whitley RJ, Lakeman F. Herpes simplex virus infections of the central nervous system: therapeutic and diagnostic considerations. Clin Infect Dis 1995;20(2): 414–20.

45. Grahn A, Studahl M. Varicella-zoster virus infections of the central nervous system—prognosis, diagnostics and treatment. J Infect 2015;71(3):281–93.

46. Koskiniemi M, Rantalaiho T, Piiparinen H, et al. Infections of the central nervous system of suspected viral origin: a collaborative study from Finland. J Neurovirol 2001;7(5):400–8.
47. Whitley RJ. Herpes simplex encephalitis: clinical assessment. JAMA 1982; 247(3):317.
48. Deresiewicz RL, Thaler SJ, Hsu L, et al. Clinical and neuroradiographic manifestations of eastern equine encephalitis. N Engl J Med 1997;336(26):1867–74.
49. Hayes EB, Sejvar JJ, Zaki SR, et al. Virology, pathology, and clinical manifestations of West Nile virus disease. Emerg Infect Dis 2005;11(8):1174–9.
50. Whitley RJ, Gnann JW. Viral encephalitis: familiar infections and emerging pathogens. Lancet 2002;359(9305):507–13.
51. Domingues R, Fink MC, Tsanaclis AM, et al. Diagnosis of herpes simplex encephalitis by magnetic resonance imaging and polymerase chain reaction assay of cerebrospinal fluid. J Neurol Sci 1998;157(2):148–53.
52. Ibitoye RT, Sarkar P, Rajbhandari S. Pitfalls in the management of herpes simplex virus encephalitis. BMJ Case Rep 2012;2012.
53. Sili U, Kaya A, Mert A, et al. Herpes simplex virus encephalitis: clinical manifestations, diagnosis and outcome in 106 adult patients. J Clin Virol 2014;60(2): 112–8.
54. Raschilas F, Wolff M, Delatour F, et al. Outcome of and prognostic factors for herpes simplex encephalitis in adult patients: results of a multicenter study. Clin Infect Dis 2002;35(3):254–60.
55. Poissy J, Wolff M, Dewilde A, et al. Factors associated with delay to acyclovir administration in 184 patients with herpes simplex virus encephalitis. Clin Microbiol Infect 2009;15(6):560–4.
56. Stehman CR, Buckley RG, DosSantos FL, et al. Bedside estimation of patient height for calculating ideal body weight in the emergency department. J Emerg Med 2011;41(1):97–101.
57. Brouwer MC, Coutinho JM, van de Beek D. Clinical characteristics and outcome of brain abscess: systematic review and meta-analysis. Neurology 2014;82(9): 806–13.
58. Nicolosi A, Hauser WA, Musicco M, et al. Incidence and prognosis of brain abscess in a defined population: Olmsted County, Minnesota, 1935-1981. Neuroepidemiology 1991;10(3):122–31.
59. Helweg-Larsen J, Astradsson A, Richhall H, et al. Pyogenic brain abscess, a 15 year survey. BMC Infect Dis 2012;12:332.
60. Brouwer MC, Tunkel AR, McKhann GM, et al. Brain abscess. N Engl J Med 2014; 371(5):447–56.
61. Rath TJ, Hughes M, Arabi M, et al. Imaging of cerebritis, encephalitis, and brain abscess. Neuroimaging Clin N Am 2012;22(4):585–607.
62. Biondi EA, Byington CL. Evaluation and management of febrile, well-appearing young infants. Infect Dis Clin North Am 2015;29(3):575–85.
63. Aronson PL, Thurm C, Alpern ER, et al. Variation in care of the febrile young infant <90 days in US pediatric emergency departments. Pediatrics 2014;134(4): 667–77.
64. Pantell RH, Newman TB, Bernzweig J, et al. Management and outcomes of care of fever in early infancy. JAMA 2004;291(10):1203–12.
65. Baker MD, Bell LM, Avner JR. Outpatient management without antibiotics of fever in selected infants. N Engl J Med 1993;329(20):1437–41.

66. Baskin MN, O'Rourke EJ, Fleisher GR. Outpatient treatment of febrile infants 28 to 89 days of age with intramuscular administration of ceftriaxone. J Pediatr 1992; 120(1):22–7.

67. Jaskiewicz JA, McCarthy CA, Richardson AC, et al. Febrile infants at low risk for serious bacterial infection–an appraisal of the Rochester criteria and implications for management. Febrile Infant Collaborative Study Group. Pediatrics 1994;94(3): 390–6.

68. van Rossum AMC, Wulkan RW, Oudesluys-Murphy AM. Procalcitonin as an early marker of infection in neonates and children. Lancet Infect Dis 2004;4(10): 620–30.

69. James SH, Kimberlin DW. Neonatal herpes simplex virus infection: epidemiology and treatment. Clin Perinatol 2015;42(1):47–59, viii.

70. Domingo P, Pomar V, de Benito N, et al. The spectrum of acute bacterial meningitis in elderly patients. BMC Infect Dis 2013;13:108.

71. Wang AY, Machicado JD, Khoury NT, et al. Community-acquired meningitis in older adults: clinical features, etiology, and prognostic factors. J Am Geriatr Soc 2014;62(11):2064–70.

72. Magazzini S, Nazerian P, Vanni S, et al. Clinical picture of meningitis in the adult patient and its relationship with age. Intern Emerg Med 2012;7(4):359–64.

73. Lai W-A, Chen S-F, Tsai N-W, et al. Clinical characteristics and prognosis of acute bacterial meningitis in elderly patients over 65: a hospital-based study. BMC Geriatr 2011;11:91.

74. Hjalmarsson A, Blomqvist P, Sköldenberg B. Herpes simplex encephalitis in Sweden, 1990-2001: incidence, morbidity, and mortality. Clin Infect Dis 2007; 45(7):875–80.

75. Bacon RM, Kugeler KJ, Mead PS, et al. Surveillance for Lyme disease–United States, 1992-2006. MMWR Surveill Summ 2008;57(10):1–9.

76. Tan IL, Smith BR, von Geldern G, et al. HIV-associated opportunistic infections of the CNS. Lancet Neurol 2012;11(7):605–17.

77. Arribas JR. Cytomegalovirus encephalitis. Ann Intern Med 1996;125(7):577.

78. Müller M, Wandel S, Colebunders R, et al. Immune reconstitution inflammatory syndrome in patients starting antiretroviral therapy for HIV infection: a systematic review and meta-analysis. Lancet Infect Dis 2010;10(4):251–61.

79. Ghanem KG. REVIEW: Neurosyphilis: a historical perspective and review. CNS Neurosci Ther 2010;16(5):e157–68.

80. Ghanem KG, Moore RD, Rompalo AM, et al. Neurosyphilis in a clinical cohort of HIV-1-infected patients. AIDS 2008;22(10):1145–51.

81. González-Duarte A, López ZM. Neurological findings in early syphilis: a comparison between HIV positive and negative patients. Neurol Int 2013;5(4):e19.

82. Davis JA, Horn DL, Marr KA, et al. Central nervous system involvement in cryptococcal infection in individuals after solid organ transplantation or with AIDS. Transpl Infect Dis 2009;11(5):432–7.

83. Ohara H, Kataoka H, Nakamichi K, et al. Favorable outcome after withdrawal of immunosuppressant therapy in progressive multifocal leukoencephalopathy after renal transplantation: case report and literature review. J Neurol Sci 2014; 341(1–2):144–6.

84. Yehia BR, Blumberg EA. Mycobacterium tuberculosis infection in liver transplantation. Liver Transpl 2010;16(10):1129–35.

85. Simon TD, Hall M, Riva-Cambrin J, et al. Infection rates following initial cerebrospinal fluid shunt placement across pediatric hospitals in the United States. Clinical article. J Neurosurg Pediatr 2009;4(2):156–65.

86. Wallace AN, McConathy J, Menias CO, et al. Imaging evaluation of CSF shunts. AJR Am J Roentgenol 2014;202(1):38–53.

87. Garton HJ, Kestle JR, Drake JM. Predicting shunt failure on the basis of clinical symptoms and signs in children. J Neurosurg 2001;94(2):202–10.

88. Rogers EA, Kimia A, Madsen JR, et al. Predictors of ventricular shunt infection among children presenting to a pediatric emergency department. Pediatr Emerg Care 2012;28(5):405–9.

89. Piatt JH, Garton HJL. Clinical diagnosis of ventriculoperitoneal shunt failure among children with hydrocephalus. Pediatr Emerg Care 2008;24(4):201–10.

90. Boyle TP, Nigrovic LE. Radiographic evaluation of pediatric cerebrospinal fluid shunt malfunction in the emergency setting. Pediatr Emerg Care 2015;31(6): 435–40.

Diagnosis of Acute Neurologic Emergencies in Pregnant and Postpartum Women

Andrea G. Edlow, MD, MSc[a], Brian L. Edlow, MD[b],
Jonathan A. Edlow, MD[c],*

KEYWORDS

- Eclampsia • Posterior reversible encephalopathy syndrome
- Reversible cerebrovascular constriction syndrome
- Cerebral venous sinus thrombosis • Pregnancy

KEY POINTS

- Pregnant and postpartum patients with headache and seizures are often diagnosed with preeclampsia or eclampsia because they are the most common conditions; however, other etiologies must be considered.
- Most cases of cerebral venous sinus thrombosis present in the early postpartum period.
- Although stroke and other cerebrovascular diseases are uncommon in pregnant women, the incidence is higher than in age and sex-matched nonpregnant individuals.
- Computed tomography scanning is insensitive to many of the acute neurologic conditions that affect pregnant and postpartum women.

INTRODUCTION

Acute neurologic symptoms in pregnant and postpartum women may be owing to an exacerbation of a preexisting neurologic condition (eg, multiple sclerosis or a known seizure disorder) or to the initial presentation of a non–pregnancy-related problem

Disclosures: None.
Contributors: Dr J.A. Edlow wrote the first draft and assumes overall responsibility for the article. All of the authors helped to organize the information, write and edit subsequent drafts of the article.
Conflicts of Interest: Dr J.A. Edlow receives fees for expert testimony; however, none is felt to represent a conflict for this article.
[a] Division of Maternal-Fetal Medicine, Department of Obstetrics and Gynecology, Mother Infant Research Institute, Tufts Medical Center, 800 Washington Street, Box 394, Boston, MA 02111, USA; [b] Division of Neurocritical Care and Emergency Neurology, Department of Neurology, Massachusetts General Hospital, 175 Cambridge Street, Suite 300, Boston, MA 02114, USA; [c] Department of Emergency Medicine, Beth Israel Deaconess Medical Center, Harvard Medical School, One Deaconess Place, West Clinical Center, 2nd Floor, Boston, MA 02215, USA
* Corresponding author.
E-mail address: jedlow@bidmc.harvard.edu

Emerg Med Clin N Am 34 (2016) 943–965
http://dx.doi.org/10.1016/j.emc.2016.06.014
0733-8627/16/© 2016 Elsevier Inc. All rights reserved.

(eg, a new brain tumor). Alternatively, patients can present with new, acute onset neurologic conditions that are either unique to or precipitated by pregnancy.

In this review, we focus on these latter conditions. The most common diagnostic tool used in emergency medicine to evaluate many of these symptoms—noncontrast head computed tomography (CT)—is often nondiagnostic or falsely negative. Misdiagnosis can result in morbidity or mortality in young, previously healthy individuals. Therefore, if a poor outcome occurs, the medical, social, and medicolegal impact is usually high. For all of these reasons, prompt diagnosis is imperative.

The unique pathophysiologic states of pregnancy and the puerperium have been reviewed.[1–4] Increasing concentrations of estrogen stimulate the production of clotting factors, increasing the risk of thromboembolism. Increases in plasma and total blood volumes increase the risk of hypertension. Elevated progesterone levels in pregnancy increase venous distensibility and, potentially, leakage from small blood vessels. The high estrogen levels decrease in the postpartum period. Combined, these hormonal changes can result in increased permeability of the blood–brain barrier and vasogenic edema.

Preeclampsia, the new onset of hypertension and proteinuria or laboratory abnormalities after 20 weeks in a previously normotensive woman, occurs in 2% to 8% of pregnancies.[5] The incidence of preeclampsia has increased by 25% in the United States over the last 20 years,[6] which has been attributed in part to the increase in maternal obesity and maternal age.[7] Diagnostic criteria for preeclampsia were recently revised.[8] Whereas previously preeclampsia was defined by systolic blood pressures of 140/90 mm Hg or greater and proteinuria of 0.3 g or greater of protein in a 24-hour urine specimen, the new criteria allow for the diagnosis of preeclampsia without proteinuria, permit the use of a spot protein/creatinine ratio or urine dip to diagnose preeclampsia, and rename what was previously called "mild preeclampsia" as "preeclampsia without severe features," among other changes. Preeclampsia is now defined as blood pressures of 140/90 mm Hg or greater on 2 occasions at least 4 hours apart after 20 weeks of gestation in a woman with a previously normal blood pressure, plus either proteinuria, or in the absence of proteinuria, thrombocytopenia, renal insufficiency, impaired liver function, pulmonary edema, or new-onset neurologic symptoms such as visual changes or headache. In practical terms, this means any woman with persistently increased blood pressure and a persistent new headache meets diagnostic criteria for preeclampsia, and the headache would confer the diagnosis of preeclampsia with severe features. However, other neurologic conditions requiring significantly different management than preeclampsia should be considered in these cases. Of note, the revised criteria state that severe range blood pressures (those $\geq$ 160/110 mm Hg) "can be confirmed within a short interval (minutes) to facilitate timely antihypertensive therapy,"[8] to stress that antihypertensive therapy should not be delayed in these women to confirm a diagnosis.

Eclampsia is defined as preeclampsia plus a generalized tonic–clonic seizure in the absence of other conditions that could account for the seizure. Eclamptic seizures occur in up to 0.6% of women with preeclampsia without severe features, and in 2% to 3% of women with preeclampsia with severe features.[9] Of note, eclampsia rarely can present atypically, without elevated pressures or proteinuria so it should remain on the differential for women with new-onset seizures in pregnancy even if the classic criteria of hypertension and proteinuria or laboratory abnormalities are not satisfied.[10–12] Maternal mortality rates for eclamptic women have been reported to be as high as 14% over the past few decades, with the highest rates in developing countries.[13] Although the most common causes of death in eclamptic women are brain ischemia and hemorrhage, most eclampsia-related neurologic events are transient, and long-term deficits are rare in properly managed patients.[14]

However, other conditions, which overlap with eclampsia and with each other, can present similarly.[15,16] These include acute ischemic stroke (AIS), intracerebral hemorrhage (ICH), subarachnoid hemorrhage (SAH), and cerebral venous sinus thrombosis (CVT). Severe vasoconstriction often develops in women with preeclampsia, especially when the blood pressure is poorly controlled. This vasoconstriction can cause brain infarction and/or hemorrhage. A reversible cerebral vasoconstriction syndrome (RCVS)—also referred to as postpartum angiopathy and Call–Fleming syndrome—can develop during the puerperium without hypertension or other features of preeclampsia. Preeclampsia, eclampsia and RCVS can all be complicated by the posterior reversible encephalopathy syndrome (PRES). In fact, 8% to 39% of patients with RCVS have PRES as well.[17,18] PRES is a clinical (headache, seizures, encephalopathy, and visual disturbances) and imaging (reversible vasogenic edema) syndrome that may occur in preeclampsia/eclampsia, RCVS, and other conditions. It is essential to recognize the significant overlap between these various etiologies, which can occur independently or simultaneously. Whereas eclampsia is specific to pregnancy, PRES, RCVS, and CVT also occur in nonpregnant individuals.

This review is intended to help clinicians avoid misdiagnosis in these high-risk patients. We therefore limit the review to clinical manifestations and diagnosis, because once a given diagnosis is established, specific treatments should naturally follow. We have organized the data by presenting symptoms as well as by specific diagnosis. Finally, we have created clinical algorithms based on our interpretation of the existing literature and our practice.

HEADACHE

Roughly 40% of postpartum women have headaches, often during the first week. Primary headache disorders—tension type and migraine—are the most common causes in both pregnant and postpartum women.[19–21] This can paradoxically make correct diagnosis more difficult unless physicians pay careful attention to "red flags" that suggest a secondary cause (**Fig. 1**B). In 1 series, among 95 patients with severe postpartum headache, one-half had tension type (39%) or migraine (11%), followed by preeclampsia/eclampsia (24%) and postdural puncture headache (PDPH; 16%).[22] Pituitary hemorrhage, mass lesions, and CVT each accounted for another 3%. This study was skewed toward sicker, hospitalized patients whose headaches were "resistant to usual therapy."

In general, migraine improves during pregnancy and returns postpartum as estrogen levels decrease.[23–25] Pregnant patients with new, worsening headaches, positional headaches, or headaches that have changed in character suggest the possibility of secondary causes. Although new migraines can develop during pregnancy,[26] migraine should be considered a diagnosis of exclusion. Implicit in the diagnosis of migraine and tension-type headache is the presence of multiple episodes ($\geq$5 episodes for migraine and $\geq$10 for tension-type headache). Therefore, one cannot definitively diagnose a first new headache that develops during pregnancy or the puerperium—or in any other patient for that matter—as a manifestation of a primary headache disorder.

Preeclamptic patients often have bilateral throbbing headaches accompanied by blurred vision and scintillating scotomata. Pregnant women with new headaches must be screened carefully for preeclampsia. Hypertension, epigastric or right upper quadrant abdominal pain, edema, increased deep tendon reflexes, proteinuria, and occasionally agitation or restlessness may accompany the headache.[27–29] Laboratory findings that increase the concern for preeclampsia include thrombocytopenia,

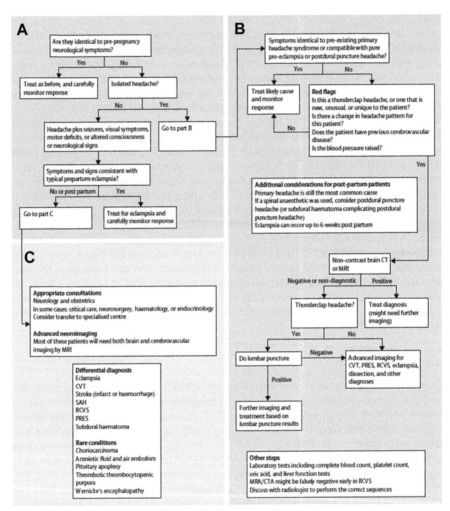

Fig. 1. Diagnostic algorithm for pregnant and postpartum patients presenting with acute neurologic symptoms. (A) Pregnant and post partum women with acute neurologic symptoms. (B) Pregnant and post partum women with isolated headache. (C) Patients with other neurologic symptoms or signs (with or without headache and not thought to be pure eclampsia) or eclamptic patterns not responding to treatment. CT, computed tomography; CVT, cerebral venous thrombosis; PRES, posterior reversible encephalopathy syndrome; RCVS, reversible cerebral vasoconstriction syndrome; SAH, subarachnoid hemorrhage.

hemoconcentration, transaminitis, elevated creatinine, and elevated uric acid. Unfortunately, despite considerable research and progress, there is no current routinely available biomarker to definitively diagnose preeclampsia.[30,31]

Patients with abrupt onset of a severe, unusual headache ("thunderclap headache") require urgent investigation.[32] Large studies evaluating the possible increased incidence of SAH in pregnant and postpartum patients report mixed results, possibly owing to varying methods of case acquisition, as well as the fact that some instances of SAH in these patients are nonaneurysmal.[33–36] Hormonal changes affecting cerebral blood vessels and surges in blood pressure from pushing during labor are

2 potential mechanisms for an increased incidence of aneurysmal SAH.[34] All patients presenting with a thunderclap headache require a thorough evaluation to exclude SAH, usually a head CT scan followed by lumbar puncture if the CT scan is nondiagnostic.

However, if the workup for SAH is negative, disorders such as PRES, CVT, RCVS, and cervicocranial arterial dissections must be considered in pregnant and postpartum patients who present with thunderclap headache (**Fig. 1**). Because CT and lumbar puncture may both be negative in these latter conditions, physicians should strongly consider following up a nondiagnostic CT and lumbar puncture with MRI sequences including diffusion-weighted images as well as vascular studies of the arteries (MR angiogram) and veins (MR venogram). If arterial dissection is suspected, acquisition of T1 fat-saturated images should be considered to increase the sensitivity for detecting a thrombus within a dissection flap.[37]

In patients who have had a spinal or epidural anesthetic, PDPH is an important consideration, and has been estimated to occur in 0.5% to 1.5% of these patients.[38–40] Caused by low intracranial pressure owing to a cerebrospinal fluid leak, headaches, often nuchal and occipital, typically begin 1 to 7 days postpartum, rapidly worsen upon standing, and resolve upon lying flat over 10 to 15 minutes.[20,39] Tinnitus, diplopia, and hypacusia may occur.[20] Symptoms usually resolve within 48 hours of a blood patch. Patients who have not had a spinal or epidural anesthetic may also develop postpartum low-pressure headaches, presumably owing to dural tears from labor-related pushing.

Rare complications of PDPH include subdural hematoma, PRES, and CVT.[41–43] Low intracranial pressure can cause subdural hematoma from the tearing of bridging veins that become taut as the brain sags.[39] Clues to this complication include loss of the postural component of headache (owing to the offsetting effects of low intracranial pressure from the dural puncture and elevated pressure from the subdural hematoma) and lack of response to a blood patch.

Most serious causes of headache are more common postpartum than during pregnancy. Therefore, if migraine or PDPH is not likely based on the history and neurologic examination, physicians must consider these other etiologies.

ACUTE NEUROLOGIC SYMPTOMS AND DEFICITS

Pregnant or postpartum patients who present with acute motor, sensory, or visual findings (with or without headache) may have more serious causes and require urgent, thorough evaluation (see **Fig. 1**). Pregnant patients with acute neurologic deficits most often have migraine with aura, even in the absence of headache (ie, acephalgic migraine). Two studies using different methods both found that of pregnant patients referred for transient motor, sensory or visual symptoms, the vast majority could be ultimately attributed to migraine with aura.[44,45]

Historical clues for a migrainous etiology include gradual onset of the neurologic symptoms and positive phenomenon (such as brightness or shimmering) as opposed to negative ones (blackness or loss of vision).[23] The gradual onset and slow progression over 15 to 30 minutes differentiates migrainous symptoms from those attributable to cerebral ischemia, which are typically maximal at onset, and seizure, which spread more rapidly (ie, over seconds). Another clue that may help to differentiate migraine from vascular thromboembolic disease is the pathophysiologic process of cortical spreading depression that is believed to cause migrainous neurologic deficits often crosses vascular territories. Migrainous positive phenomena (brightness or sparkling in vision, tingling or prickling feelings in the limbs or body) often leave in their wake transient loss of function (scotoma or numbness). Symptoms affecting 1 modality (eg, vision) may clear and then involve another modality (eg, sensation).

Because visual symptoms are common with preeclampsia, one must be cautious not to make that diagnosis without considering other possibilities such as PRES, pituitary apoplexy or tumor growth, and strokes affecting the visual pathways. Because pituitary adenomas (micro or macro) may grow during pregnancy, any woman with a known pituitary tumor and new onset of headache with or without diplopia and a bitemporal field cut should undergo emergent pituitary imaging.[46] Another consideration is orbital hemorrhage, which presents as acute diplopia, proptosis, and eye pain, and can occur during the first trimester (from hyperemesis) or during labor (from pushing).[46,47]

Overall, stroke in pregnant and postpartum women is rare; however, the risk is increased compared with nonpregnant age-matched controls, especially in late pregnancy and the early puerperium.[33,48] Recent evidence suggests that the rate of pregnancy- and postpartum-associated strokes is increasing.[49,50] This epidemiologic trend is true for patients with and without pregnancy-related hypertensive disorders.[50] The event rates per 100,000 deliveries range from 4 to 11 (AIS), 3.7 to 9 (ICH), 2.4 to 7 (SAH), and 0.7 to 24 (CVT).[33,48,49,51–54] These epidemiologic studies varied in their methodology (**Table 1**). The wide range for CVT likely reflects variability in the case-finding definitions and radiologic modalities. Moreover, the extremely low stroke rate in the most recent study is likely owing to the fact that postpartum patients (the period of highest risk) were not included.[55]

Preeclampsia/eclampsia plays an etiologic role in 25% to 50% of pregnant and postpartum patients with strokes: highest with ICH, lower in AIS, and lowest with CVT.[33,48,51,54,56] Other stroke risk factors in these women include older age, African American race, congenital and valvular heart disease, hypertension, caesarian delivery, migraine, thrombophilia, systemic lupus erythematosus, sickle cell disease, and thrombocytopenia.[49,50,52,53] In an analysis of 347 cases of fatal pregnancy-related strokes over a 30-year period in the United Kingdom, these patients accounted for 1 in 7 maternal deaths.[57] Themes that emerged from analysis of these 347 fatal cases were failure to recognize and treat hypertension, delays in imaging owing to concerns about radiation exposure, delays in senior physician involvement, and diagnostic anchoring of "hysteria" or drug-seeking behavior.[57]

Thrombocytopenia also suggests the HELLP syndrome (hemolysis, elevated liver enzymes, low platelets) and thrombotic thrombocytopenic purpura (TTP), whose incidence is elevated in pregnancy and which can present with strokelike symptoms.[58] These 2 conditions have very different clinical courses and management, so maternal–fetal medicine and hematology experts should be involved immediately in the evaluation, particularly if TTP is on the differential. One study of 1166 deliveries found 12 cases of HELLP syndrome of which 8 had neurologic complications—namely, seizures (4 patients), focal deficits (2 patients), and encephalopathy (2 patients).[59] On imaging, 6 patients had PRES (3 with associated hemorrhages) and 2 had isolated ICH.[59]

Another unusual cause of stroke in pregnant and postpartum women is cervicocranial arterial dissection. There may be an increasing frequency in pregnant and postpartum women, although comprehensive epidemiologic data are lacking.[60] Patients with cervicocranial arterial dissections often present with isolated headache and/or neck pain without neurologic deficit,[61] but they can also present with focal deficits owing to embolic strokes.[62,63] There may be a predisposition for multiple vessel dissections.[64] In the largest series of 8 postpartum cases, the only differences between postpartum cases and those occurring in nonpregnant/postpartum women were that

Table 1
Incidence of stroke in pregnant and postpartum women, per 100,000 deliveries

Study, Year Published	AIS	ICH	SAH	CVT	Eclampsia	Comments (Methods, Total Deliveries, Years of Analysis)
Sharshar et al,[54] 1995	4.3	4.6	—	—	47% of AIS 44% of ICH	Population-based regional French study 348,295 deliveries 1989–1991
Kittner et al,[48] 1996	11	9	Excluded	—	25% of AIS 15% of ICH	Population-based regional US study 141,243 deliveries 1988–1991
Jaigobin & Silver,[51] 2000	11.1	3.7	4.3	6.9	23% of AIS 38% of CVT 17% of ICH 0% of SAH	Referral single-center Canadian study 50,700 deliveries 1980–1997
Lanska & Kryscio,[53] 2000[b]	13[a]	[a]	[a]	12.1	Not reported	US national inpatient database 1,408,015 deliveries 1993–1994
Salonen Ros et al,[33] 2001	4.0	3.8	2.4	—	Not reported	Population-based national Swedish study 1,003,489 deliveries 1987–1995
James et al,[52] 2005[b]	9.2	8.6	—	0.7	15.7[c]	US national inpatient database 8,322,799 deliveries 2000–2001
Kuklina et al,[49] 2011[b]	11	7	7	24	Not reported	US national inpatient database 8,786,475 deliveries 2006–2007
Scott et al,[55] 2012 Note: included prenatal events only; see text	0.9[d]	0.4[e]	—	—	11% of AIS 33% of ICH (preeclampsia and eclampsia)	United Kingdom national population-based cohort and nested case-control study 1,958,203 deliveries 2007–2010

Abbreviations: AIS, acute ischemic stroke; CVT, cerebral venous thrombosis; ICH, intracerebral hemorrhage; SAH, subarachnoid hemorrhage.
[a] The 13 includes AIS, ICH and SAH in this study.
[b] Intrinsic to the studies using the US national database is a sampling of approximately 20% of patients. Therefore, the reported number of deliveries is an extrapolated number.
[c] The authors do not directly state which strokes are eclampsia-related but do include an International Classification of Disease, 9th edition (ICD-9) code for "pregnancy-related cerebrovascular events" separate from the ICD-9 codes for AIS, ICH, or CVT.
[d] Includes CVT.
[e] Includes SAH.

simultaneous PRES, RCVS, and SAH were more often seen in the postpartum cases, again emphasizing the theme of overlapping clinical syndromes in these patients.[61] The vast majority of these dissections occur postpartum.[65]

Data from a small case series suggests that women with a prior cervical artery dissection without an underlying connective tissue disorder may not be at significantly increased risk for subsequent pregnancy-related dissections.[66] Still, this series included only 11 women with completed pregnancies after the index event, only 1 of 11 had the initial event in the peripartum period, and 7 subsequent pregnancies were delivered by cesarean, suggesting possible confounding by indication, so the data must be interpreted with caution.

In patients with ICH and SAH, underlying structural lesions such as vascular malformations and aneurysms are relatively common.[48,51,54,56] SAH that occurs around the circle of Willis suggests an aneurysm, whereas convexal SAH suggests RCVS or CVT (with or without an associated cortical vein thrombosis). Brain infarction and hemorrhage can result from many of the vasculopathies, including RCVS and preeclampsia. Finally, TTP, pituitary apoplexy, choriocarcinoma, amniotic fluid embolism, air embolism, and cardioembolism from postpartum cardiomyopathy are rare causes of stroke in this population.[16,67] Sufficient diagnostic testing including vascular imaging must be performed in these patients to identify specific treatable causes.

SEIZURES

Pregnant or postpartum women with seizures can be grouped into 3 categories. The most common are patients with an established seizure disorder before pregnancy.[68] Of note, again demonstrating the frequency of overlapping clinical syndromes, women with epilepsy before pregnancy have an increased likelihood of developing preeclampsia, and of progressing to eclampsia.[69] The second group includes patients with a new non–pregnancy-related seizure disorder, such as a new seizure from an undiagnosed brain tumor or hypoglycemia. These pregnant and postpartum patients require the same systematic approach to a new seizure as in all seizure patients, but are not the focus of this review.

The third group has new seizures that are pregnancy related. Important causes include eclampsia, ICH, CVT, RCVS, PRES, and TTP. Seizures are very common in PRES and usually occur at presentation in the absence of prodromal symptoms, whereas in CVT seizures usually occur later and nearly always after headache.[16] Head CT scans can be normal in each of these conditions. Seizures are much less common in RCVS.[70]

Data are lacking to direct the initial workup in these patients. However, because of this wide differential diagnosis and lack of sensitivity of CT scanning, we believe that pregnant and postpartum patients with new-onset seizures, even those who have returned to baseline and are neurologically intact, should undergo sufficient workup, which usually includes MRI, to establish the cause of the seizure. Postpartum women, even those who are breastfeeding, should undergo the same neuroimaging study that would be done in any other patient for the same indication. For antepartum patients whose optimal neuroimaging would normally involve gadolinium, maternal–fetal medicine should be consulted to discuss the risks versus benefits of gadolinium administration in this setting.

INDIVIDUAL CONDITIONS

The clinical presentations of the specific conditions have considerable overlap and can coexist. However, the details (eg, characteristics of headache, evolution of symptoms over time, and frequency of some symptoms such as seizures or visual problems) can often help to distinguish among them (**Table 2**).

CEREBRAL VENOUS SINUS THROMBOSIS

A rare cause of stroke overall, CVT is an important consideration in pregnant and post-partum women.[71–74] There is a spike in the incidence during the first trimester, probably owing to women with an underlying thrombophilia who become pregnant[56]; however, more than 75% of cases occur postpartum.[75] Although the greatest risk for postpartum thromboembolism is in the first 6 weeks, the risk probably extends out to 12 weeks.[76] Risk factors include caesarian section, dehydration, traumatic delivery, anemia, increased homocysteine levels, and low cerebrospinal fluid pressure owing to dural puncture.[42,53] CVT is posited to be more common in developing countries owing to the increased frequency of poor nutrition, infections, and dehydration.[77,78] CVT owing to pregnancy or oral contraceptive use tend to have better long-term outcomes than men or women with CVT unrelated to pregnancy.[75]

Most patients with CVT present with a progressive, diffuse, constant headache, although in 10% it is a thunderclap headache.[79,80] However, 10% of patients with CVT may have no headache at all.[81] Other findings include dizziness, nausea, seizures, papilledema, lateralizing signs, lethargy, and coma. The specific presentation depends on the extent and location of the involved dural sinuses and draining veins, collateral circulation, effects on intracranial pressure, and presence of associated hemorrhage.[82] Symptoms vary and may fluctuate over time.[42,71,78] Neurologic deficits do not follow arterial distributions.

Although D-dimer is usually increased in patients with CVT, most do not recommend its use in pregnant and postpartum women.[83,84] These patients are often D-dimer positive, especially late in pregnancy and in the early puerperium.[85] Pending further studies, we do not recommend using a negative D-dimer in pregnant or postpartum women to exclude CVT. Noncontrast CT scans are often negative, but may show a hyperdense venous clot or signs of infarction in 30% of cases[84] (**Fig. 2**). Ischemic infarcts often undergo hemorrhagic transformation owing to venous hypertension. CT venography often shows the clot, but MRI with MR venogram, gradient recalled echo, and contrast-enhanced magnetization-prepared rapid gradient echo sequences is typically diagnostic and considered the imaging study of choice.[84]

REVERSIBLE CEREBRAL VASOCONSTRICTION SYNDROME

RCVS is characterized by abrupt onset of usually multiple thunderclap headaches and multifocal, reversible cerebral vasoconstriction, typically occurring during the first week after delivery.[86] Recurring daily thunderclap headaches over several weeks that follow a single thunderclap headache may be pathognomonic.[86–88] When related to pregnancy, two-thirds of patients with RCVS develop symptoms within 1 week of delivery and after a normal pregnancy.[18] RVCS is also associated with use of immunosuppressive drugs, vasoactive medications (eg, serotonin reuptake inhibitors and phenylpropanolamine), recreational drugs (eg, cocaine and marijuana), blood products, catecholamine-secreting tumors, craniocervical arterial dissections, and various other miscellaneous conditions.[18] In a review of a large series of RCVS and arterial dissections designed to identify patients with both conditions simultaneously, the postpartum state emerged as an association of this overlap.[89] Vomiting, confusion, photophobia, and blurred vision often accompany the headaches. When seizures or focal neurologic deficits develop, they nearly always follow the headache.

Table 2
Distinguishing clinical and imaging features of selected conditions

	PRES	RCVS	CVT	Eclampsia
Mode of onset	Rapid (over hours), usually postpartum	Abrupt, usually postpartum	Third trimester or postpartum. Symptoms often progress over days.	Antepartum, intrapartum or postpartum (10%–50%)
Prominent findings	Early prominent seizures. Usually seizures plus at least other symptoms (stupor, visual loss, visual hallucinations). HA dull and throbbing, not thunderclap	Thunderclap HA, multiple episodes. Seizures occur but much less so than in PRES. Transient focal deficits (may become permanent in cases with ICH or infarction)	HA nearly universal at onset, generally progressive and diffuse; thunderclap in small minority. Seizures occur in ~40%. Focal signs may develop later	Seizure, frequent visual symptoms and abdominal pain, hyperreflexia, hypertension, proteinuria
Evolution over time	Symptoms resolve over days to a week if blood pressure controlled	Dynamic process over time; as a general rule, HAs are common during first week, ICH during the second week and ischemic complications during the third week	Evolves over several days; nonarterial territorial infarcts and hemorrhages may develop	Can evolve (from preeclampsia) gradually or abruptly
CSF findings	Usually normal, may have slightly elevated protein	Often normal (unless complicated by SAH) but 50% will have slight pleocytosis and protein elevations	Opening pressure elevated ~80% of cases ~35%-50% will have slight elevations of protein or cells	Usually normal unless complicated by hemorrhage
Imaging aspects	CT positive in ~50% of cases. MR prominent T2-weighted and FLAIR abnormalities nearly always in the parietooccipital lobes but can involve other parts of the brain. ICH in ~15% of patients	CT usually normal (if no SAH). MR ~20% with localized convexal SAH. CTA, MRA usually shows typical "string of beads" constriction of cerebral arteries. DSA is more sensitive. May have associated cervical arterial dissection. Initial arteriogram may be negative	CT often negative. MR may show nonarterial territorial infarcts. Hemorrhage common. MRV shows intraluminal clot flow voids. Although MRV is preferred, CTV is also sensitive	Same as for PRES. Some patients may have coincident AIS or ICH

Abbreviations: CSF, cerebrospinal fluid; CT, computed tomography; CTA, CT angiogram; CTV, CT venogram; CVT, cerebral venous thrombosis; DSA, digital subtraction angiogram; FLAIR, fluid-attenuated inversion recovery; HA, headache; ICH, intracerebral hemorrhage; MRA, MR angiogram; MRI, magnetic resonance imaging; MRV, MR venogram; PRES, posterior reversible encephalopathy syndrome; RCVS, reversible cerebral vasoconstriction syndrome.

Symptoms usually subside over several weeks.[70,86,87,90] Although most patients have good outcomes, there is considerable variability in disease progression and fatal outcomes have been reported in postpartum patients with RCVS.[17,91] The reversibility refers to the angiographic vasospasm, not to the clinical outcomes. Complications include nonaneurysmal convexal SAH, ICH, and AIS.[70,86–88,90,92,93] Convexal SAH is more common than parenchymal ICH.[93] Hemorrhagic complications usually precede ischemic ones.[86] In patients without infarction, the disease resolves over time. Up to 10% of patients with RCVS may also have cervicocranial arterial dissections.[89] Unless there is a complicating hemorrhage, the cerebrospinal fluid is usually normal, but may show small numbers of lymphocytes and mildly elevated protein.[70,86]

Absent a hemorrhage, the CT scan is usually normal. With regard to vascular testing, it is important to recognize that RCVS is a dynamic process. Transcranial Doppler ultrasonography and various forms of angiography are useful tools; however, they may be normal early in the course of the disease. Angiography and transcranial Doppler ultrasonography may be discordant.[18] Angiography reveals multifocal segmental arterial constriction and can also detect arterial dissections.[92] By definition, focal areas of arterial constriction on catheter angiography are always present. However, it is important to recognize 2 limitations of noninvasive angiography (MR angiogram or CTA): (1) these modalities are only positive in approximately 80% of patients, showing the diagnostic pattern of alternating dilatation and constriction, simulating a "string of beads" (see **Fig. 2**)[86,94]; and (2) CTA and MR angiogram may be normal in the first 5 to 6 days of RCVS.[18,94] Transcranial Doppler ultrasonography can be used to follow resolution of the vasoconstriction.[95]

POSTERIOR REVERSIBLE ENCEPHALOPATHY SYNDROME

PRES is a syndrome characterized by headache, seizures, encephalopathy, and visual disturbances in the setting of reversible vasogenic edema on CT scan or MRI.[96,97] PRES occurs in patients with acute hypertension, preeclampsia or eclampsia, renal disease, sepsis, exposure to immunosuppressant drugs, and numerous other conditions and drug exposures.[98–100] In a single-center series, 46 of 47 patients with eclampsia (98%) had PRES, suggesting that in the setting of eclampsia, PRES is an integral part of the pathophysiology.[101] Early diagnosis and management may improve outcomes.[102]

Symptoms develop without prodrome and progress rapidly over 12 to 48 hours. Seizures, which occur in approximately 75% to 90% of patients, may be focal initially, then become generalized tonic–clonic. Severe symptoms can occur even in the absence of severe hypertension.[97,103] Headache occurs in roughly 50% of patients.[97] The headache is generally dull, bilateral, and not thunderclap in nature. Some degree of encephalopathy, ranging from mild confusion to stupor and coma, is present in 50% to 80% of patients.[97]

Because the vasogenic edema typically involves the occipital lobes, approximately 40% of patients have visual symptoms, including visual hallucinations, blurred vision, scotomata, and diplopia.[97,104] Transient cortical blindness occurs in 1% to 15% of patients. The retina and pupils are normal. Consider electroencephalographic monitoring to detect electrical seizure activity in encephalopathic patients without overt seizure activity (ie, nonconvulsive status epilepticus).[97] CT scans will show edema in about 50% to 60% of patients.[105,106] However, MRI should be performed when PRES is suspected because of its increased sensitivity for detecting vasogenic edema, microhemorrhages, and other PRES-related intracranial pathology.

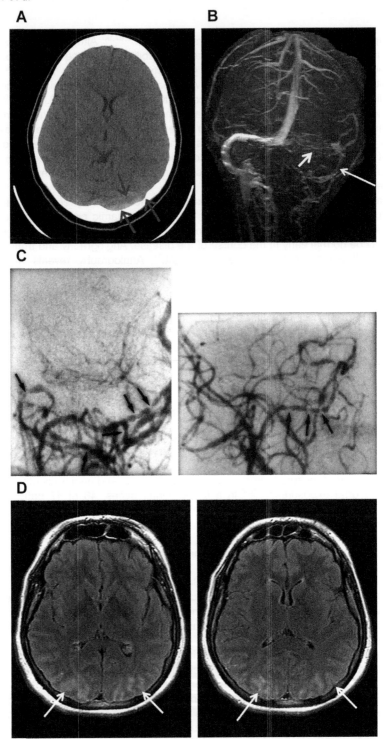

Fig. 2. Selected patient images. (*A*) Noncontrast CT scan of a 21-year-old woman who presented with 7 days of increasing left-sided headache. A subtle increased density (*black arrows*) that is consistent with clot in the left transverse sinus can be seen. (*B*) The MR

MRI reveals focal edema, nearly always in the parietooccipital lobes (see **Fig. 2**). Although the mechanism of this posterior predominance has not been fully elucidated, it is hypothesized that the posterior cerebrovascular circulation has less autoregulatory capacity than does the anterior circulation in the setting of increased cerebral perfusion pressure. Nevertheless, regions of the brain supplied by the anterior cerebrovascular circulation are often involved concomitantly.[107,108] The visual symptoms often resolve completely in hours to days; resolution of the edema on imaging lags behind.[109,110] In eclamptic patients, PRES is not the only potential explanation for seizures. Although most pregnant or postpartum women with PRES have eclampsia, other contributing factors (such as medication use or RCVS) are also possible.

Studies comparing clinical and radiological features of PRES in nonpregnant versus pregnant patients have reported mixed results. One small study (21 patients) found no differences.[111] In a larger study (96 patients), eclamptic or preeclamptic patients with PRES more commonly presented with headache, and were less likely to be confused and more likely to have visual symptoms.[112] A third study (38 patients) also found less alteration in mental status in pregnant versus nonpregnant patients with PRES, as well as overall lower systolic blood pressures.[113] On imaging, pregnant patients had less edema, fewer hemorrhages, and more complete resolution.[112] In another study of 70 patients with "severe" PRES admitted to an intensive care unit, pregnancy or postpartum states (23% of the patients) were associated with better 90-day outcomes than other patients with PRES.[114] Given the small numerators (pregnant and postpartum patients) and denominators (total PRES patients) of these studies, it is difficult to draw firm conclusions about the impact of pregnancy on presentation or prognosis.

NEUROLOGIC COMPLICATIONS OF ECLAMPSIA

Seizures are the hallmark of eclampsia. Eclamptic seizures are usually tonic–clonic and last approximately 1 minute. Symptoms that can precede seizures include persistent frontal or occipital headache, blurred vision, photophobia, right upper quadrant or epigastric pain and altered mental status. In up to one-third of cases, there is no proteinuria or blood pressure is less than 140/90 mm Hg before the seizure.[10]

Although the exact mechanism of eclamptic seizures is unknown, several hypotheses have been proposed.[115] Overactivity of cerebrovascular autoregulation in response to hypertension can lead to cerebral arterial vasospasm and ischemia, resulting in cytotoxic edema. Alternatively, loss of autoregulation in response to hypertension leads to endothelial dysfunction, capillary leak, and vasogenic edema.[9,115,116] This vasculopathy can also result in PRES or regions of infarction and hemorrhage.[117]

---

venogram from the same patient shows a clot in the left transverse sinus (*short wide arrow*) and in the sigmoid sinus (*long thin arrow*). (*C*) Selected images from a digital subtraction angiogram of a patient with reversible cerebral vasoconstriction syndrome who presented with a thunderclap headache. The image on the left shows the diffuse nature of the vasoconstriction. The image on the right shows the classic "string of beads" appearance (*black arrows* show the focal areas of vasoconstriction). Similar findings are seen in most patients with noninvasive (compute tomography or MR) angiography. (*D*) Two images from the T2-weighted fluid-attenuated inversion recovery (FLAIR) sequence on an MRI show increased signal in the bilateral parietooccipital regions (*white arrows*), slightly more on the right, in a 29-year-old patient with posterior reversible encephalopathy syndrome. Diffusion-weighted imaging on this same patient was normal. Note that the bilateral FLAIR hyperintensities, indicating vasogenic edema, spare the medial occipital lobe and calcarine cortex, which distinguishes this finding from posterior cerebral artery ischemic lesions.

Although focal vasogenic edema is characteristic of eclampsia, up to one-quarter of patients have areas of persistent cytotoxic edema consistent with infarction or focal hemorrhage.[116] In 1 study, one-third of patients with "eclamptic encephalopathy" had cytotoxic edema.[118] Thus, components of PRES, areas of ischemia or hemorrhage, and even RCVS may also contribute to eclamptic seizures.

Approximately 90% of eclampsia occurs at or after 28 weeks of gestation.[13] Just more than one-third of eclamptic seizures occur at term, developing intrapartum or within 48 hours of delivery.[13] Although a large population-based study in California suggests that the incidence of eclampsia in the United States is decreasing,[119] recent data suggest an increase in "late" postpartum eclampsia (>48 hours after delivery).[13] In 1 large study of postpartum diagnoses of preeclampsia/eclampsia, two-thirds of patients had been discharged and were readmitted because of late postpartum preeclamptic symptoms, most commonly headache.[120] Of these 151 patients with delayed postpartum preeclampsia, approximately 16% of those readmissions were complicated by eclampsia. The proportion of preeclampsia/eclampsia diagnosed postpartum ranges from 11% to 55% and may be increasing owing to improved antepartum recognition.[121–124] Postpartum patients sometimes ignore early symptoms, such as headache or abdominal pain, and only seek medical care later, after a seizure.[121,125]

Patients with postpartum eclampsia, especially those with late postpartum eclampsia, have an higher incidence of CVT, ICH, and AIS.[13,126] If an experienced clinician thinks that a woman has typical eclampsia, brain imaging is not necessarily indicated.[13] However, in postpartum eclamptic patients, those with focal neurologic deficits, persistent visual disturbances, and symptoms refractory to magnesium and antihypertensive therapy or in patients for whom there is any diagnostic uncertainty, a thorough diagnostic workup, preferably including MRI, is recommended. Imaging may also reveal areas of vasoconstriction consistent with RCVS. Rarely, pregnant patients, especially those with RCVS, develop craniocervical arterial dissections.[61–63,127] Thus, the spectrum of neurologic imaging findings in preeclamptic/eclamptic patients includes infarction, hemorrhage, vasoconstriction, dissection, and both vasogenic and cytotoxic edema.

RARE CONDITIONS CAUSING ACUTE NEUROLOGIC SYMPTOMS IN PREGNANT AND POSTPARTUM WOMEN

Amniotic fluid embolism and metastatic choriocarcinoma are 2 rare pregnancy-specific conditions that can present with acute neurologic symptoms. In a single-center series, only 10 cases of amniotic fluid embolism were found over 30 years.[128] One-half of these cases presented with postpartum hemorrhage and one-half presented with cardiovascular collapse.[128] The latter presentation is associated with agitation, confusion, seizures, and encephalopathy with cardiopulmonary collapse occurring during or immediately after labor.[129,130] Choriocarcinoma, a rare malignancy of trophoblastic tissue, metastasizes to the brain in 20% of patients.[131,132] Because the tumor can cause hemorrhage, mass effect, and invasion of cerebral vessels, its clinical and imaging manifestations are variable.[132,133]

Air embolism occurs when air that enters the myometrium during delivery is absorbed into the venous circulation and right ventricle, reducing cardiac output. Nearly any focal or generalized neurologic symptom can occur owing right-to-left intracardiac shunting of air via a patent foramen ovale.[134] Alternatively, air may enter the left-sided arterial circulation via transpulmonary shunting of blood. Air emboli may then occlude the cerebral microvasculature, resulting in cerebral ischemia and/or seizures during or just after delivery.[134] The presence of air in the retinal veins and a "mill wheel" cardiac murmur suggest the diagnosis.

Another important consideration is Wernicke's encephalopathy, which, although classically associated with alcohol use and malnutrition, can also complicate hyperemesis gravidarum. Among 625 nonalcoholic patients with Wernicke's encephalopathy, 76 (12%) were in women with hyperemesis.[135] Abnormal eye movements are nearly always present; however, the classic triad of confusion, ocular findings (diplopia and nystagmus), and gait abnormalities occurs in a minority of patients.[136] Some patients have an otherwise unexplained metabolic acidosis.[137] Neither biochemical confirmation nor MRI is necessary, the simplest test being the response to intravenous thiamine.[135–137] It is essential to administer intravenous thiamine before administration of glucose-containing intravenous fluids in pregnant women with severe hyperemesis to avoid provoking neurologic injury in the setting of thiamine deficiency.

Pregnant women are at particular risk for TTP, which most commonly presents late in the second or early third trimesters.[58,138] The classic pentad includes thrombocytopenia, microangiopathic hemolytic anemia, fever, and neurologic and renal dysfunction.[139] Neurologic manifestations, occurring in more than one-half of patients, include fluctuating headache, seizures, and generalized and focal neurologic deficits. Coexistent PRES is common.[140] Because the treatments are so different, distinction between TTP (plasma exchange) and HELLP (magnesium and delivery of the fetus) is important.[58,138,140] Given that there is no single distinguishing feature, hematologic and maternal–fetal medicine consultation is strongly recommended.

Pituitary apoplexy, acute infarction, or hemorrhage of the gland, usually in the setting of a (previously undiagnosed) adenoma, presents with headache, visual loss, varying degrees of ophthalmoplegia, and decreased level of consciousness. Although the pituitary gland enlarges during pregnancy, pregnancy is a rare precipitant for pituitary apoplexy.[141,142] Pituitary apoplexy must be distinguished from Sheehan syndrome (hypopituitarism presenting indolently, weeks to months after severe postpartum hemorrhage)[143] and lymphocytic hypophysitis (presents in pregnant patients with headache and visual symptoms but typically with a slower onset).[144]

NEUROIMAGING AND MULTIDISCIPLINARY COORDINATION OF CARE

Most of these patients require brain imaging to make a specific diagnosis. Several basic principles should be kept in mind. First, the emergency physician should discuss the differential diagnosis with the other consultants (including the radiologist) before imaging. The goals of imaging are to minimize ionizing radiation and intravenous contrast exposure, and ensure that, when MRI is being performed, the correct sequences are obtained the first time to optimize the diagnostic yield. Second, the fetal radiation exposure from a noncontrast brain CT scan is negligible.[145] Although CT scanning is safe to perform in this population, clinicians must realize its diagnostic limitations for many of the target conditions. Third, because many of these conditions that cause acute neurologic symptoms and signs in pregnant and postpartum patients require MRI to establish the diagnosis, the clinician's threshold for proceeding directly to MRI must be accordingly low. MRI in pregnant patients is generally thought to be safe, although conclusive data are lacking.[145–147] Until recently, there were no reported teratogenic or other adverse fetal effects of iodinated contrast.[148–150] In September 2015, a report was published describing thyroid dysfunction in 5 of 212 Japanese neonates born to women who underwent hysterosalpingogram with ethiodized oil (an iodinated contrast medium) before becoming pregnant.[151] Given that this is a single report in the medical literature, as well as the lack of clarity as to how pre-pregnancy hysterosalpingogram exposure to ethiodized oil relates to pregnant women receiving intravenous iodinated contrast, this report must be interpreted very cautiously. Because repeated supraclinical doses of gadolinium have been associated with fetal demise and malformations in animal studies, gadolinium is best avoided unless the physician believes that the information to be gained by its use exceeds its potential risk.[145,152]

Authorities recommend obtaining informed consent before these procedures and use of intravenous contrast agents.[145,146,152] However, in an emergent situation, necessary imaging should not be delayed if the patient is unable to give consent and a surrogate decision maker is not readily available. Last, because only minute amounts of both iodinated contrast and gadolinium are secreted in breast milk and because similarly minutes quantities are absorbed across an infant's gut, both types of contrast are considered to be safe in postpartum with respect to breast feeding.[145,152]

No data address the effects on outcomes of location of care of pregnant and postpartum patients with acute neurologic emergencies. Our opinion is that because these situations are uncommon and inherently multidisciplinary, these patients are ideally cared for in hospitals that have neurologic, neurosurgical, advanced radiological, obstetric, and critical care expertise. Even in such centers, close coordination of care across various disciplines is key.

SUMMARY

Pregnant and postpartum patients who present with acute neurologic symptoms require a thorough diagnostic evaluation that targets a broad range of pathologic conditions that are either unique to or occur more frequently in this population. Once an accurate diagnosis is made, specific therapy can follow. Because of the multidisciplinary nature and relative infrequency of most of these conditions, we recommend that emergency physicians work closely with various consultants to coordinate care in these patients. Early transfer of these patients to a center capable of delivering the full range of diagnostic testing and potential care should be considered.

REFERENCES

1. Sidorov EV, Feng W, Caplan LR. Stroke in pregnant and postpartum women. Expert Rev Cardiovasc Ther 2011;9(9):1235–47.
2. Cipolla MJ. Cerebrovascular function in pregnancy and eclampsia. Hypertension 2007;50(1):14–24.
3. Cipolla MJ, Bishop N, Chan SL. Effect of pregnancy on autoregulation of cerebral blood flow in anterior versus posterior cerebrum. Hypertension 2012;60(3): 705–11.
4. Hammer ES, Cipolla MJ. Cerebrovascular dysfunction in preeclamptic pregnancies. Curr Hypertens Rep 2015;17(8):575.
5. Duley L, Meher S, Abalos E. Management of pre-eclampsia. BMJ 2006; 332(7539):463–8.
6. Wallis AB, Saftlas AF, Hsia J, et al. Secular trends in the rates of preeclampsia, eclampsia, and gestational hypertension, United States, 1987-2004. Am J Hypertens 2008;21(5):521–6.
7. Ananth CV, Keyes KM, Wapner RJ. Pre-eclampsia rates in the United States, 1980-2010: age-period-cohort analysis. BMJ 2013;347:f6564.

8. ACOG Task Force on Hypertension and Pregnancy. Hypertension in Pregnancy. American College of Obstetrics and Gynecology; 2013. Available at: www.acog.org/resources-and-publications/task force-hypertension-and-pregnancy. Accessed November 26, 2015.

9. Norritz E. Eclampsia. UpToDate: Wolters Kluwer Health; 2012.

10. Douglas KA, Redman CW. Eclampsia in the United Kingdom. BMJ 1994; 309(6966):1395–400.

11. Sibai BM, Stella CL. Diagnosis and management of atypical preeclampsia-eclampsia. Am J Obstet Gynecol 2009;200(5):481.e1-7.

12. Walker JJ. Pre-eclampsia. Lancet 2000;356(9237):1260–5.

13. Sibai BM. Diagnosis, prevention, and management of eclampsia. Obstet Gynecol 2005;105(2):402–10.

14. Sibai BM, Spinnato JA, Watson DL, et al. Eclampsia. IV. Neurological findings and future outcome. Am J Obstet Gynecol 1985;152(2):184–92.

15. Shainker SA, Edlow JA, O'Brien K. Cerebrovascular emergencies in pregnancy. Best Pract Res Clin Obstet Gynaecol 2015;29(5):721–31.

16. Edlow JA, Caplan LR, O'Brien K, et al. Diagnosis of acute neurological emergencies in pregnant and post-partum women. Lancet Neurol 2013;12(2): 175–85.

17. Fugate JE, Ameriso SF, Ortiz G, et al. Variable presentations of postpartum angiopathy. Stroke 2012;43(3):670–6.

18. Ducros A. Reversible cerebral vasoconstriction syndrome. Lancet Neurol 2012; 11(10):906–17.

19. Goldszmidt E, Kern R, Chaput A, et al. The incidence and etiology of postpartum headaches: a prospective cohort study. Can J Anaesth 2005;52(9): 971–7.

20. Klein AM, Loder E. Postpartum headache. Int J Obstet Anesth 2010;19(4): 422–30.

21. Von Wald T, Walling AD. Headache during pregnancy. Obstet Gynecol Surv 2002;57(3):179–85.

22. Stella CL, Jodicke CD, How HY, et al. Postpartum headache: is your work-up complete? Am J Obstet Gynecol 2007;196(4):318.e1-7.

23. Goadsby PJ, Goldberg J, Silberstein SD. Migraine in pregnancy. BMJ 2008; 336(7659):1502–4.

24. Sances G, Granella F, Nappi RE, et al. Course of migraine during pregnancy and postpartum: a prospective study. Cephalalgia 2003;23(3):197–205.

25. Melhado E, Maciel JA Jr, Guerreiro CA. Headaches during pregnancy in women with a prior history of menstrual headaches. Arq Neuropsiquiatr 2005;63(4): 934–40.

26. Chancellor AM, Wroe SJ, Cull RE. Migraine occurring for the first time in pregnancy. Headache 1990;30(4):224–7.

27. Steegers EA, von Dadelszen P, Duvekot JJ, et al. Pre-eclampsia. Lancet 2010; 376(9741):631–44.

28. Martin SR, Foley MR. Approach to the pregnant patient with headache. Clin Obstet Gynecol 2005;48(1):2–11.

29. Bushnell C, Chireau M. Preeclampsia and stroke: risks during and after pregnancy. Stroke Res Treat 2011;2011:858134.

30. Warrington JP, George EM, Palei AC, et al. Recent advances in the understanding of the pathophysiology of preeclampsia. Hypertension 2013;62(4):666–73.

31. Jadli A, Sharma N, Damania K, et al. Promising prognostic markers of preeclampsia: new avenues in waiting. Thromb Res 2015;136(2):189–95.

32. Schwedt TJ, Matharu MS, Dodick DW. Thunderclap headache. Lancet Neurol 2006;5(7):621–31.

33. Salonen Ros H, Lichtenstein P, Bellocco R, et al. Increased risks of circulatory diseases in late pregnancy and puerperium. Epidemiology 2001;12(4):456–60.

34. Selo-Ojeme DO, Marshman LA, Ikomi A, et al. Aneurysmal subarachnoid haemorrhage in pregnancy. Eur J Obstet Gynecol Reprod Biol 2004;116(2):131–43.

35. Tiel Groenestege AT, Rinkel GJ, van der Bom JG, et al. The risk of aneurysmal subarachnoid hemorrhage during pregnancy, delivery, and the puerperium in the Utrecht population: case-crossover study and standardized incidence ratio estimation. Stroke 2009;40(4):1148–51.

36. Bateman BT, Olbrecht VA, Berman MF, et al. Peripartum subarachnoid hemorrhage: nationwide data and institutional experience. Anesthesiology 2011; 116(2):324–33.

37. Schievink WI. Spontaneous dissection of the carotid and vertebral arteries. N Engl J Med 2001;344(12):898–906.

38. Choi PT, Galinski SE, Takeuchi L, et al. PDPH is a common complication of neuraxial blockade in parturients: a meta-analysis of obstetrical studies. Can J Anaesth 2003;50(5):460–9.

39. Sachs A, Smiley R. Post-dural puncture headache: the worst common complication in obstetric anesthesia. Semin Perinatol 2014;38(6):386–94.

40. Van de Velde M, Schepers R, Berends N, et al. Ten years of experience with accidental dural puncture and post-dural puncture headache in a tertiary obstetric anaesthesia department. Int J Obstet Anesth 2008;17(4):329–35.

41. Ho CM, Chan KH. Posterior reversible encephalopathy syndrome with vasospasm in a postpartum woman after postdural puncture headache following spinal anesthesia. Anesth Analg 2007;105(3):770–2.

42. Lockhart EM, Baysinger CL. Intracranial venous thrombosis in the parturient. Anesthesiology 2007;107(4):652–8 [quiz: 87–8].

43. Zeidan A, Farhat O, Maaliki H, et al. Does postdural puncture headache left untreated lead to subdural hematoma? Case report and review of the literature. Int J Obstet Anesth 2006;15(1):50–8.

44. Ertresvg JM, Stovner LJ, Kvavik LE, et al. Migraine aura or transient ischemic attacks? A five-year follow-up case-control study of women with transient central nervous system disorders in pregnancy. BMC Med 2007;5:19.

45. Liberman A, Karussis D, Ben-Hur T, et al. Natural course and pathogenesis of transient focal neurologic symptoms during pregnancy. Arch Neurol 2008; 65(2):218–20.

46. Digre KB, Kinard K. Neuro-ophthalmic disorders in pregnancy. Continuum (Minneap Minn) 2014;20(1 Neurology of Pregnancy):162–76.

47. Digre KB. Neuro-ophthalmology and pregnancy: what does a neuro-ophthalmologist need to know? J Neuroophthalmol 2011;31(4):381–7.

48. Kittner SJ, Stern BJ, Feeser BR, et al. Pregnancy and the risk of stroke. N Engl J Med 1996;335(11):768–74.

49. Kuklina EV, Tong X, Bansil P, et al. Trends in pregnancy hospitalizations that included a stroke in the United States from 1994 to 2007: reasons for concern? Stroke 2011;42(9):2564–70.

50. Leffert LR, Clancy CR, Bateman BT, et al. Hypertensive disorders and pregnancy-related stroke: frequency, trends, risk factors, and outcomes. Obstet Gynecol 2015;125(1):124–31.

51. Jaigobin C, Silver FL. Stroke and pregnancy. Stroke 2000;31(12):2948–51.

52. James AH, Bushnell CD, Jamison MG, et al. Incidence and risk factors for stroke in pregnancy and the puerperium. Obstet Gynecol 2005;106(3):509–16.
53. Lanska DJ, Kryscio RJ. Risk factors for peripartum and postpartum stroke and intracranial venous thrombosis. Stroke 2000;31(6):1274–82.
54. Sharshar T, Lamy C, Mas JL. Incidence and causes of strokes associated with pregnancy and puerperium. A study in public hospitals of Ile de France. Stroke in Pregnancy Study Group. Stroke 1995;26(6):930–6.
55. Scott CA, Bewley S, Rudd A, et al. Incidence, risk factors, management, and outcomes of stroke in pregnancy. Obstet Gynecol 2012;120(2 Pt 1):318–24.
56. Cantu-Brito C, Arauz A, Aburto Y, et al. Cerebrovascular complications during pregnancy and postpartum: clinical and prognosis observations in 240 Hispanic women. Eur J Neurol 2011;18(6):819–25.
57. Foo L, Bewley S, Rudd A. Maternal death from stroke: a thirty year national retrospective review. Eur J Obstet Gynecol Reprod Biol 2013;171(2):266–70.
58. McCrae KR. Thrombocytopenia in pregnancy. Hematology Am Soc Hematol Educ Program 2010;2010:397–402.
59. Paul BS, Juneja SK, Paul G, et al. Spectrum of neurological complications in HELLP syndrome. Neurol India 2013;61(5):467–71.
60. Tettenborn B. Stroke and pregnancy. Neurol Clin 2012;30(3):913–24.
61. Arnold M, Camus-Jacqmin M, Stapf C, et al. Postpartum cervicocephalic artery dissection. Stroke 2008;39(8):2377–9.
62. Borelli P, Baldacci F, Nuti A, et al. Postpartum headache due to spontaneous cervical artery dissection. Headache 2011;51(5):809–13.
63. McKinney JS, Messe SR, Pukenas BA, et al. Intracranial vertebrobasilar artery dissection associated with postpartum angiopathy. Stroke Res Treat 2010; 2010:1–5.
64. Kelly JC, Safain MG, Roguski M, et al. Postpartum internal carotid and vertebral arterial dissections. Obstet Gynecol 2014;123(4):848–56.
65. Maderia LM, Hoffman MK, Shlossman PA. Internal carotid artery dissection as a cause of headache in the second trimester. Am J Obstet Gynecol 2007;196(1): e7–8.
66. Reinhard M, Munz M, von Kannen AL, et al. Risk of recurrent cervical artery dissection during pregnancy, childbirth and puerperium. Eur J Neurol 2015; 22(4):736–9.
67. Davie CA, O'Brien P. Stroke and pregnancy. J Neurol Neurosurg Psychiatry 2008;79(3):240–5.
68. Stead LG. Seizures in pregnancy/eclampsia. Emerg Med Clin North Am 2011; 29(1):109–16.
69. MacDonald SC, Bateman BT, McElrath TF, et al. Mortality and morbidity during delivery hospitalization among pregnant women with epilepsy in the United States. JAMA Neurol 2015;72(9):981–8.
70. Singhal AB, Hajj-Ali RA, Topcuoglu MA, et al. Reversible cerebral vasoconstriction syndromes: analysis of 139 cases. Arch Neurol 2011;68(8):1005–12.
71. Cantu C, Barinagarrementeria F. Cerebral venous thrombosis associated with pregnancy and puerperium. Review of 67 cases. Stroke 1993;24(12):1880–4.
72. Jeng JS, Tang SC, Yip PK. Incidence and etiologies of stroke during pregnancy and puerperium as evidenced in Taiwanese women. Cerebrovasc Dis 2004; 18(4):290–5.
73. Ruiz-Sandoval JL, Chiquete E, Banuelos-Becerra LJ, et al. Cerebral venous thrombosis in a Mexican multicenter registry of acute cerebrovascular disease: the RENAMEVASC Study. J Stroke Cerebrovasc Dis 2011;21(5):395–400.

74. Srinivasan K. Cerebral venous and arterial thrombosis in pregnancy and puerperium. A study of 135 patients. Angiology 1983;34(11):731–46.
75. Coutinho JM, Ferro JM, Canhao P, et al. Cerebral venous and sinus thrombosis in women. Stroke 2009;40(7):2356–61.
76. Kamel H, Navi BB, Sriram N, et al. Risk of a thrombotic event after the 6-week postpartum period. N Engl J Med 2014;370(14):1307–15.
77. Mas JL, Lamy C. Stroke in pregnancy and the puerperium. J Neurol 1998; 245(6–7):305–13.
78. Caplan L. Cerebral venous thrombosis. In: Caplan L, editor. Caplan's stroke: a clinical approach. Philadelphia: Saunders Elsevier; 2009. p. 554–77.
79. de Bruijn SF, Stam J, Kappelle LJ. Thunderclap headache as first symptom of cerebral venous sinus thrombosis. CVST Study Group. Lancet 1996; 348(9042):1623–5.
80. Stam J. Thrombosis of the cerebral veins and sinuses. N Engl J Med 2005; 352(17):1791–8.
81. Coutinho JM, Stam J, Canhao P, et al. Cerebral venous thrombosis in the absence of headache. Stroke 2015;46(1):245–7.
82. Masuhr F, Mehraein S, Einhaupl K. Cerebral venous and sinus thrombosis. J Neurol 2004;251(1):11–23.
83. Alons IM, Jellema K, Wermer MJ, et al. D-dimer for the exclusion of cerebral venous thrombosis: a meta-analysis of low risk patients with isolated headache. BMC Neurol 2015;15(1):118.
84. Saposnik G, Barinagarrementeria F, Brown RD Jr, et al. Diagnosis and management of cerebral venous thrombosis: a statement for healthcare professionals from the American Heart Association/American Stroke Association. Stroke 2011;42(4):1158–92.
85. Epiney M, Boehlen F, Boulvain M, et al. D-dimer levels during delivery and the postpartum. J Thromb Haemost 2005;3(2):268–71.
86. Ducros A, Bousser MG. Reversible cerebral vasoconstriction syndrome. Pract Neurol 2009;9(5):256–67.
87. Calabrese LH, Dodick DW, Schwedt TJ, et al. Narrative review: reversible cerebral vasoconstriction syndromes. Ann Intern Med 2007;146(1):34–44.
88. Chen SP, Fuh JL, Lirng JF, et al. Recurrent primary thunderclap headache and benign CNS angiopathy: spectra of the same disorder? Neurology 2006;67(12): 2164–9.
89. Mawet J, Boukobza M, Franc J, et al. Reversible cerebral vasoconstriction syndrome and cervical artery dissection in 20 patients. Neurology 2013;81(9): 821–4.
90. Sattar A, Manousakis G, Jensen MB. Systematic review of reversible cerebral vasoconstriction syndrome. Expert Rev Cardiovasc Ther 2010;8(10):1417–21.
91. Fugate JE, Wijdicks EF, Parisi JE, et al. Fulminant postpartum cerebral vasoconstriction syndrome. Arch Neurol 2012;69(1):111–7.
92. Ducros A, Boukobza M, Porcher R, et al. The clinical and radiological spectrum of reversible cerebral vasoconstriction syndrome. A prospective series of 67 patients. Brain 2007;130(Pt 12):3091–101.
93. Ducros A, Fiedler U, Porcher R, et al. Hemorrhagic manifestations of reversible cerebral vasoconstriction syndrome: frequency, features, and risk factors. Stroke 2010;41(11):2505–11.
94. Ducros A. Reversible cerebral vasoconstriction syndrome. Handb Clin Neurol 2014;121:1725–41.

95. Chen SP, Fuh JL, Chang FC, et al. Transcranial color Doppler study for reversible cerebral vasoconstriction syndromes. Ann Neurol 2008;63(6):751–7.
96. Fugate JE, Claassen DO, Cloft HJ, et al. Posterior reversible encephalopathy syndrome: associated clinical and radiologic findings. Mayo Clin Proc 2010; 85(5):427–32.
97. Fugate JE, Rabinstein AA. Posterior reversible encephalopathy syndrome: clinical and radiological manifestations, pathophysiology, and outstanding questions. Lancet Neurol 2015;14(9):914–25.
98. Bartynski WS. Posterior reversible encephalopathy syndrome, part 1: fundamental imaging and clinical features. AJNR Am J Neuroradiol 2008;29(6): 1036–42.
99. Hauser RA, Lacey DM, Knight MR. Hypertensive encephalopathy. Magnetic resonance imaging demonstration of reversible cortical and white matter lesions. Arch Neurol 1988;45(10):1078–83.
100. Raroque HG Jr, Orrison WW, Rosenberg GA. Neurologic involvement in toxemia of pregnancy: reversible MRI lesions. Neurology 1990;40(1):167–9.
101. Brewer J, Owens MY, Wallace K, et al. Posterior reversible encephalopathy syndrome in 46 of 47 patients with eclampsia. Am J Obstet Gynecol 2013;208(6): 468.e1-6.
102. Postma IR, Slager S, Kremer HP, et al. Long-term consequences of the posterior reversible encephalopathy syndrome in eclampsia and preeclampsia: a review of the obstetric and nonobstetric literature. Obstet Gynecol Surv 2014;69(5): 287–300.
103. Roth C, Ferbert A. The posterior reversible encephalopathy syndrome: what's certain, what's new? Pract Neurol 2011;11(3):136–44.
104. Weiner CP. The clinical spectrum of preeclampsia. Am J Kidney Dis 1987;9(4): 312–6.
105. Roth C, Ferbert A. Posterior reversible encephalopathy syndrome: long-term follow-up. J Neurol Neurosurg Psychiatry 2010;81(7):773–7.
106. Li Y, Gor D, Walicki D, et al. Spectrum and potential pathogenesis of reversible posterior leukoencephalopathy syndrome. J Stroke Cerebrovasc Dis 2011; 21(8):873–82.
107. Ahn KJ, You WJ, Jeong SL, et al. Atypical manifestations of reversible posterior leukoencephalopathy syndrome: findings on diffusion imaging and ADC mapping. Neuroradiology 2004;46(12):978–83.
108. McKinney AM, Short J, Truwit CL, et al. Posterior reversible encephalopathy syndrome: incidence of atypical regions of involvement and imaging findings. AJR Am J Roentgenol 2007;189(4):904–12.
109. Cunningham FG, Fernandez CO, Hernandez C. Blindness associated with preeclampsia and eclampsia. Am J Obstet Gynecol 1995;172(4 Pt 1):1291–8.
110. Pande AR, Ando K, Ishikura R, et al. Clinicoradiological factors influencing the reversibility of posterior reversible encephalopathy syndrome: a multicenter study. Radiat Med 2006;24(10):659–68.
111. Roth C, Ferbert A. Posterior reversible encephalopathy syndrome: is there a difference between pregnant and non-pregnant patients? Eur Neurol 2009;62(3): 142–8.
112. Liman TG, Bohner G, Heuschmann PU, et al. Clinical and radiological differences in posterior reversible encephalopathy syndrome between patients with preeclampsia-eclampsia and other predisposing diseases. Eur J Neurol 2012; 19(7):935–43.

113. Marrone LC, Gadonski G, Diogo LP, et al. Posterior reversible encephalopathy syndrome: differences between pregnant and non-pregnant patients. Neurol Int 2014;6(1):5376.
114. Legriel S, Schraub O, Azoulay E, et al. Determinants of recovery from severe posterior reversible encephalopathy syndrome. PLoS One 2012;7(9):e44534.
115. Morriss MC, Twickler DM, Hatab MR, et al. Cerebral blood flow and cranial magnetic resonance imaging in eclampsia and severe preeclampsia. Obstet Gynecol 1997;89(4):561–8.
116. Zeeman GG, Fleckenstein JL, Twickler DM, et al. Cerebral infarction in eclampsia. Am J Obstet Gynecol 2004;190(3):714–20.
117. Zeeman GG. Neurologic complications of pre-eclampsia. Semin Perinatol 2009; 33(3):166–72.
118. Junewar V, Verma R, Sankhwar PL, et al. Neuroimaging features and predictors of outcome in eclamptic encephalopathy: a prospective observational study. AJNR Am J Neuroradiol 2014;35(9):1728–34.
119. Fong A, Chau CT, Pan D, et al. Clinical morbidities, trends, and demographics of eclampsia: a population-based study. Am J Obstet Gynecol 2013;209(3): 229.e1-7.
120. Matthys LA, Coppage KH, Lambers DS, et al. Delayed postpartum preeclampsia: an experience of 151 cases. Am J Obstet Gynecol 2004;190(5):1464–6.
121. Chames MC, Livingston JC, Ivester TS, et al. Late postpartum eclampsia: a preventable disease? Am J Obstet Gynecol 2002;186(6):1174–7.
122. Katz VL, Farmer R, Kuller JA. Preeclampsia into eclampsia: toward a new paradigm. Am J Obstet Gynecol 2000;182(6):1389–96.
123. Leitch CR, Cameron AD, Walker JJ. The changing pattern of eclampsia over a 60-year period. Br J Obstet Gynaecol 1997;104(8):917–22.
124. Shah AK, Rajamani K, Whitty JE. Eclampsia: a neurological perspective. J Neurol Sci 2008;271(1–2):158–67.
125. Isler CM, Rinehart BK, Terrone DA, et al. Maternal mortality associated with HELLP (hemolysis, elevated liver enzymes, and low platelets) syndrome. Am J Obstet Gynecol 1999;181(4):924–8.
126. Lubarsky SL, Barton JR, Friedman SA, et al. Late postpartum eclampsia revisited. Obstet Gynecol 1994;83(4):502–5.
127. Williams TL, Lukovits TG, Harris BT, et al. A fatal case of postpartum cerebral angiopathy with literature review. Arch Gynecol Obstet 2007;275(1):67–77.
128. Yoneyama K, Sekiguchi A, Matsushima T, et al. Clinical characteristics of amniotic fluid embolism: an experience of 29 years. J Obstet Gynaecol Res 2014; 40(7):1862–70.
129. Gist RS, Stafford IP, Leibowitz AB, et al. Amniotic fluid embolism. Anesth Analg 2009;108(5):1599–602.
130. Moore J, Baldisseri MR. Amniotic fluid embolism. Crit Care Med 2005;33(10 Suppl):S279–85.
131. Brass SD, Copen WA. Neurological disorders in pregnancy from a neuroimaging perspective. Semin Neurol 2007;27(5):411–24.
132. Huang CY, Chen CA, Hsieh CY, et al. Intracerebral hemorrhage as initial presentation of gestational choriocarcinoma: a case report and literature review. Int J Gynecol Cancer 2007;17(5):1166–71.
133. Saad N, Tang YM, Sclavos E, et al. Metastatic choriocarcinoma: a rare cause of stroke in the young adult. Australas Radiol 2006;50(5):481–3.
134. Muth CM, Shank ES. Gas embolism. N Engl J Med 2000;342(7):476–82.

135. Galvin R, Brathen G, Ivashynka A, et al. EFNS guidelines for diagnosis, therapy and prevention of Wernicke encephalopathy. Eur J Neurol 2010;17(12):1408–18.
136. Chiossi G, Neri I, Cavazzuti M, et al. Hyperemesis gravidarum complicated by Wernicke encephalopathy: background, case report, and review of the literature. Obstet Gynecol Surv 2006;61(4):255–68.
137. Selitsky T, Chandra P, Schiavello HJ. Wernicke's encephalopathy with hyperemesis and ketoacidosis. Obstet Gynecol 2006;107(2 Pt 2):486–90.
138. Martin JN Jr, Bailey AP, Rehberg JF, et al. Thrombotic thrombocytopenic purpura in 166 pregnancies: 1955-2006. Am J Obstet Gynecol 2008;199(2): 98–104.
139. Austin S, Cohen H, Losseff N. Haematology and neurology. J Neurol Neurosurg Psychiatry 2007;78(4):334–41.
140. Burrus TM, Wijdicks EF, Rabinstein AA. Brain lesions are most often reversible in acute thrombotic thrombocytopenic purpura. Neurology 2009;73(1):66–70.
141. Biousse V, Newman NJ, Oyesiku NM. Precipitating factors in pituitary apoplexy. J Neurol Neurosurg Psychiatry 2001;71(4):542–5.
142. Bonicki W, Kasperlik-Zaluska A, Koszewski W, et al. Pituitary apoplexy: endocrine, surgical and oncological emergency. Incidence, clinical course and treatment with reference to 799 cases of pituitary adenomas. Acta Neurochir (Wien) 1993;120(3–4):118–22.
143. Kelestimur F. Sheehan's syndrome. Pituitary 2003;6(4):181–8.
144. Flanagan DE, Ibrahim AE, Ellison DW, et al. Inflammatory hypophysitis - the spectrum of disease. Acta Neurochir (Wien) 2002;144(1):47–56.
145. Klein JP, Hsu L. Neuroimaging during pregnancy. Semin Neurol 2011;31(4): 361–73.
146. ACOG Committee on Obstetric Practice. ACOG Committee Opinion. Number 299, September 2004 (replaces No. 158, September 1995). Guidelines for diagnostic imaging during pregnancy. Obstet Gynecol 2004;104(3):647–51.
147. Kanal E, Barkovich AJ, Bell C, et al. ACR guidance document for safe MR practices: 2007. AJR Am J Roentgenol 2007;188(6):1447–74.
148. Tirada N, Dreizin D, Khati NJ, et al. Imaging pregnant and lactating patients. Radiographics 2015;35(6):1751–65.
149. Chen MM, Coakley FV, Kaimal A, et al. Guidelines for computed tomography and magnetic resonance imaging use during pregnancy and lactation. Obstet Gynecol 2008;112(2 Pt 1):333–40.
150. Tremblay E, Therasse E, Thomassin-Naggara I, et al. Quality initiatives: guidelines for use of medical imaging during pregnancy and lactation. Radiographics 2012;32(3):897–911.
151. Satoh M, Aso K, Katagiri Y. Thyroid dysfunction in neonates born to mothers who have undergone hysterosalpingography involving an oil-soluble iodinated contrast medium. Horm Res Paediatr 2015;84(6):370–5.
152. Cohan R. American College of Radiology Manual on Contrast Media. In: Medium ACoDaC, editor. Sections on pregnant and breast-feeding women. Version 7. American College of Radiology; 2010. p. 59–63.

Neuro-Ophthalmology in Emergency Medicine

J. Stephen Huff, MD*, Everett W. Austin, MD

KEYWORDS

• Anisocoria • Ptosis • Diplopia

KEY POINTS

- Understanding the anatomy and physiology of the eye, the orbit, and the central connections is key to understanding neuro-ophthalmologic emergencies.
- Anisocoria is an important sign that requires a systematic approach to avoid misdiagnosis of serious conditions, including carotid dissection (miosis) and aneurysmal third nerve palsy (mydriasis).
- Ptosis may be a sign of either Horner syndrome or third nerve palsy.
- An explanation should be pursued for diplopia since the differential diagnosis ranges from the trivial to life-threatening causes.

INTRODUCTION

Neuro-ophthalmologic emergencies are inexactly defined but may be thought of as neurologic emergencies where findings of the eyes or vision predominate and there is some urgency for evaluation or treatment. There is overlap with other neurologic and ophthalmologic disorders. This discussion is a brief overview directed at the emergency physician. Findings on the neuro-ophthalmologic system do not exist in isolation and must be viewed in context of the entire presentation of the patient. A patient's level of consciousness, comorbidities, and associated conditions or injuries frequently direct the tempo of evaluation.

Examination of the neuro-ophthalmologic system allows a sampling of the general neurologic examination. Motor function, sensory findings, coordination, several of the cranial nerves, and even cortical and higher cerebral functions are tested. Although the neuro-ophthalmologic examination is often straightforward, it is occasionally perplexing. Like the general neurologic examination, the history informs the key portions of the physical examination and these clinical findings together suggest the anatomic localization of abnormalities within the central nervous system, which is critical to

---

Department of Emergency Medicine, University of Virginia, PO Box 800699, Charlottesville, VA 22902, USA
* Corresponding author.
E-mail address: jshuff@virginia.edu

Emerg Med Clin N Am 34 (2016) 967–986
http://dx.doi.org/10.1016/j.emc.2016.06.016
0733-8627/16/© 2016 Elsevier Inc. All rights reserved.

determine if addition work-up is necessary. Funduscopic examination allows visualization of blood vessels and the neural tissue in the optic disc.

With neuro-ophthalmologic emergencies, the emergency physician is faced with determining the need for prompt consultation, imaging, or hospital admission. This article presents examination techniques and findings as well as summaries of several clinical entities that are encountered in emergency medicine practice. Emphasis is on do-not-miss causes.

ANATOMY AND PHYSIOLOGY

An understanding of anatomy aids both with examination and formulation of a clinical impression. The eye developmentally is an amalgam of neural elements and connective tissues. The globes are moved by the extraocular muscles, and disorders of muscles or the neuromuscular junction may affect eye movements. Because muscles are controlled by the nervous system, disorders of cranial nerves, the cranial nerve nuclei, and neural systems controlling the cranial nerve nuclei may also affect eye movements. The coordination needed to maintain visual fixation of 2 eyes simultaneously in a moving environment is complex, and the interaction and coordination of extraocular movements and conscious interpretation of visual information is complex as well as involving extra-ocular muscles, their innervation, cerebellum and cerebellar pathways, and cortical and subcortical structures.

Vision involves light entering the pupil, having an impact on the retina with photochemical conversion of light energy to electrical impulses and transmission of the visual information by the optic nerves via the optic chasm and optic tracts to the thalamus. At the optic chiasm, partially crossing fibers form the optic tracts in route to the lateral geniculate bodies of the thalamus (**Fig. 1**). Pupillary reactivity with efferent responses through parasympathetic and sympathetic systems is supplied by specialized ganglion cells, which leave the optic tract to reach the pupillary centers in the dorsal midbrain. Transmission via the optic radiations through the temporal lobes to the occipital cortex is the pathway for conscious awareness of vision and

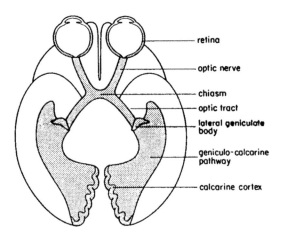

Fig. 1. Visual pathway with light impacting the retina where it is converted to electrical energy prior to being transmitted along the optic nerve, partially crossing at the chiasm, and down the optic tract to the lateral geniculate bodies. (*From* Pellock JM, Myer EC. Neurologic emergencies in infancy and childhood. 2nd edition. Philadelphia: Butterworth-Heinemann; 1993; with permission.)

higher cerebral processing. Interpretation of the imagery involves interaction with other cortical areas.

Pupillary testing involves provoking a reflex arc involving receptors on the retina, the afferent optic nerve (cranial nerve II), and fibers to the midbrain pupillary nuclei, brainstem interneuronal connections, and then efferent parasympathetic response. The parasympathetic pupilloconstrictors originating in the Edinger-Westphal complex of the third nerve nucleus take a direct route from the midbrain to the globes along the third cranial nerves (inferior division). The proximity of the third nerve with its pupilloconstrictors to the tentorium cerebelli is the basis for the pupillary dilatation in patients with uncal herniation. The sympathetic pupillodilators take a circuitous route from the supraoptic nuclei in the hypothalamus via the intermediolateral column through the brainstem, along the intermediolateral portion of the cervical and upper thoracic spinal cord, and reach the orbit along blood vessels (**Fig. 2**).

CLINICAL FINDINGS/PHYSICAL EXAMINATION TECHNIQUES

The sequence of the neuro-ophthalmologic examination varies from patient to patient. In most patients, the best fit is with cranial nerves testing during the neurologic examination. For primary ophthalmologic issues, a physician might start with examination directed at the visual system. It is axiomatic that visual acuity should be tested and recorded in every patient with a visual problem. Best corrected visual acuity using glasses or a pinhole (if patients do not have their glasses) should be obtained. The

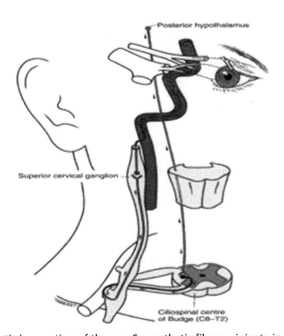

Fig. 2. Sympathetic innervation of the eye. Sympathetic fibers originate in the hypohthalamus with second-order neurons exiting the spinal cord traveling along the sympathetic chain to the superior cervical ganglion. Third-order neurons then travel back along the carotid arteries. (*From* Bowling B. Kanski's clinical ophthalmology. 8th edition. Philadelphia: Saunders; 2016; with permission.)

eye does not exist in isolation. Each of these findings must be interpreted in context. For example, the clinical implication of a large, nonreactive pupil is much different in an alert interactive patient than in a comatose patient.

Inspection of the Pupils and Pupillary Reactivity

The jargon PERRLA (pupils equal, round, reactive to light and accommodation) should be broken down to different components. First of all, are the pupils equal? Physiologic anisocoria is common in the population. One millimeter of asymmetry may occur but in less than 5% of the population. It is equally important to determine whether both pupils react normally. A sluggish reaction (or no reaction) may be important especially if involving the larger pupil. The ability of casual observers to note differences in pupillary size is not clear. It is a common occurrence in the resuscitation area for 1 caregiver to be calling out pupillary sizes that on closer inspection are simply not accurate. Additionally, pupillary size and asymmetry vary with lighting, becoming more noticeable in lower ambient lighting. The dim room phenomena may explain some of the different assessments at different times by observers because pupillary asymmetry often becomes more noticeable in low ambient lighting.

The response of the pupil to light has both a direct and consensual component. A bright light directed at 1 pupil should cause constriction of that pupil (the direct response) as well as constriction of the other pupil (the consensual response). Failure of a pupil to constrict to direct stimulation may represent a problem of light conduction or reception by the retina; dysfunction of the optic nerve, tract, or chiasm; brainstem interneurons; cranial nerve nuclei; or the efferent limb of the reflex with cranial nerve III. The magnitude of constriction of both pupils should be relatively similar; this is the basis of the so-called swinging flashlight test. A bright light directed at 1 pupil should cause constriction; after the light is shifted to stimulate the other eye, that pupil should remain the same size. If that pupil enlarges after the light is swung to it, seemingly paradoxically dilating in the face of a bright light, this is a positive swinging flashlight test (**Fig. 3**). This is indicative of an afferent pupillary defect, most frequently indicating a problem with that optic nerve.

The "A" in PERRLA, stands for accommodation. If a visual target is moved closer to the patient while the patient continues to track the target, the pupil is observed constrict. There currently is interest in convergence pupilloconstriction in concussion evaluation. Because this is infrequently tested in common practice, the "A" in that acronym should be a dropped if not performed. In common practice, testing a pupil accommodative response is only indicated if the pupil does not react to light. If it does react to a near stimulus, then the differential of light-near dissociation should be explored.

Examination of the optic disc is frequently perplexing to emergency physicians. This examination is limited by time, confidence, and experience of the examiner and because in most ED settings it is performed with a pupil that has not been pharmacologically dilated. Funduscopic detail is difficult to discern in patients given these limitations. With practice, an emergency physician should be able to make some assessment of the quality of the view of the posterior pole (possibly indicating a cataract or other media problem), sharpness of the optic disc, possible presence of disc edema or optic atrophy, a comment on the blood vessels (narrowed, dilated, or sclerotic), the presence of exudate, or the presence of hemorrhage. With practice, the presence of retinal venous pulsations may be appreciated, which has implications regarding intracranial pressure (ICP). Portable retinal cameras may have an impact on funduscopic assessment in the future.

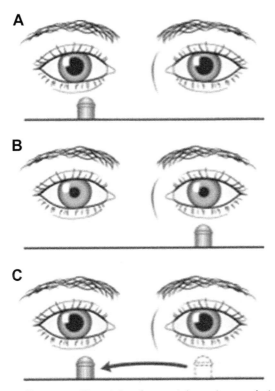

Fig. 3. Right relative afferent pupillary defect from a right optic nerve lesion. (*A*) Poor direct and consensual reaction with illumination of the right eye. (*B*) Excellent direct and consensual reaction with illumination of the left eye. (*C*) Poor direct and consensual reaction, manifest as redilation of both pupils when the light is swung back to the right eye. (*From* Daroff RB, Jankovic J, Mazziotta JC, et al. Bradley's neurology in clinical practice. 6th edition. Philadelphia: Elsevier; 2016; with permission.)

Extraocular Movements

Evaluation of extraocular movements is sometimes thought to only test different cranial nerve functions. Because there are multiple other causes of motility disruption, start by examining movement of each eye (ductions) in all directions. Assessment of versions examines whether the 2 eyes move together. Assessment of cranial nerves, in particular, cranial nerves III and VI, are commonly done during evaluation of extraocular movements testing. By way of review, the sixth cranial nerve innervates the lateral rectus of each globe, responsible for lateral movement or abduction of each globe. The fourth cranial nerve (the most difficult to assess) innervates the superior oblique muscle responsible for depression in adduction and intorsion of each globe. The third cranial nerve innervates the other extraocular muscles and controls adduction, elevation, and depression of each globe. Associated parasympathetic fibers with cranial nerve III are involved with pupilloconstriction. Frequently, several cranial nerves and extraocular muscles are involved with eye motions. The H-shaped tracing examination pattern and knowledge of the principal direction of movement of the individual muscles attempts to isolate these different motions, allowing assessment of specific extraocular muscles and cranial nerve functions **(Fig. 4)**.

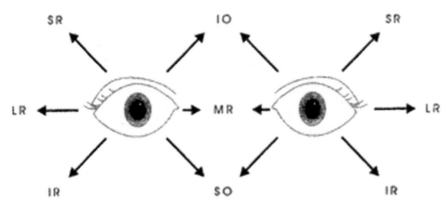

Fig. 4. Cranial nerve testing with extraocular movements. IO, inferior oblique; IR, inferior rectus; LR, lateral rectus; MR, medial rectus; SO, superior oblique; SR, superior rectus. (*From* Richardson LD, Joyce DM. Diplopia in the emergency department. Emerg Med Clin North Am 1997;15(3):652; with permission.)

Like other voluntary muscle movements, some assessment of coordination is possible analogous to assessing cerebellar functions. Asking a cooperative patient to slowly track a moving finger or other object assesses smooth pursuit functions. An observation of breakup or irregularity of smooth pursuit movement may indicate a cerebellar system problem. Directing patients to direct their eyes back-and-forth between different objects — typically an examiner's nose and finger — may show over or undershoot phenomena (saccadic dysmetria) — the eyes are seen to overshoot the target then quickly correct. Again, this frequently represents a cerebellar system lesion. These fast movements are part of the saccadic system. Saccades are rapid eye movements that shift the line of sight between successive points of fixation. Abnormalities of saccadic movements may occur from cerebellar or cerebellar pathway lesions but also occur from midbrain or other problems in the nervous system.

Vestibular-Ocular and Caloric Testing

Extraocular movements can also be assessed with rapid motion of the head or by irrigation of the auditory canal, provoking thermal stimulation to the vestibular system. Probably the most common use of this in contemporary practice is for brain death determination. Focusing on cold water irrigation of the right auditory canal, the response for a comatose patient with a functional vestibular system, efferent cranial VIII intact, functional interneurons and pathways, and functional cranial nerves III and VI is for tonic deviation of the eyes toward the side of cold water irrigation (**Fig. 5**). Nystagmus is not observed in the comatose patient because this requires a functioning cerebral cortex. Should nystagmus be observed in a seemingly comatose patient, this is evidence of a functional cortex and suggests pseudocoma. The old mnemonic, cold opposite, warm same (COWS), refers to the direction of induced nystagmus for the alert patient, not eye movement direction in the patient with altered mental status. More useful in emergency practice is cold same, warm opposite (CSWO), the direction of the slow, tonic movement of eye direction in a comatose patient. In a patient with brain death or severely depressed brainstem functioning from any cause, including some toxicologic or metabolic causes, there is no reaction.

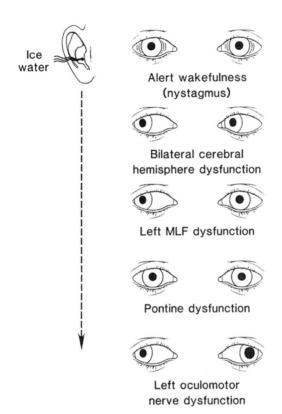

Ice water

Alert wakefulness (nystagmus)

Bilateral cerebral hemisphere dysfunction

Left MLF dysfunction

Pontine dysfunction

Left oculomotor nerve dysfunction

Fig. 5. Cold water caloric testing. Using CSWO, slow deviation of eyes to the side of cold water irrigation suggestive of bilateral cerebral dysfunction. MLF, medial longitudinal fasciculus. (*Data from* Pellock JM, Myer EC, Neurologic emergencies in infancy and childhood. 2nd edition. Butterworth-Heinemann; 2013.)

Corneal Reflex

Sensation to the globe is supplied by cranial nerve V; the corneal reflex reflects a cranial V–VII reflex arc. Although not strictly a neuro-ophthalmologic test, it may be useful in some patients. Much like the pupillary response, the corneal reflex has both direct and consensual responses. Abnormalities may result from the afferent cranial nerve V, interneuron connections, or from the efferent motor function of cranial nerve VII.

Visual Fields

Visual field testing is often used to detect cortical abnormalities, but lesions anywhere along the optic paths may cause different patterns of visual field loss. Bedside testing performed with confrontation maneuvers, 1 eye at a time, comparing an examiner's fields to those of the patient, is the usual method in the ED. Visual field testing with confrontation maneuvers has limitations compared with quantitative perimetric testing. Even so, some distinctive patterns may be detected. The classic bitemporal hemianopsia pattern results from chiasmal lesions reflecting the partial decussation of fibers at the optic chiasm. Pathologic processes between the optic chiasm and the occipital cortex cause variable degrees of homonymous visual field losses.

Unilateral occipital cortex lesions show contralateral homonymous hemianopsia. A summary is presented in (**Fig. 6**). In some patients, the visual field deficit may seem pronounced if a parietal lobe lesion adds an element of cortical neglect to the visual field loss.

Patients with Altered Mental Status or Coma

For a patient with altered mental status or coma, the examination is brief. Note if the eyes are open or closed and if there is resistance to eye opening. Pupillary size, reactivity, and globe alignment are noted. Alignment of the globes should be noted to detect a cranial nerve issue, such as third or sixth nerve dysfunction (discussed later). Frequently in patients with altered mental status, the alignment is off — skew gaze — and may correct with stimulation and alerting. The eyes should be observed for any spontaneous movements. Corneal responses may be assessed. Visualization of the discs may be easier than in alert patients who are moving. Caloric testing (described previously) may be indicated in some cases. In this situation, if nystagmus is present, the cortex is functioning. Abnormal eye movements, however, such as vertical ocular bobbing in comatose patients or rhythmic eye movements that at times are present in patients with status epileptics, may cause confusion. On careful observation, these movements differ from nystagmus in eye movement speed and magnitude and can be termed *nystagmoid* or the examiner can simply describe the movements in words.

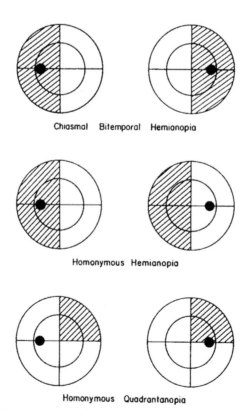

Chiasmal Bitemporal Hemianopia

Homonymous Hemianopia

Homonymous Quadrantanopia

Fig. 6. Chiasmal and posterior visual fields cuts. (*From* Pellock JM, Myer EC. Neurologic emergencies in infancy and childhood. 2nd edition. Philadelphia: Butterworth-Heinemann; 1993; with permission.)

SPECIFIC CLINICAL ISSUES
Visual Loss

Visual loss is a common presentation to an emergency department (ED). The clinician should first determine what the patient means by the chief complaint. Is the loss monocular or binocular; is there a total loss of vision or a dimming or blurring of vision? Historical factors, such as tempo and progression as well as patient comorbidities, enter the diagnostic process. Monocular visual loss points to a problem anterior to the optic chiasm that is either in the globe or the optic nerve. Emergency physicians are aware of retinal detachment but should also keep in mind optic neuropathies, which might to be ischemic, demyelinating, or any of myriad other causes. Ischemic optic neuropathies most commonly result from hypoperfusion and infarct of the optic disc. Other risk factors include hypotension, hypertension, severe anemia, and sleep apnea. In elderly patients, giant cell (temporal) arteritis should be considered. Funduscopy should be attempted to assess for swelling or hemorrhage. Pallor indicating the development of optic atrophy takes weeks to months to occur. Because arteritic ischemic optic neuropathies are potentially treatable causes of blindness (at least to prevent frequent involvement of the opposite eye), rapid assessment and consultation should occur. For the older patient, investigation should include erythrocyte sedimentation rate, C-reactive protein, and platelet count as a screen for giant cell (temporal) arteritis. More importantly, patients should be asked about temporal pain, temporal discomfort when chewing, polymyalgia symptoms, and recent weight loss. Temporal artery biopsy should be arranged but, importantly, high-dose oral steroids should be started in the ED. This does not affect biopsy results for a week or more and can prevent subsequent vision loss.

Multiple sclerosis may also present as monocular visual loss. Optic disc abnormalities may be present on inspection; however, in retrobulbar optic neuritis, the disc appears normal. Prompt consultation should be obtained for further ophthalmologic evaluation in all cases of acute monocular vision loss.

Binocular vision loss points to a problem of both optic nerves or more commonly posterior to the optic chiasm, such as infarcts involving the occipital lobes. Patients with cortical blindness from bilateral occipital lobe injury are unusual and may seem puzzling at presentation. Pupillary reactivity remains intact, and patients with so-called cortical blindness sometimes have small islands or tunnels of vision remaining. Patients are largely blind but oddly able to move around some objects. Hemorrhage or tumor with edema may cause similar problems. With the possibility of ischemia, diagnostic work-up is directed along the pathway of stroke diagnosis with cranial CT, perhaps CT angiography (CTA), and neurologic consultation. MRI and magnetic resonance angiography may be indicated.

Lesions at the optic chiasm, although infrequent, are encountered in emergency medicine practice. The most dramatic presentation is rapidly expanding tumor or hemorrhage into a pituitary tumor compressing the optic chiasm — so-called pituitary apoplexy. Patients may have a severe headache and the visual loss maybe profound. Other clinical findings may dominate, such as mental status changes, diplopia (due to involvement of the ocular motor nerves in the cavernous sinus), and hypotension from hypopituitarism with resultant adrenal insufficiency. Compression of the optic chiasm may also cause visual field cuts (discussed later). Imaging by either CT or MRI should be obtained followed by prompt neurosurgical consultation if a tumor or hemorrhage is discovered.

Visual Field Loss

Visual field deficits often accompany visual loss (discussed previously). Again, the clinician should start by assessing whether the visual loss is monocular or binocular. Subcortical and cortical lesions posterior to the chiasm may result in a variety of bilateral hemianopsia patterns. Generally, the more posterior the lesion, the more similar or congruous are the field cuts. If a neglect syndrome from parietal lobe injury is also present, the field cut may seem exaggerated, or in extreme cases, the patient is unaware of the visual field loss and may bump or even drive into objects. This may occur with nondominant hemispheric lesions, typically right hemispheric, and the patient loses appreciation of the existence of the left visual world.

Lesions compressing the chiasm classically cause bitemporal defects but in some settings arcuate defects or central scotomas or even homonymous defects (when there is a replaced chiasm and the optic tract is affected) may be seen. Visual field deficits from lesions compressing the optic chiasm usually do not reduce central acuity but may produce blindness.

The causes of visual field loss vary with age and comorbidities of the patient, but ischemic stroke, hemorrhage, and tumor with edema are the causes commonly encountered in the ED. Diagnostic approach after bedside assessment for complaint of isolated field cut is neuroimaging and consultation. Anatomic correlates with visual filed cuts are summarized in image (**Fig. 7**).

Unequal Pupils — Anisocoria

The clinical condition of a patient always must be considered when interpreting physical examination findings. The presence of a large unreactive pupil in the presence of severe headache or altered mental status is much more serious than a large pupil in a patient awake, alert, interactive, and with no other issues. Other physical examination findings, such as additional cranial nerve deficits or focal findings, direct the work-up elsewhere. A dilated pupil with other third cranial nerve findings is discussed later.

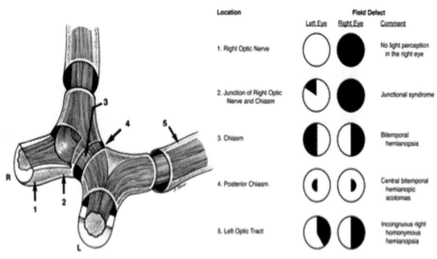

Fig. 7. Visual field deficits with associated lesions of the optic nerve, chiasm, or tract. (*From* Liu GT. Disorders of the eyes and eyelids. In: Samuels MA, Feske S (eds): The Office Practice of Neurology, p 46. New York, Churchill Livingstone, 1996, with permission. Adapted from Hoyt WF, Luis O, Arch Ophthalmol 1963;70:69–85.)

A large unreactive or sluggishly reactive pupil in a patient with new headache, altered mental status, or coma is a cause for alarm. The fear is that of third nerve compression from an expanding or ruptured aneurysm or another mass lesion (**Fig. 8**). The parasympathetic pupilloconstrictors are more susceptible to injury from compression than other elements of the third nerve and may become impaired before other signs of third nerve dysfunction are present. With the pupilloconstrictors impaired, pupillary dilation predominates. This is the basis of the model of uncal herniation syndrome where an expanding mass with brainstem shifting compresses the third nerve against the tentorium cerebelli. In a majority of cases of uncle herniation syndrome, the large pupil is ipsilateral to the expanding mass. In approximately 10% of cases, the dilated pupil is contralateral to the mass (Kernohan notch phenomenon) and said to be falsely localizing. Again, examination should determine if this finding is present in isolation or if additional signs and symptoms are present. Possible causes are mass lesions of any type — subdural hematoma, intracerebral hematoma, ischemic stroke, intracranial tumor, and stroke with edema.

A large, unreactive pupil in an awake, alert patient ambulatory to the ED without other complaints or findings is not infrequent and almost never of clinical significance. Careful physical examination should confirm that this is an isolated finding specifically that no other elements of third nerve dysfunction are present. Typically there is a history of handling scopolamine motion sickness patches or other anticholinergic substances. Less common is surreptitious installation of pupillodilating medication to feign illness.

The large pupil is not always the abnormal one. In some patients with anisocoria, the abnormal pupil is the smaller one. Horner syndrome of ptosis, miosis, and anhidrosis (focal loss of sweating) does not always present with the complete syndrome — miosis may predominate. Perhaps the most serious emergency clinical

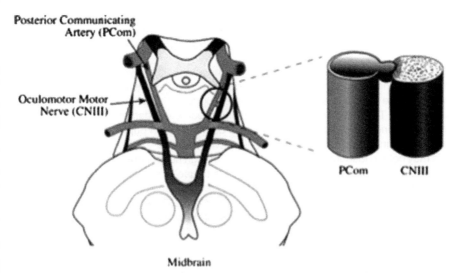

Fig. 8. Third cranial nerve compression due to an aneurysm of the posterior communicating artery. Injury to the parasympathetic pupilloconstrictors with resultant pupillary dilation. (*From* Woodruff MM, Edlow JA. Evaluation of third nerve palsy in the emergency department. J Emerg Med 2008;35:242; with permission.)

condition is carotid artery dissection, which has associated headache or facial pain. Abnormal taste (dysgeusia) is unusual but a suggestive sign. The arterial dissection damages the sympathetic pupillodilators running along the vessel to the orbit. Ipsilateral pupillary constriction follows with the unopposed parasympathetic innervation. If carotid dissection is suspected, immediate imaging is indicated. CTA or magnetic resonance angiography documents blood flow through the vessels but blood in the wall of the vessel is demonstrated by MRI. Some centers may use specialized MRI techniques, such as fat-suppression magnetic resonance, or prefer ultrasound.

Diplopia, Cranial Nerve Palsies

The definition of diplopia (seeing double) describes the phenomenon of the same object seen in 2 different points in space. Further clarification of the chief complaint may be useful. Is the diplopia only present in with 1 eye? Monocular diplopia is usually form a refractive problem in 1 globe (high astigmatism). Are the images of equal clarity? Patients may articulate blurry vision or may report seeing multiple ghostlike images. Typically, the "false" image is of lesser clarity and may localize the problem to 1 eye. Are the symptoms always present or intermittent? Are there any exacerbating factors or is there a history of fatigability? The causes of diplopia range from trivial to life threatening. Tables in textbooks list many causes of diplopia that are not directly applicable to emergency medicine practice because they often reflect ascertainment and referral bias to ophthalmology clinics.

As with other neuro-ophthalmologic problems, this complaint may not exist in isolation and other clinical findings might direct attention toward a different work-up. Particularly important is the presence of additional neurologic problems or cranial nerve findings involving nerves other than III, IV, and VI. The presence of pain may be a red flag and numbness often indicates significant pathology. Recent trauma, fever, altered mental status, nausea, or vomiting might suggest another process that directs the investigation. Injection of the globe, proptosis, or asymmetric swelling may suggest an orbital (or retro-orbital) infectious or infiltrative process. Multiple cranial nerve abnormalities may be a particular worrisome sign suggesting cavernous sinus involvement. Isolated, intermittent diplopia may be with myasthenia gravis.

In the setting of double vision relieved by covering either eye, the goal is to determine the abnormally moving eye. Gross defects may be detected by examining ductions. Failure to completely move the eye suggests either a paretic or restrictive component. The first step is to use a point light source in a darkened room. The reflection of the bright light should appear in the center of each pupil to the examiner with normally aligned eyes. If one is abnormally deviated with the light reflection not central, this may help to identifying a weak muscle. Although not generally done by emergency physicians, the oldest method of doing this is to use a red glass placed in front on 1 eye. If the eyes have a tendency to deviate the red light and the white light will not overlap. By identifying in which of the 9 cardinal positions of gaze (straight, right, left, up, down, up right, up left, down right, and down left) the objects are furthest apart, the abnormally moving eye (see **Fig. 4**) can be identified. One examination rule is that the false image is projected laterally to the true image.

A cranial nerve III lesion may result in ptosis, dilated pupil, and deviation of the globe laterally from the unopposed action of the lateral rectus (**Fig. 9**). The patient also demonstrates an ipsilateral hypertropia on down gaze and a contralateral hypertropia on upward gaze due to limitation in vertical eye movement. When a third nerve palsy involves the pupil, the concern is always for an aneurysm of the posterior

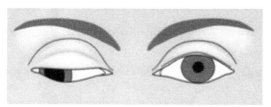

Fig. 9. Complete third cranial nerve palsy. The classic down-and-out position due to unopposed input from cranial nerves VI and IV. The pupil is dilated and ptosis is present. (*From* Woodruff MM, Edlow JA. Evaluation of third nerve palsy in the emergency department. J Emerg Med 2008;35:241; with permission.)

communicating artery compressing the third nerve.[1] The differential diagnosis is, however, broad. Other differential diagnoses that may mimic a third nerve palsy include myasthenia, botulism, thyroid orbitopathy, orbital infections, trauma, and others.

A key point is that of pupillary reactivity. A diabetic third nerve palsy (better termed a vasculopathic third nerve palsy because many patients do not have diabetes) is also in the differential diagnosis of a third nerve palsy. The axiom is that cranial nerve III palsy resulting from diabetes or microvascular dysfunction preserves the action of the pupil (pupillary sparing). Older literature suggests that if an isolated third nerve palsy spares the pupil (the pupil reacts normally to light), imaging may be deferred unless the pupil becomes involved or the patient fails to improve. This older approach was suggested in an era where formal catheter angiography was required to find an aneurysm. Now that easy noninvasive vascular imaging, such as CTA, is commonplace, a safer approach is to either perform CTA or consult neurology in all patients with a new third nerve palsy because emergency physicians generally do not see this problem frequently.

A lateral rectus weakness results in abduction failure of the globe-on observation the affected eye appears to pause in motion when tracking horizontally to lateral. Lateral rectus palsy from cranial nerve VI dysfunction is a common finding in patients with increased ICP. Neuroimaging is recommended on presentation even with this isolated finding.

Cranial nerve IV lesions — supplying the superior oblique muscle — may be difficult to detect on inspection. Careful attention directed at observing inward rotation of the eye with abduction — watching scleral small vessels may help — may help detect an isolated fourth nerve palsy. Failure of the globe to intort is characteristic of superior oblique/cranial nerve IV palsy. Patients may show a head tilt to the side of the IV palsy to compensate. Although trochlear nerve palsies may be secondary to microvascular disease in older patients, head trauma is the common cause.

How do these findings translate to emergency medicine practice? Few studies are based on presentation to EDs. A recent study from an Italian ED enrolled adult patients over a 3-year period who presented to the ED with binocular diplopia[2] (**Box 1**). Emergency physicians gathered information about the physical examination, cardiovascular risk factors, smoking history, hypertension, and other factors. Physical examination evaluation included assessment of gait, speech, coordination, and observation for papilledema, nystagmus, and anisocoria. All patients underwent noncontrast CT scan in the ED. A majority of patients were admitted and additional tests, including MRI, were performed. The gold standard for determining the cause of diplopia was a neurologist and an internist with adjudication if needed by the senior emergency physician. Diplopia without any discernible cause (primary diplopia) was present in approximately two-thirds of total cases. For this group of patients, no cause could

> **Box 1**
> **Causes of binocular diplopia in adult patients presenting to an emergency department**
>
> All patients in study had binocular diplopia.
>
> 167 (64%) Determined to have primary diplopia (including migraine with aura) — no detectable cause
>
> 93 (35.8%) Secondary diplopia — diplopia identified from another process
>
> Of this group with secondary diplopia
> - Stroke 45%
> - Multiple sclerosis 18%
> - Brain tumors 12%
> - Aneurysms 9%
> - Myasthenia gravis 6%
> - Miller Fisher variant Guillain-Barré syndrome 2%
> - Pseudotumor 2%
> - Intracranial hypotension 2%
> - Brain abscess 1%
> - Arteritis 1%
> - Cavernous sinus thrombosis 2%
>
> *Adapted from* Nazerian P, Vanni S, Tarocchi C, et al. Causes of diplopia in the emergency department: diagnostic accuracy of clinical assessment and head computed tomography. Eur J Emerg Med 2014;21(2):118–24.

be identified after a battery of tests, and this was a diagnosis of exclusion. In approximately one-third of cases in this study, diplopia was from some disease process (secondary diplopia). Of patients with secondary diplopia, the most frequent diagnoses were ischemic or hemorrhagic stroke (45% of the secondary cause group), multiple sclerosis (18%), intracranial tumors (12%), and aneurysms (9%). Most of these patients had other neurologic symptoms or signs. Those patients with secondary diplopia where the diplopia was the only sign and symptom represented only 11% of the secondary cases of diplopia.

Again, red flags to prompt further imaging and consultation are patients with binocular diplopia and multiple cranial nerve involvement, third nerve palsy with pupil involvement possibly suggesting intracranial nerve compression, painful or progressive third nerve involvement, or cranial nerve VI palsy.

A condition that may present with diplopia with distinctive findings on physical examination is an internuclear ophthalmoplegia (INO). The lesion is in the pontine medial longitudinal fasciculus, a medulla to midbrain neural tract connecting the cranial nerve nuclei responsible for eye movements. This is an anatomically small structure and the finding of an isolated INO anatomically localizes the lesion to the medial longitudinal fasciculus. The hallmark is adduction failure of a globe on examination with gaze directed laterally and most commonly with nystagmus of the abducting eye. In the authors' small experience, the adduction failure may predominate. INO may be unilateral or bilateral. With right INO, the adduction failure is observed as failure of the right globe to adduct, that is, to move medially toward the nose. Bilateral INO demonstrates bilateral adduction failure. Etiology in younger patients is often from multiple sclerosis, whereas older patients often have a small vessel stroke. Imaging with CT or preferably MRI should occur along with appropriate consultation.

Ptosis

Ptosis is an occasional presentation in ED patients and may be unilateral or bilateral. Ptosis may result from issues of muscles or cranial nerves III or VII. Again, the physician should determine if additional signs or symptoms are present. Ptosis is present in a III nerve lesion and other signs of oculomotor nerve dysfunction (discussed previously) are present. The degree of ptosis from a Horner syndrome is much less marked than ptosis from a third nerve palsy. Myopathic ptosis is discussed further.

Nystagmus

There are dozens of different descriptive terms for different varieties of nystagmus, which involves the saccadic system and fast eye movements (discussed previously). The presence of nystagmus implies an abnormality in the vestibular or pursuit pathways. Nystagmus as it relates to the acutely dizzy patient is covered (See Andrea Morotti and Joshua N. Goldstein's article, "Diagnosis and Management of Acute Intracerebral Hemorrhage," in this issue). A few simple principles should be kept in mind. The presence of nystagmus implies a functioning cortex. Comatose patients do not have nystagmus, although at times they may have other abnormal repetitive eye movements. Nystagmus may be rotary, horizontal, or vertical or chronic or acute. In emergency medicine practice, horizontal nystagmus is commonly observed. This may be normal with extreme lateral gaze (gaze paretic) but is exaggerated with various medication (chiefly alcohol or antiepileptic medications). The emergency physician also commonly observes nystagmus in patients with peripheral vertigo. Typically, this is brief, usually horizontal, and provoked by positional changes.

One approach in evaluating nystagmus is for the examiner to first note if nystagmus is present in primary gaze, that is, with the patient looking at an object straight ahead. Nystagmus present with primary gaze is always abnormal most commonly due to vestibular pathology. Then note if the nystagmus is provoked by looking in 1 direction or if provoked by movements. Vertical or torsional diagnosis is usually of central origin and represents a pathologic process.

Although currently uncommonly used in the ED, provoking optokinetic nystagmus may be useful in some clinical conditions. Presented with large repetitive patterns, such as contrasting squares or stripes, normally the eyes appear to track objects and then quickly move back to pick up trailing objects. The quick movement is observed as nystagmus by the examiner. The observation of provoked optokinetic nystagmus implies that visual impulses are being received, information is being presented to the retina, optic nerve and chasmal structures are functional, transmission to the thalamus is intact, some cortical visual areas are functional, cerebellar systems are functioning, and provoked horizontal movements show that the third and sixth cranial nerves are working. This test is useful in establishing vision in infants and young children and at times in demonstrating that some element of vision is present in patients that may be subjectively reporting no vision.

Acute nystagmus found on examination of course must be viewed in context with other history and physical examination findings. Generally, acute nystagmus with patients with altered mental status other than from simple intoxications, vertical or torsional nystagmus, or associated with other physical findings requires further work-up and consultation.

Increased Intracranial Pressure

Increased ICP from a variety of causes may be suspected or confirmed with findings on the neuro-ophthalmologic examination. Causes include any intracranial mass lesion, idiopathic intracranial hypertension (pseudotumor cerebri), cerebral venous thrombosis, and many others. Tumors or masses may cause abnormal findings on examination by either direct impairment of structures, surrounding edema, or indirectly by the effects of increased ICP.

Increased ICP results in a typical syndrome of headaches, nausea, or vomiting, and sometimes focal findings, such as cranial nerve IV or VI palsy. Again, the tempo and location of the pathologic process cause wide variation in presentation. Cranial nerve VI is particularly susceptible to the effects of increased ICP. This may cause unilateral or bilateral lateral rectus palsy with failure of 1 globe or both to abduct and move laterally usually causing diplopia.

The presence of papilledema may be useful in detection of increased ICP (discussed previously). Papilledema may take some hours to develop, and patients with acute increased in ICP may not have this finding. The assessment of blurring and abnormal elevation of the optic disc may be technically difficult, particularly with a nondilated pupil. Additionally, some anatomic variants simulate papilledema. The presence of retinal venous pulsations indicate that ICP is not elevated at that moment and may be an important finding. Bedside ultrasound is increasingly used in detection of papilledema and shows great promise; however, prospective evaluation in large number of patients with acute increased ICP is lacking at this time.

In patients with suspected increased ICP, additional work-up, such as imaging or ICP assessment with LP or even ICP monitor, is indicated. Neuroimaging and consultation helps direct the work-up. If a mass lesion has been excluded, lumbar puncture may be performed to assess CSF pressures. If a mass lesion is detected or ICP is confirmed to be elevated, further evaluation and consultation should follow.

Coma and Altered Mental Status

A variety of abnormal eye movements have been described in comatose patients, such as ocular dipping and ocular bobbing. These recurrent vertical downward movements have some localizing value but perhaps are best used by emergency physicians as an indication for emergent imaging.

Prompt assessment of cranial nerve function is valuable in all patients presenting in coma. As discussed previously, a large pupil in a comatose patient is suggestive of cranial nerve III dysfunction possibly from uncal herniation. A picture of full cranial nerve III paresis may be present with the eye laterally deviated from unopposed lateral rectus activity in addition to being dilated (see **Fig. 9**). Likewise, cranial nerve VI dysfunction may be suspected if medial deviation of a globe is noted.

Toxins

In general, the physical examination signs of toxidromes are symmetric; asymmetry suggests structural causes. In a profoundly unresponsive patient, however, the absence of a sign on physical examination does not allow determination of a structural versus metabolic or toxicologic coma. The cholinergic and anticholinergic toxidromes, and their effects on pupillary size, respectively small and large, are well known to emergency physicians. A variety of other toxins may affect the neuro-opthalmalogic system. Many of the effects are nonspecific for sedation. A few medications have been noted to cause toxic ophthalmoplegia and include carbamazepine, doxepin, amitriptyline, and others.

Seizures

Most patients with seizures have open eyes. During an apparent generalized seizure, there should not be any resistance to eye-opening and certainly resistance should not increase as the effort to open the lids increases. This is a quick and excellent screening maneuver for nonepileptic spells, also known as pseudoseizures.

The most common seizure type in adults is partial-onset seizures with secondary generalization. Frequently, eye movements just before or during the generalized convulsion are useful to confirm the seizure and possibly add localization information. The eyes may conjugately deviate to 1 side, which predicts a seizure focus in the contralateral frontal hemisphere. Frequently the eyes conjugately move in brisk rhythmic movements — not true nystagmus, perhaps best termed nystagmoid movements — again, predicting a seizure focus of the contralateral hemisphere.

Status epilepticus, particularly transformed or subtle status epilepticus, at times may be suspected only from eye signs. Generalized convulsions have appeared to ceased, yet the patient remains unresponsive. Inspection at times may show repetitive nystagmoid movements (discussed previously) or tonic deviation of the eyes in 1 direction and may suggest the diagnosis of nonconvulsive status.

A variety of postictal eye movement abnormalities are also observed. Perhaps the most common is a skew gaze, a nonspecific marker for altered consciousness. The eyes appear inexactly aligned. A postictal Todd phenomenon is also observed with the eyes, seemingly fatigued, no longer driven contralaterally from the seizure focus, and the eyes drift toward the hemisphere of origin of the seizure.

Generalized-onset seizures, such as absence seizures, may produce frequent eye blinks with brief interruptions of consciousness. These may occur frequently in some patients.

Carotid Cavernous Fistula

Although uncommon, patients with carotid cavernous fistula can present with a cluster of neuro-ophthalmologic findings. Most of these fistulae are due to trauma, but other causes include rupture of an intracavernous carotid artery aneurysm and various collagen vascular diseases that weaken the arterial wall. Most of the fistulae produce a high-pressure phenomenon due to arterial pressure being introduced into a venous sinus. These present with acute-onset proptosis, chemosis, conjunctival injection ocular bruits, headache, and altered function of the nerves that traverse the cavernous sinus (3, 4, and 6). Oddly, some patients present with a lower pressure variant that leads to the same findings but with a much more insidious onset. The conjunctival injection in this group is often misdiagnosed as conjunctivitis. All of the other findings (proptosis, diplopia, cranial bruit, and decreased vision) not found in conjunctivitis.

Nutritional Deficiency

No discussion of neuro-ophthalmologic emergencies is complete without a mention of Wernicke disease, which results from thiamine deficiency. The complete clinical triad of confusion, gait ataxia, and oculomotor abnormalities is imperfect with an estimated 10% of patients having the complete syndrome. The cornerstone is a history of malnutrition or malabsorption. Typically this is found in alcoholics with poor diets but there is likely a component of malabsorption in this patient group. Patients with a history of bariatric surgery or severe hyperemesis gravidarum and those on long-term parenteral nutrition are other groups at risk. A wide variety of oculomotor findings have been reported in Wernicke disease, including, in approximate descending order, nystagmus, bilateral sixth nerve palsy, conjugate gaze abnormality, pupillary abnormality, retinal hemorrhage, and ptosis.[3] These may be difficult to assess in the intoxicated individual. Emergency medical service (EMS) systems in the past commonly administered thiamine routinely to patients with altered mental status, but in many systems thiamine is no longer carried by EMS. When in doubt, if the clinical situation suggests the possibility of Wernicke disease, particularly in the presence of oculomotor abnormalities, thiamine should be administered intravenously.

Myasthenia Gravis

The presentation of myasthenia gravis is sometimes overlooked in the ED. Because of the high metabolic activity of the extraocular muscles, weakness of an extraocular muscle often leads to diplopia. Fatigability is the key historical in the weakness of myasthenia gravis. The clinical findings may vary with activity and time of the day and at times are seemingly inconsistent. Prolonged or repeated movements may provoke abnormalities on examination. Diplopia or ptosis are frequent presenting complaints. Patients presenting with generalized weakness or dysphagia may have ptosis giving a clue to a new presentation of myasthenia gravis. In some patients, the clinical findings are limited to the ocular system and the condition is referred to as ocular myasthenia.

Sustained upward gaze is an examination maneuver to bring out fatigability, with ptosis increasing as the upward gaze effort continues. Neuromuscular transmission is improved with cooling. The ice pack test — placing an ice pack (with a gauze pad for comfort) to cool the lid sometimes causes the ptosis to improve and may be a diagnostic clue. Tensilon (used in the tensilon test), rarely used in the ED, is no longer manufactured in the United States. Definitive diagnosis is by serologic testing.

Stroke

Depending on the site of injury, stroke may cause many findings on neuro-ophthalmologic examination. Often there are additional findings that make localization possible. Large vessel stroke or large intracranial hemorrhages often show deviation of the eyes toward the side of the destructive lesion. Smaller strokes reflect injuries to the different areas injured.

Pontine destruction, whether from ischemic stroke or hemorrhage, may have the distinct finding of truly pinpoint pupils. These extraordinarily small pupils in an acutely comatose patient with eye movement abnormalities are pathognomonic of pontine destruction. Other stroke syndromes, in particular posterior fossa strokes, may show a variety of abnormal eye movement abnormalities. Basilar artery occlusion desires special mention. These patients have other findings of hemiparesis, quadriparesis, or abnormal consciousness. A variety of abnormal eye movements may be present, including unilateral or bilateral horizontal gaze palsy, INO, or combinations of these signs. In this era of thrombolytic and clot extraction therapies, rapid identification of suitable patients for interventional therapies is important.

A particular area of recent interest is eye findings in posterior fossa stroke. For patients awake and alert, perhaps with vertigo, head impulse, nystagmus type, test of skew gaze (HINTS) is said be useful in distinguishing peripheral vertigo from causes of stroke. A recent a combined the ABCD^2 (age, blood pressure, clinical features, duration of TIA, and presence of diabetes) rule with HINTS testing for increased sensitivity.[4,5] Readers are referred to the articles on vertigo and stroke for further details.

Functional Neuro-Ophthalmologic Problems

Functional problems presenting with neuro-ophthalmologic issues are not infrequent. Any diagnosis of conversion disorder or malingering, however, should be established on the basis of the certainty that the finding represents a nonanatomic and nonphysiologic presentation, not the inability to define the problem. Visual loss or blindness might be reported. Tunnel vision that remains limited with distance from objects — that is, perhaps like seeing through a pipe rather than an expanding cone — is reported.

Oculomotor abnormalities are sometimes reported and may take the appearance of convergence spasm, essentially a voluntary crossing of the eyes while looking medially. At times unilateral convergence spasm may mimic a sixth nerve palsy medial deviation of an eye and seeming failure of abduction. A key finding is to observe the pupils — the pupils constrict during convergence maneuver; with a sixth nerve paresis there is no pupillary constriction.

In an unresponsive patient, a variety of observations may suggest functional coma. The presence of nystagmus is discussed previously as is volitional eye clenching. If the patient's eyes deviate toward the floor as the head is turned to either side in the supine patient, this is a non-anatomic voluntary response. These geotropic, literally ground-going, eyes suggest functional unresponsiveness. Resistance to eye opening is another clue to feigned unresponsiveness. As discussed previously, induced nystagmus — true nystagmus with rapid eye corrections — implies an awake intact cortex.

For suspected functional neuro-ophthalmologic issues in the ED, liberal consultation and referral are recommended for diagnostic confirmation.

SUMMARY

The neuro-ophthalmologic system and examination do not exist in isolation from the general physical examination and neurologic examinations. Findings should be considered in the context of a patent's history and other findings.

There are several chief complaints primarily of the neuro-ophthalmologic that are emergencies and demand prompt action. The emergency physician must know basics of examination and interpretation of examination findings, when to obtain additional diagnostic studies or imaging, and when to consult or refer.

ACKNOWLEDGMENTS

The authors would like to thank Dr Steven Newman and Dr William Woods, both of the University of Virginia, for reviewing early versions of the article.

REFERENCES

1. Woodruff MM, Edlow JA. Evaluation of third nerve palsy in the emergency department. Journal Emerg Med 2008;35:239–46.
2. Nazerian P, Vanni S, Tarocchi C, et al. Causes of diplopia in the emergency department: diagnostic accuracy of clinical assessment and head computed tomography. Eur J Emerg Med 2014;21(2):118–24.
3. Donning MW, Vega J, Miller J, et al. Myths and misconceptions of Wernicke's encephalopathy: what every emergency physician should know. Ann Emerg Med 2007;50:715–21.
4. Kerber KA, Meurer WJ, Brown DL, et al. Stroke risk stratification in acute dizziness presentations. Neurology 2015;85:1869–78.
5. Newman-Toker DE. Comment: diagnosing stroke in acute dizziness- the "eyes" have it. Neurology 2015;85:1877.

FURTHER READINGS

Biller J, Gruener G, Brazis P. DeMyer's the neurologic examination: a programmed text. New York: McGraw-Hill; 2011.
Henry G, Jagoda A, Little NE, et al. Neurologic emergencies: a symptom-oriented approach. New York: McGraw-Hill; 2003.
Huff JS. Special neurologic tests and procedures [Chapter 61]. In: Roberts and Hedges' clinical procedures in emergency medicine. Philadelphia: WB Saunders; 2013. p. 1243–58.

Pellock JM, Myer ED. Neurologic emergencies in infancy and childhood. Boston (MA): Butterworth-Heineman; 1993.

Leigh RJ, Zee DS. The neurology of eye movements. New York: Oxford University Press; 2006.

Index

Note: Page numbers of article titles are in **boldface** type.

Emerg Med Clin N Am 34 (2016) 987–994
http://dx.doi.org/10.1016/S0733-8627(16)30089-X
0733-8627/16/$ – see front matter

emed.theclinics.com

UNITED STATES POSTAL SERVICE®

Statement of Ownership, Management, and Circulation
(All Periodicals Publications Except Requester Publications)

1. Publication Title	2. Publication Number	3. Filing Date
EMERGENCY MEDICINE CLINICS OF NORTH AMERICA	000 – 714	9/18/2016

4. Issue Frequency	5. Number of Issues Published Annually	6. Annual Subscription Price
FEB, MAY, AUG, NOV	4	$298

7. Complete Mailing Address of Known Office of Publication (Not printer) (Street, city, county, state, and ZIP+4®)
ELSEVIER INC.
360 PARK AVENUE SOUTH
NEW YORK, NY 10010-1710

Contact Person
STEPHEN R. BUSHING

Telephone (Include area code)
215-239-3688

8. Complete Mailing Address of Headquarters or General Business Office of Publisher (Not printer)
ELSEVIER INC.
360 PARK AVENUE SOUTH
NEW YORK, NY 10010-1710

9. Full Names and Complete Mailing Addresses of Publisher, Editor, and Managing Editor (Do not leave blank)
Publisher (Name and complete mailing address)
LINDA BELFUS, ELSEVIER INC.
1600 JOHN F KENNEDY BLVD. SUITE 1800
PHILADELPHIA, PA 19103-2899

Editor (Name and complete mailing address)
PATRICK MANLEY, ELSEVIER INC.
1600 JOHN F KENNEDY BLVD. SUITE 1800
PHILADELPHIA, PA 19103-2899

Managing Editor (Name and complete mailing address)
ADRIANNE BRIGIDO, ELSEVIER INC.
1600 JOHN F KENNEDY BLVD. SUITE 1800
PHILADELPHIA, PA 19103-2899

10. Owner (Do not leave blank. If the publication is owned by a corporation, give the name and address of the corporation immediately followed by the names and addresses of all stockholders owning or holding 1 percent or more of the total amount of stock. If not owned by a corporation, give the names and addresses of the individual owners. If owned by a partnership or other unincorporated firm, give its name and address as well as those of each individual owner. If the publication is published by a nonprofit organization, give its name and address.)

Full Name	Complete Mailing Address
WHOLLY OWNED SUBSIDIARY OF REED/ELSEVIER, US HOLDINGS	1600 JOHN F KENNEDY BLVD. SUITE 1800 PHILADELPHIA, PA 19103-2899

11. Known Bondholders, Mortgagees, and Other Security Holders Owning or Holding 1 Percent or More of Total Amount of Bonds, Mortgages, or Other Securities. If none, check box → ☐ None

Full Name	Complete Mailing Address
N/A	

12. Tax Status (For completion by nonprofit organizations authorized to mail at nonprofit rates) (Check one)
The purpose, function, and nonprofit status of this organization and the exempt status for federal income tax purposes:
☐ Has Not Changed During Preceding 12 Months
☐ Has Changed During Preceding 12 Months (Publisher must submit explanation of change with this statement)

PS Form 3526, July 2014 [Page 1 of 4 (see instructions page 4)] PSN: 7530-01-000-9931   PRIVACY NOTICE: See our privacy policy on www.usps.com.

---

13. Publication Title	14. Issue Date for Circulation Data Below
EMERGENCY MEDICINE CLINICS OF NORTH AMERICA	MAY 2016

15. Extent and Nature of Circulation		Average No. Copies Each Issue During Preceding 12 Months	No. Copies of Single Issue Published Nearest to Filing Date
a. Total Number of Copies (Net press run)		404	508
b. Paid Circulation (By Mail and Outside the Mail)	(1) Mailed Outside-County Paid Subscriptions Stated on PS Form 3541 (Include paid distribution above nominal rate, advertiser's proof copies, and exchange copies)	180	264
	(2) Mailed In-County Paid Subscriptions Stated on PS Form 3541 (Include paid distribution above nominal rate, advertiser's proof copies, and exchange copies)	0	0
	(3) Paid Distribution Outside the Mails Including Sales Through Dealers and Carriers, Street Vendors, Counter Sales, and Other Paid Distribution Outside USPS®	76	104
	(4) Paid Distribution by Other Classes of Mail Through the USPS (e.g., First-Class Mail®)	0	0
c. Total Paid Distribution [Sum of 15b (1), (2), (3), and (4)]	▶	256	368
d. Free or Nominal Rate Distribution (By Mail and Outside the Mail)	(1) Free or Nominal Rate Outside-County Copies included on PS Form 3541	45	70
	(2) Free or Nominal Rate In-County Copies Included on PS Form 3541	0	0
	(3) Free or Nominal Rate Copies Mailed at Other Classes Through the USPS (e.g., First-Class Mail)	0	0
	(4) Free or Nominal Rate Distribution Outside the Mail (Carriers or other means)	45	70
e. Total Free or Nominal Rate Distribution (Sum of 15d (1), (2), (3) and (4))	▶	45	70
f. Total Distribution (Sum of 15c and 15e)	▶	301	438
g. Copies not Distributed (See Instructions to Publishers #4 (page 83))	▶	103	70
h. Total (Sum of 15f and g)	▶	404	508
i. Percent Paid (15c divided by 15f times 100)		85%	84%

* If you are claiming electronic copies, go to line 16 on page 3. If you are not claiming electronic copies, skip to line 17 on page 3.

16. Electronic Copy Circulation	Average No. Copies Each Issue During Preceding 12 Months	No. Copies of Single Issue Published Nearest to Filing Date
a. Paid Electronic Copies ▶	0	0
b. Total Paid Print Copies (Line 15c) + Paid Electronic Copies (Line 16a) ▶	256	368
c. Total Print Distribution (Line 15f) + Paid Electronic Copies (Line 16a) ▶	301	438
d. Percent Paid (Both Print & Electronic Copies) (16b divided by 16c × 100) ▶	85%	84%

☒ I certify that 50% of all my distributed copies (electronic and print) are paid above a nominal price.

17. Publication of Statement of Ownership
☒ If the publication is a general publication, publication of this statement is required. Will be printed in the NOVEMBER 2016 issue of this publication. ☐ Publication not required.

18. Signature and Title of Editor, Publisher, Business Manager, or Owner	Date
STEPHEN R. BUSHING - INVENTORY DISTRIBUTION CONTROL MANAGER	9/18/2016

I certify that all information furnished on this form is true and complete. I understand that anyone who furnishes false or misleading information on this form or who omits material or information requested on the form may be subject to criminal sanctions (including fines and imprisonment) and/or civil sanctions (including civil penalties).

PS Form 3526, July 2014 (Page 3 of 4)   PRIVACY NOTICE: See our privacy policy on www.usps.com.

Printed and bound by CPI Group (UK) Ltd, Croydon, CR0 4YY

08/05/2025

01864687-0001